Practical Issues in Geriatrics

Series Editor
Stefania Maggi
Aging Branch
CNR-Neuroscience Institute
Padua, Italy

This practically oriented series presents state of the art knowledge on the principal diseases encountered in older persons and addresses all aspects of management, including current multidisciplinary diagnostic and therapeutic approaches. It is intended as an educational tool that will enhance the everyday clinical practice of both young geriatricians and residents and also assist other specialists who deal with aged patients. Each volume is designed to provide comprehensive information on the topic that it covers, and whenever appropriate the text is complemented by additional material of high educational and practical value, including informative video-clips, standardized diagnostic flow charts and descriptive clinical cases. Practical Issues in Geriatrics will be of value to the scientific and professional community worldwide, improving understanding of the many clinical and social issues in Geriatrics and assisting in the delivery of optimal clinical care.

More information about this series at http://www.springer.com/series/15090

Jacopo Demurtas • Nicola Veronese
Editors

The Role of
Family Physicians
in Older People
Care

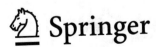 Springer

Editors
Jacopo Demurtas
Primary Care Department USL
Toscana Sud Est
Grosseto, Italy

Nicola Veronese
Department of Internal Medicine and
Geriatrics
University of Palermo
Palermo, Italy

ISSN 2509-6060   ISSN 2509-6079   (electronic)
Practical Issues in Geriatrics
ISBN 978-3-030-78925-1   ISBN 978-3-030-78923-7   (eBook)
https://doi.org/10.1007/978-3-030-78923-7

This Springer imprint is published by the registered company Springer Nature Switzerland AG
The registered company address is: Gewerbestrasse 11, 6330 Cham, Switzerland

To Claudia, and Sara
hoping to grow old together
JD & NV

Foreword

Dear Reader,

In my capacity of the Academic Director of the European Geriatric Medicine Society (EuGMS), I am glad to recommend this book, entitled *The Role of Family Physicians in Older People Care*, in which Dr Nicola Veronese and Dr Jacopo Demurtas, two active members of the EuGMS, discuss the most important aspects and scenarios of care for older people in which geriatricians and general practitioners are, often together, involved.

On the one side, the population is overall getting older, with new challenges for physicians involved in primary care and in geriatric medicine; on the other side, the problematics are rapidly changing. For these reasons, Dr Veronese and Dr Demurtas treated some important issues in older people, such as frailty and comprehensive geriatric assessment, psychiatric conditions in older people, end of life and many others, equally important topics. In addition, they also decided to deal with the recent COVID-19 pandemic, in which older people were dramatically involved.

I am confident that this book will be useful in better understanding of the current state of the art in the field of care for older people in which geriatricians and general practitioners are together involved on a daily basis.

Enjoy your reading!

Mirko Petrovic
Ghent University
Ghent, Belgium

Preface

This book was born from our educational needs in the field of geriatrics.

These pages arise from a simple question: "What would I, as a Family Doctor, like to learn to improve my way of caring for my older patients, wherever they are and whatever is afflicting them?"

On this basis, we drafted and then defined the table of contents, keeping in mind that as family physicians we have a role in counselling and advising our healthy older patients, not just the sick ones. This is why we included several chapters regarding healthy ageing and its importance.

We have also tried to describe new scenarios which seem to be more and more interesting in older people medicine, notably the potentially disruptive impact of new technologies on ageing. Then we described, for the benefit of younger practitioners and colleagues who may not be particularly familiar with geriatrics scores, the main ones.

As it is normal and somehow due, we then focused on macro-areas of illness in the third section, while in the fourth we analyse the contexts in which more often our patients live and their peculiarities, dedicating our attention also to the role of family/informal caregivers. In our opinion, it was important to involve an expert patient and caregiver in the writing process since she shared her insights on the topic, helping us build the chapter as a whole.

The next section of the book thoroughly (at least we hope) explores the role of family physicians in palliative care for older people and describes also the often-forgotten dignity of the dying patient, keeping as a compass the humanistic approach which may encompass several disciplines and that can help us shape a better medicine and better physicians.

Finally, without research and innovation, there is no way to strengthen or at least keep safe the primary care setting. Research should be comprehensive and our work evidence-based. Therefore, we dared to present two chapters, one regarding the importance of meta-research in geriatrics, a topic which keeps us "busy", and the other regarding the deep and crucial role that qualitative research may and, in our opinion has to play, in defining priorities in older people care.

This book has been delayed, due to Covid-19 and the way it brutally hit us. We dedicate it to the many, many colleagues that died because of this pandemic.

Capalbio, Italy
Palermo, Italy

Jacopo Demurtas
Nicola Veronese

Contents

Family Doctors and the Silver Tsunami: Team up to Survive the Storm

1

Jacopo Demurtas, Alessandro Mereu, Nicola Veronese, and Jan De Maeseneer

Abstract

Growing older populations, sometimes referred to as gray (or silver or aging) tsunami, are an increasingly serious health and socioeconomic concern for modern societies. To face the challenge posed by this phenomenon, strategies at several levels must be planned.

Primary care doctors and family physicians can have a pivotal role in this situation, helping to address and manage the strategies to withstand the tasks and guarantee health coverage to this population. Notably, older population cannot be assessed and managed with a one-size-fits-all model or tool. Among older adults we can find healthy people, frail or disabled people, people with palliative or supportive needs, and people needing end of life care.

To help family doctor dealing with this complex scenario, team-working is crucial and also a redistribution of the healthcare burden through mechanisms of task shifting and adopting a complex adaptive leadership model.

J. Demurtas (✉)
Primary Care Department, USL Toscana Sud Est, Grosseto, Italy
e-mail: jacopo.demurtas@unimore.it

A. Mereu
Primary Care Department, Azienda USL Toscana Centro, Sesto Fiorentino, Italy

N. Veronese
Department of Internal Medicine and Geriatrics, University of Palermo, Palermo, Italy

J. De Maeseneer
Department of Public Health and Primary Care, Ghent University, Ghent, Belgium

Family physicians should recognize the peculiarities of this evolving scenario, keeping in mind the social determinants of health and acting with the person-centered and the community-centered approach at the same time.

Keywords

Aging · Family doctor · Task shifting · Teamwork · Complex adaptive leadership Social determinants of health · Comprehensive healthcare · Universal health coverage

1.1 Introduction

The ability of primary care systems to provide comprehensive healthcare is crucial in dealing with complex health problems.

The aging population, in strong growth in terms of numbers and in terms of care needs [1], represents a paradigmatic target to which to apply comprehensive care.

In the USA, for instance, aging adults will comprise 25% of the population by 2050 [2].

This will be due to increased longevity; baby boomer surge, starting in 2025–2030; and demographic shift [2].

This has consequences for health, social, and family care in any modern society.

Thus, a response from the society to the question of how we will care for all these older persons is more and more urgently needed [1]. It should be mentioned that this is not always approached only in positive ways, but many different negative opinions are also circulating, culminating in so-called ageism or partial exclusion of older adults from society.

1.2 The Silver Tsunami

The unprecedented potential burden on society of this aging population is what is called the "gray tsunami" or "silver tsunami" or "aging tsunami" [1].

It is about a growing number of people all together older than the previous generation with increased health, social, and other needs without a youngest robust (e.g., welfare, work opportunities, etc.) at its back.

In the silver tsunami metaphor, older persons represent the great walls of water that destroy or displace everything in their path and then recede, leaving nothing behind but rubble, salty mud, and broken lives [3], while we, intended as society, are the coast on which the wave will exercise its destructive power.

Charise pointed out that this definition "testifies to the barely conscious figurative language that serves to construct perceptions of an aging population" [4].

The conditions that brought this extraordinary demographic situation were social protection and welfare, improved diagnostic and therapeutic performance, and a disruptive economic development.

Neglecting to consider this scenario makes this perception limited, inaccurate, and damaging [3].

This scenario is what is synthesized, together with its consequences with the name "silver tsunami."

The family, social, urban, welfare, and health systems will not be able to give enough answers but will respond in some way. Those ways will be more effective if we prepare and adapt our systems to the "storm."

1.3 Peculiarities of Geriatric Care

The word *geriatrics* was coined in 1901 by Doctor Ignatz Nascher that proposed that adult aging is considered as a distinct stage in life span development. This stage encompasses several dimensions, namely, physiological, psychological, and social aspect. More and more research studies are focusing also on existential dimensions [5]. Also the geriatric definition is debatable [6]. What elements define "geriatric" a patient if the age cannot do it? At the same time, older population needs cannot be addressed with just a *one-size-fits-all* tool [7]. Since its definitions, it is clear how the multimodal and multidimensional approach is the basis of geriatric care.

The need for care and the planning of care plans in people where it is possible to foresee a functional decline require multiple tools and different resources to be activated in forecast or at the time of need, and working with aging adults requires specific knowledge and skills.

Aging population is not unique but is composed of several clusters of people with different conditions, including people at the end of their lives, people with one or more organ shortages, people with disabilities, and older people in good health.

In all these categories, it is important to promote healthy aging to a weighted extent to the specific conditions of everyone. Furthermore, the older population has some peculiar characteristics on which social and health systems must reflect and modulate their activity.

1.3.1 Characteristics of Aging Population and Families

The older people are for the most part retired, without formal work constraints, but may have family or social relationships and commitments that can modulate their quality of life.

An older widower who lives alone in a gentrificated[1] city, lacking in personal services such as shops or offices, even in the absence of frank organic pathology, can be considered as a person with welfare needs.

---

[1] https://dictionary.cambridge.org/dictionary/english/gentrification.

An older couple in an urban suburb involved in the care of their grandchildren and in the community in an active way, despite the presence of a relevant organic disease, can enjoy a good level of functioning and have little need for assistance. Geography also has its meaning in the analysis of needs. Older people living in areas with low human settlement can have different needs with the same biological conditions and economic resources of older people living in highly anthropized environments. Another important determinant, common to so-called "westernized" civilizations, is the atomization of family units.

The fragmentation of family units over the past 70 years has produced, to varying degrees, a different way of caring for needy older people. The extended family, living in spaces and congruous environments, guaranteed a high level of care for the older in difficulty and at the same time allowed the older to maintain a social function in the family. Today the nuclear family is organized without the sharing of homes and social environments among the older people, children, and grandchildren. This slow, but progressive reformulation of family relationships has imposed on the services a welfare approach, inventing residential and semi-residential structures or developing the private home care system. These services, variably constituted in the different countries, are at high cost for families or for the social-health service both in terms of economic resources and in terms of human resources.

In function of this model, without moving negative criticisms to the operations or to the quality of the services, a series of further problems of difficult resolution or economic and human stress was produced. Those who do not have resources or cannot access them risk social and welfare exclusion until the conditions deteriorate. Caregivers, family members or hired individuals, are subjected to great stress provoking burnout, moral injuries, and sometimes real pathological conditions.

1.4   Dealing with the Silver Tsunami

A possible operational model for dealing with "silver tsunami" is the comprehensive and integrated management of needs and their early detection and further planning and the allocation of resources in a respectful and fair manner.

Moreover, there is a need—certainly in people with multi-morbidity—for a paradigm shift from "disease-oriented" towards "goal-oriented" care, focusing on the achievement of the life goals of the patient. Very often these life goals are related to "being able to function" and "social participation."

Goals focus on what "matters" to the patient.

However, this model requires an active and not only bureaucratic-administrative collaboration between professionals; therefore it requires the organization of the team.

The team allows to share the competences to be activated on individual cases and on groups of people (territorial areas, population clusters), allows a concrete integration of activities and planning, and allows the multiplicity of interventions.

1.4.1 Task Shifting

Assembling the right team in modern healthcare is challenging, given its complexity. A mechanism through which teamwork activities can be improved is **task shifting** [8–10].

Task shifting can contribute to the flexibility necessary to respond when the system is under pressure. Within health systems this is necessary for at least four reasons, as reported by the Expert Panel on Effective Ways of Investing in Health (EXPH) board [11, 12].

The first is that task shifting **can contribute to the sustainability of the health workforce** [9, 13].

Health systems in all countries are facing shortages of health workers [13], with different groups affected to greater or lesser degrees. Inward migration and increased training capacity helped meeting these shortages in high-income countries, yet challenges are still open. It makes little sense in these conditions that scarce health workers' forces keep some roles that can be easily undertaken by others. Moreover, these strategies could also help reducing burnout rates among healthcare workers [14–17].

Second, task shifting can **contribute to the financial sustainability of health system** [13, 18].

Many health professionals spend a considerable amount of their time undertaking activities for which they are overqualified. If it is possible to transfer these responsibilities to less qualified and, consequently, less highly paid health workers, it will reduce costs without affecting health outcomes, therefore improving the efficiency of the health system. The saved resources can contribute to sustainability of health spending and/or be re-invested in other valuable healthcare. In other circumstances, transferring roles to a higher qualified health worker, even if more expensive to employ, may be more efficient if their greater expertise means that they use fewer resources or achieve better health outcomes. Task shifting may also support social sustainability, meaning the maintenance of a health system that societies trust and want to use. These changes may involve the transfer of responsibility for an entire package of care, for example, where a doctor's role is taken over by a nurse or a nurse's role is taken over by a healthcare assistant.

Third, task shifting can be a means to **improve quality of care**, with evidence showing that activities are performed better by one group than another, e.g., routine management of uncomplicated chronic disease can be performed with outstanding results by nurses [8]. Finally, task shifting can **enhance the resilience of the health system**, especially where different professional groups can substitute for one another in emergencies. However, this requires the existence of established, and tested, systems and mechanisms through which task shifting can be adopted and supported in a timely manner. Assembling the right mix of skills in the right place is challenging, given the complexity of modern healthcare. Task shifting can contribute to the flexibility necessary to respond when the system is under pressure.

1.4.2 Comprehensive Care and Teamwork for Aging Societies: A Leadership Revolution

Comprehensive care is a milestone inside the Primary Health Care definition since the famous 1978 WHO Alma-Ata Declaration [19].

Thinking to aging people and societies leads health professionals to set comprehensive health strategies in order to ensure an holistic approach inside an echo-bio-psycho-social framework. This is not a solo-professional commitment or a policy statement. Comprehensive care is the strategy which permits health professionals to afford valued and equitable care for aging people [20]. It permits health professionals to connect multiple elements (not just medical ones) and follow their complex and dynamic links.

A comprehensive approach cannot be accomplished by a professional [19]. A comprehensive approach requires a multidisciplinary team that works in an inter-professional way with a commitment and social involvement, in a political-ethical positioning [21]. This is the connotation of family medicine [22], as Starfield demonstrated that this is the approach which guarantees quality and equity and sustainability in different national health systems [22, 23].

If comprehensive care is about complex framework and is about teamwork, it is important to look at the team functioning.

There are many examples of teams, their structure, and how they work. There is probably no single winning model. At the same time, there are numerous obstacles to the establishment and functioning of the team.

As described by Obolensky [24], there is an important difference between two main leadership approaches, the "command-and-control" in which obeying *unempowered* people simply waits for a master to command (wait to be said what to do) [24] and **complex adaptive leadership (CAL)**, derived from the complex adaptive system (CAS) model. It moves from the consideration that systems are complex and share at least four common aspects: self-organization, inter-relatedness, adaptive, and emergence [24].

Complex adaptive leadership is a continuous balance of diagnosis and intervention, which requires the involvement and commitment of the parties in the problem being faced. Thus it cannot be limited to the "top-down" application of technical knowledge or decisions taken by those in positions of authority as in a command-and-control model but is sensitive to each change at every level and requires proactiveness.

In a wider vision, in the geriatric field as the same for general population, it is possible to frame it in three layers, each one interconnected with the only bureaucratic hierarchy between them.

The "micro" layer concerns the primary care unit that deals with the health and disease of the population (in the specific case of the older individuals and its epiphenomena about health promotion, prevention from primary to quaternary, diagnostic processes – therapeutic and rehabilitative). This complex and permanent set of actions begins in the pre-geriatric era and continues until death and cure of family mourning.

The "meso" layer concerns the network of social and health services in which the micro layer is inserted, and of which it is a fundamental fiber, where the empowerment activities of the primary care unit and support activities for the person are placed with services that can be customized but aimed at collectively and with high economic or social cost technologies.

The "macro" layer crosses the two previous layers providing them with the political structures and policies that support their actions, referring to the principles of fairness and solidarity that govern the welfare and healthcare processes.

The CAL described here moves in this multi-layered complex, where leaders inhabit all three layers and connect with each other.

The leadership exercised is trans-stratum; the effects are realized in the skills allocated in the functions of proximity to the person and the collective of the individual professionals or in the level of coordination and integration as well as in the level of policy-making.

Building multidisciplinary workforce capacity to better deliver integrated care models and meet the needs of older people is a key recommendation of the WHO World Report on Ageing and Health [25] and consistent with emerging evidence for delivering integrated care for older people with complex health needs. In a recent review, most intervention was commonly directed toward building capacity in nurses, physiotherapists, general practitioners, and social workers to deliver integrated care [26].

1.4.3 Intersection among Clinical and Social Issues Affecting Health Status of Older People

As described by the social determinants of health (SDH) theory, adopted by WHO [27], health status is affected by several interconnected factors. Just a few of them are under control of health systems, and inside this narrow field, the clinical power of health professionals is too small facing the broader framework [28].

Setting a teamwork in this framework, ask to recognize how big and complex it is; otherwise, it lead to ineffective intervention or blind leadership. How health professionals can take care about an old man with diabetes who is a homeless living in its car? How primary care unit can prevent COPD exacerbations in a polluted smog area? How social workers can help a deprived old woman without family support?

SDH must be addressed by the whole society, where professionals and political institutions could have advocacy skills and proactive approach in order to promote health and protect from disease. This desirable scenario put the family medicine team approach to the macro-level as a primary care unit shall advocate for patients and its community and the professional community shall advocate for healthy societies in a healthy world.

A team could be more powerful than a solo professional in order to address social determinants of health in the community level. Training of professionals' team member is a crucial determinant of health. Trained skilled professionals in the field of interprofessional collaboration, community-oriented commitment, and political-ethic positioning are needed. Social accountability training could play a key role inside a team member [29].

Team member composition can change all over different countries due to local labor market and professional status. It is not so important the administrative connection among members; it is important if they are able to cooperate and to have a unique mission with different health objectives reachable by multiple skills sometimes shifted among themselves. In this way the team can assess goal-oriented care because of the multiple points of view already settled.

1.4.4 System's Accountability and Sustainability in Older People Care

In recent years, not only Western countries but also developing countries started with "chronic disease management programs" to improve care. The design of those programs includes most frequently:

- Strategies for case finding.
- Protocols describing what should be done and by whom, the importance of information and empowerment of the patient, and the definition of process.
- Outcome indicators that may contribute to the monitoring of care.

In the context of multimorbidity, there is a need for a shift from "chronic disease management" toward "participatory patient management," with the patient at the center of the process.

For many people, giving meaning to the chronic illness process they are going through is of the utmost importance. Safety and avoiding side effects (not having to suffer more from the treatment than from the disease) are very important. Patients expect comprehensiveness in their care instead of fragmentation.

1.4.5 Multimorbidity, Goal-Oriented Care, and Equity

When implementing goal-oriented care, there may be a threat to equity, as the way goals are formulated by patients may be determined by, for example, social class.

Moreover, integrating "contextual evidence" implies the risk of taking the context for granted: people living in poverty will generally have been obliged to take on lower expectations in terms of quantity and quality of life than well-educated people.

So, "goal-oriented medical care" could contribute to an increase in social inequities in health. This challenges primary healthcare providers with the question of how to deal with an "unhealthy" and "inequitable" context. It is obvious that this cannot be the responsibility only of primary care providers. They may have an important "signaling" role to document and draw attention to the problems that patients are facing.

This is where **community-oriented primary care (COPC)** comes into the picture. COPC integrates individual and population-based care, blending clinical skills of practitioners with epidemiology, preventive medicine, and health promotion [13].

Starting from observations in daily patient care, COPC makes a systematic assessment of healthcare needs in practice populations; identifies community health problems; implements systematic interventions, involving a target population (e.g., modification of practice procedures and improvement of living conditions); and monitors the effect of changes to ensure that health services are improved and congruent with the needs of individual patients and of the community.

COPC designs specific interventions to address priority health problems. Teams consisting of primary healthcare workers and community members assess resources and develop strategic plans to deal with problems that have been identified. So, COPC is an essential part of a strategy to re-orientate care toward the needs and the goals of the individual and of the community. It will help to identify the "upstream causes" that lead to social inequities in health.

Creating greater awareness of health is an essential investment in an equal and fair society and of the centrality of it as a value to achieving universal health coverage [12].

This process needs to:

- Provide clear narratives setting out how the financial sustainability of existing: progress toward universal health coverage is endangered by waste and low-value care;
- Develop a long-term strategy for a step-by-step value-based approach toward change of culture. This strategy should encompass the definition of a series of goals that support the long-term objective of change, moving forward in small steps (work plans), including the implementation and monitoring of effects by use of existing data sources and methodologies as well as the creation of mechanisms to further guide the direction of change toward high-value care;
- Support research and development of methodologies on appropriateness and unwarranted variation by exchanging robust methodologies for measuring and monitoring patterns of clinical practice, regional variation, and appropriateness research, by stimulating data collections (incl. Real-world evidence and big data) and by defining and aligning goal-oriented outcomes that matter to patients [14];
- Encourage health professionals to take responsibility and feel accountable for increasing value in healthcare, which may require freeing resources from low-value care to re-invest in high-value care encompassing the training of "change agents" (leaders) that feel accountable for the health of the population, including equitable distribution of resources across diseases. Health professionals hold a key role in advocating a change of culture toward social cohesion and connectedness;
- Support the creation of learning communities, including communities of health professionals, to bring together the best expertise, experiences, and practices, to contribute to change of attitudes, and to learn from each other by measuring, benchmarking, and implementing actions across the EU. Member states should take the lead in identifying and pinpointing the most important tasks; the EC should create a supportive and facilitating environment for the establishment of those learning communities that will contribute to a change of behavior and a change in legislation;

- Support initiatives for patients' engagement in shared decision-making, recognizing the importance of patients' goals, values, and preferences, informed by high-quality information to implement empowering practices and goal-oriented person-centered care (Fig. 1.1) [30].

Box 1.1 Jennifer and Her Goals - Modified from [31]

Jennifer is 75 years old. Fifteen years ago she lost her husband. She has been a patient at the practice for 15 years now. During these 15 years, she has been through a difficult medical history: hip replacement surgery for osteoarthritis, hypertension, type 2 diabetes, and COPD.

She lives independently at home, with some help from her youngest daughter, Elisabeth. I visit her regularly and each time she starts by saying: "Doctor, you must help me."

Then follows a succession of complaints and feelings: sometimes it has to do with her heart, another time with lungs, then the hip,…Each time I suggest – according to the guidelines – all sorts of examinations that do not improve her condition.

Her request becomes more and more explicit; my feelings of powerlessness, inadequacy, and irritation increase.

Moreover, I have to cope with guidelines that are contradictory: for COPD she sometimes needs corticosteroids, which always worsen her diabetes control. The adaptation of the medication for the blood pressure (once too high, once too low) does not meet with her approval, and nor does my interest in her HbA1C and lung function test results. After so many contacts, Jennifer says:

> Doctor, I want to tell you what really matters to me. On Tuesday and Thursday, I want to visit my friends in the neighborhood and play cards with them. On Saturday, I want to go the supermarket with my daughter. Foremost, I just want some peace. I do not want to continually change the therapy anymore, especially not having to do this and to do that.

In the conversation that followed, it became clear to me how Jennifer had formulated the goals for her life. I felt challenged to identify how the guidelines could contribute to the achievement of Jennifer's goals. I have visited Jennifer with pleasure ever since. I know what she wants and how much I can (merely) contribute to her life.

1.4.6 The Role of Family Physicians within the Team

Approaching a patient with multimorbidity challenges practitioners' institutions for health professionals' education to train providers that are not only "experts," or excellent "professionals," but are also "change agents" that continuously improve the health system constantly questioning the reality of knowledge and care. It requires fundamental reflection on the individual provider-patient interaction, on

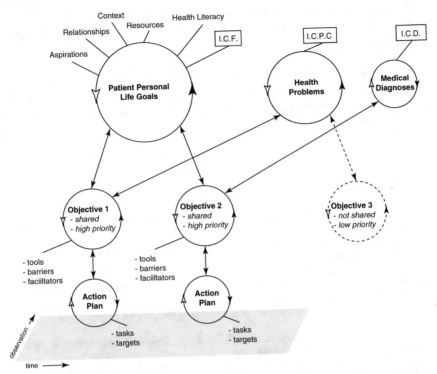

Fig. 1.1 Revised model of goal-oriented care with the patient's personal life goals in pole position. Arrows represent flows of information. ICD, ICPC, and ICF stand for the International Classification of Diseases, International Classification of Primary Care, and International Classification of Functioning [30]

the need for a paradigm shift from problem-oriented to goal-oriented care, on the organization of the healthcare services and the features of the health system.

Most fundamentally, it will also require dialogue and communication methodologies between the health sector and people in need of healthcare and with other stakeholders within society involved in healthcare at the practice, research, and policy level, in order to guarantee the essential characteristics of an effective health system: relevance, equity, quality, cost-effectiveness, sustainability, people-centeredness, and innovation.

1.5 Conclusions

Family doctors must adapt their commitment to this new scenario of silver tsunami. What will be changed is the increasing need of a proactive teamworking inside the community and close to the patients and a goal-oriented approach. Working as a GP in this scenario means to be able to address SDH and go beyond the biological health issues, adopting an eco-bio-psycho-social approach. It will be crucial to learn and act how to promote healthy aging and take care about increasing palliative and end of life care needs.

- **Gentrification:** *the buying and renovation of houses and stores in deteriorated urban neighborhoods by upper- or middle-income families or individuals, raising property values but often displacing low-income families and small businesses.*

References

1. Fulop T, Larbi A, Khalil A, Cohen AA, Witkowski JM. Are we ill because we age? Front Physiol. 2019;10:1508.
2. Masselam VS. Prepare for the surge of the silver tsunami: learning about working with the aging adult. Psychiatry. 2017;80:413–4.
3. Barusch AS. The aging tsunami: time for a new metaphor? Taylor & Francis; 2013.
4. Charise A. "Let the reader think of the burden": old age and the crisis of capacity. Occasion: Interdiscip Stud Humanities. 2012;4:1–16.
5. Forlenza OV, Vallada H. Spirituality, health and Well-being in the elderly. Int Psychogeriatr. 2018;30:1741–2.
6. Orimo H, Ito H, Suzuki T, Araki A, Hosoi T, Sawabe M. Reviewing the definition of "elderly". Geriatr Gerontol Int. 2006;6:149–58.
7. Fillit HM, Rockwood K, Woodhouse K. Introduction: aging, frailty, and geriatric medicine. Brocklehurst's textbook of geriatric medicine and gerontology. Elsevier; 2010. p. 1–2.
8. Maier CB, Aiken LH. Task shifting from physicians to nurses in primary care in 39 countries: a cross-country comparative study. Eur J Pub Health. 2016;26:927–34.
9. Aithal A, Aithal P. ABCD analysis of task shifting–an optimum alternative solution to professional healthcare personnel shortage. Int J Health Sci Pharm (IJHSP). 2017;1:36–51.
10. Joshi R, Alim M, Kengne AP, Jan S, Maulik PK, Peiris D, Patel AA. Task shifting for non-communicable disease management in low and middle income countries–a systematic review. PLoS One. 2014;9:e103754.
11. Jönsson B. Disruptive innovation and EU health policy. Springer; 2017.
12. De Maeseneer J. European expert panel on effective ways of investing in health: opinion on primary care. Prim Health Care Res Dev. 2015;16:109–10.
13. Aluttis C, Bishaw T, Frank MW. The workforce for health in a globalized context–global shortages and international migration. Glob Health Action. 2014;7:23611.
14. Ricciardi W, Boccia S. New challenges of public health: bringing the future of personalised healthcare into focus. Eur J Pub Health. 2017;27:36–9.
15. De Simone S, Vargas M, Servillo G. Organizational strategies to reduce physician burnout: a systematic review and meta-analysis. Aging Clin Exp Res. 2019;33:883.
16. Panagioti M, Panagopoulou E, Bower P, Lewith G, Kontopantelis E, Chew-Graham C, Dawson S, van Marwijk H, Geraghty K, Esmail A. Controlled interventions to reduce burnout in physicians: a systematic review and meta-analysis. JAMA Intern Med. 2017;177:195–205.
17. West CP, Dyrbye LN, Erwin PJ, Shanafelt TD. Interventions to prevent and reduce physician burnout: a systematic review and meta-analysis. Lancet. 2016;388:2272–81.
18. Buchan J, Perfilieva G. Making progress towards health workforce sustainability in the WHO European region. World Health Organization; 2015.
19. Organization WH. Declaration of Alma-Ata: International Conference on Primary Health Care, Alma-Ata, USSR, 6–12 September 1978. Retrieved February 14:2006; 1978.

20. Southey G, Heydon A. The Starfield model: measuring comprehensive primary care for system benefit. Healthcare management forum. Elsevier; 2014. p. 60–4.
21. Braveman P, Murray CJ, Starfield B, Geiger HJ. World Health Report 2000: how it removes equity from the agenda for public health monitoring and policy commentary: comprehensive approaches are needed for full understanding. BMJ. 2001;323:678–81.
22. Starfield B. Family medicine should shape reform, not vice versa. Fam Pract Manag. 2009;16:6.
23. Starfield B. Toward international primary care reform. CMAJ. 2009;180:1091–2.
24. Obolensky N. Complex adaptive leadership: embracing paradox and uncertainty. Routledge; 2017.
25. Beard JR, Officer A, De Carvalho IA, Sadana R, Pot AM, Michel J-P, Lloyd-Sherlock P, Epping-Jordan JE, Peeters GG, Mahanani WR. The world report on ageing and health: a policy framework for healthy ageing. Lancet. 2016;387:2145–54.
26. Briggs AM, Valentijn PP, Thiyagarajan JA, de Carvalho IA. Elements of integrated care approaches for older people: a review of reviews. BMJ Open. 2018;8:e021194.
27. Marmot M, Wilkinson R. Social determinants of health. OUP Oxford; 2005.
28. Marmot M, Allen J, Goldblatt P, Boyce T, McNeish D, Grady M, Geddes I. The Marmot review: fair society, healthy lives. London: UCL; 2010.
29. Mnguni LA. Theoretical framework for training socially accountable science teachers. J Educ Gifted Young Sci. 7:159–75.
30. Tange H, Nagykaldi Z, De Maeseneer J. Towards an overarching model for electronic medical-record systems, including problem-oriented, goal-oriented, and other approaches. Eur J Gen Pract. 2017;23:257–60.
31. De Maeseneer J, Boeckxstaens P. James Mackenzie Lecture 2011: multimorbidity, goal-oriented care, and equity. Br J Gen Pract. 2012;62:e522–4.

Part I

Healthy Ageing

The Consultation with Older Patients in Primary Care: Communication Management and Clinical Reasoning

2

Jacopo Demurtas and Giuseppe Parisi

> "...patient care requires offering a service that is actually suitable for the person as a whole, that is, as far as possible, to respond to his/her physical needs, his/her pathophysiological situation, but also to his/her psychological expectations and emotional needs"
>
> (Luciano Vettore) [1].

Abstract

Consultation represents a crucial task in everyday practice. Thus, it has to be properly taught, and it has to be acknowledged from scholars and clinicians as a unique, complex and potentially incredibly effective medical procedure.

In this chapter the phases of consultation will be described and discussed focusing on the peculiarities of consultation with older patients.

During the consultation the doctor will face several situations, always dealing with uncertainty.

The patient has to explain his concerns, expectations and possible limitations regarding a medical problem, and the doctor should encourage patients in this phase, facilitating it where opportune and possible. The doctor using his/her communication skills and clinical skills can convert the data given by the patient

J. Demurtas
Primary Care Department, USL Toscana Sud Est, Grosseto, Italy

G. Parisi (✉)
School of Medicine and Surgery, University of Milano Bicocca, Milan, Italy

Italian Society of Medical Education (SIPEM), Trento, Italy
e-mail: giuseppe.parisi.trento@gmail.com

© Springer Nature Switzerland AG 2022
J. Demurtas, N. Veronese (eds.), *The Role of Family Physicians in Older People Care*, Practical Issues in Geriatrics, https://doi.org/10.1007/978-3-030-78923-7_2

in information, formulate diagnostic hypotheses and suggest care advice based on this information.

Doctors should always consider patients' preferences and dignity when formulating hypotheses and making suggestions.

Some aspects of consultation with older patients are slightly different from those in average consultation with younger adults, and also the purpose of intervention can be different or perceived differently.

Keywords

Older patient · Consultation · Uncertainty · Management · Communication

2.1 Consultation as a Complex and Effective Medical Procedure

The consultation is the most common diagnostic and therapeutic procedure, and it is the usual way in which primary care is delivered. Therefore, the GP has to be skilled in conducting it, as in any medical procedure.

In managing an older patient, conducting a good quality consultation is even more important, because it is an opportunity for a unique face-to-face encounter with the patient, who usually is cared for by several professionals (who act following the dictates or the advice of the doctor), and the encounter could strongly affect the complex situation of the older patient.

The consultation is a complex procedure, which shows its exceptional potential in specific situations [2], for instance, when a decision on the treatment of a severe disease has to be shared. Sharing is possible only in the interaction with the patient, in a confidential setting and in an appropriate time, in other words, in a consultation setting [3].

The consultation can be seen as a situation composed of discrete elements emerging from "thick" interaction [4] between doctor's competences and patient's needs. We follow a consultation model grounded in the large number of operative models reported in literature over the last 50 years [5–14] (see Table 2.1).

The elements are **subjectivity** of the patient, **examination, evaluation, design** and **shared choice**. These elements are framed by two phases: an **opening phase**, (greetings and visual pre-assessment of the patient's appearance) and a **final phase** with a summary of the consultation, an enquiry about other potential health issues and farwells. The consultation itself is a part of the organization of the service, which affects the encounter.

The doctor acts to facilitate the emergence of each element, and in doing so each element contributes to organize the consultation.

How can the doctor foster the organization of the consultation?

He/she has to reach several goals in three areas: clinical, communication and management. The doctor does not simply act (communicate to the patient and manage the consultation) but he/she thinks (clinical reasoning), using clinical skills

Table 2.1 A framework of medical consultation (*modified from Parisi, Pasolli* [3])

Element	Management task	Clinical task	Communication task	Patient as…
Opening	Did you build the setting?	Did you catch the early warnings signs?	Did you put the patient at ease?	Person
Subjectivity	Did you manage the presenting problems, ideas, concerns and expectations?	Did you generate early hypotheses?	Did you collect information by allowing patient expression?	Individual
Examination	Did you manage your agenda problems?	Did you reach a working diagnosis?	Did you actively collect information?	Matter of research
Evaluation	Did you reframe the situation?	Did you perform an overall clinical judgement?	Did you inform the patient?	Partner
Design	Did you map out a plan?		Did you inform the patient about the pros and cons of each option?	Consultant
Shared choice	Did you choose an option?		Did you share the decision with the patient, and did you reach a consent, possibly involving them?	Partner
End	Did you schedule the next consultation date and inform the patient about the safety net?		Did you greet the patient?	Person

(what to ask the patient), communication skills (how to ask the patient, how to listen…) and management skills: she/he makes orders; establishes length of consultation, priorities and agenda; and defines the situation and the connections of elements. This last skill is crucial when working with multimorbid patients.

On the other hand, management problems cannot overtake clinical tasks in importance. Figuratively, we can compare the clinical task to the blue sky, which is always there, even if temporarily obscured by clouds.

As we stated, at the end of the consultation, doctor and patient should reach a shared decision. Therefore, the shared decision-making (SDM) [15] process is the core of the consultation.

The interaction during the consultation is the only way to achieve an appropriate SDM [15], and this is the reason why the other means to decide are not so effective.

There is another consideration: clinical reasoning and communication in the consultation are two different entities strictly linked together. The clinical reasoning is affected by many factors, placed on the patient's side or on the doctor's side, for instance, time, clinical setting and availability of resources (see Table 2.2), and the management of the consultation and the communication with the patient are influenced by the disease, patient's psychological profile and the scenario in which the situation can be placed [3].

Table 2.2 Factors affecting clinical reasoning

Patient side:
Environment
Reasons for encounter
Kind of requests
Style in presenting complaints
Symptoms and signs
Preferences
Doctor side:
Communication style interviewing the patient and negotiating the care plan
time
Other:
Thick interaction emerging in the consultation
Availability of resources
Availability of tests, scans and consultants
Clinical setting

We outline ta guide to consultation following these considerations, an Ariadne thread in the labyrinth of consultation with the complex patient [16], presenting the elements emerging from the interaction, subjectivity, examination, evaluation, design and shared choice, and suggesting effective intervention in the specific consultation with older patients.

Notably, in dealing with older individuals, a crucial role is played by their evolving priorities and needs, which may change in short time, making the consultation with these patients even more complex.

2.2 Organization of the Service and Opening Phase

The organization of the service affects the consultation itself: the doctor has to ensure an effective appointment system, provide enough time for each patient and privacy (see Box 2.1). The system must recognize the needs of patients and establish an appropriate waiting time.

> **Box 2.1 The Office**
> The waiting room should have comfortable chairs, and the doctor, or the staff, should inform the older patients about timing of the consultation and offer support if necessary, avoiding stress and discomfort, which could make the patient more confuse and affect the information gathering phase of the consultation, and not only for charity aims.

Older people should have a fast track in acute situations, and follow-up should be booked in advance in consultation for chronic diseases.

Also, the consultation length should be different: older patients are usually slower to describe concerns and symptoms, they have a lot of problems (see

Table 2.3 Vignette: the multiple concerns of Mr. Mario

One day, I went to Mario's home to visit him

Mario is an 83-year-old patient with several chronic diseases

Looking at me, intently he says: "I have shortness of breath, and this shortness of breath is becoming more and more disturbing. I have plenty of mucus and it affects my breathing. This mucus is used to be white, but now it is yellow or green… The medical therapy is not useful and my symptoms are worsening. The symptoms are worsening even though I am taking my medication. Five days ago, you doctor gave me five pills of furosemide instead of three, and I feel very tired. If possible, I want to stop taking this drug because I think that it makes me tired. Also, my sons never visit me anymore, and I am taking too many drugs; I can't live this way anymore… It's better to just die! I have pain at the back of my chest near my shoulder; sometimes it feels like I am being pierced with a knife in my chest, and other times it feels like a stinging pain… I tried to take paracetamol with codeine, but it was not effective. The pain remained the same. I would like something stronger, but I would prefer it not to be a NSAID (non-steroidal anti-inflammatory drug) because I have problems with my stomach! I have a distended abdomen and I have been constipated for 3 days. In addition, I had a fever 2 days ago…"

Table 2.3), many medications have to be reviewed, and sometimes they have companions, spouses or caregivers to talk on their behalf or to comment on what the patient states, making the information gathering phase longer.

Even if it seems that in the encounter we are losing (or spending) a lot of time, the attention on each care episode represents a gain of time in the long run, avoiding multiple and recurrent consultations.

In the opening phase of the consultation, it is useful to put the patient at ease, establishing a rapport, with "social behaviours" [17] connecting with the daily life of the patient and non-clinical issues.

Furthermore, to facilitate the completeness of patient disclosure, a written list of concerns, to make before the consultation, is recommended [3, 18].

Often the older patient needs to discuss about complex treatment in a "time out" consultation [19].

Before starting the consultation, the doctor has to ask the patient if he or she wants somebody else with him/her during the consultation, without taking for granted that the companions should enter in the consulting room. This attention is important to safeguard privacy and dignity of the older person.

In Table 2.4 we outline some tips useful in this phase.

2.3   Subjectivity

Subjectivity is composed by phenomena, discourses, reasoning process, emotions and feelings involved in the interaction, emerging directly from the voice of the patient. They are "symptom or condition perceived by the patient and not by the examiner" [8].

The letter of a specialist about diseases of the patient is not an example of subjectivity, whereas a letter written by the patient is. The patient is the subject, who is unique and manages his/her own life.

Table 2.4 Tips for a good organization of the service and the opening phase of the consultation with older patients

Fast track in acute situation
Effective follow-up in chronic situation
Sufficient consultation length
Comfortable waiting room
Patient at ease
Social behaviour
Companions not necessarily in the consulting room

Table 2.5 Mario's problems prioritized

1 Acute bronchitis attack
2 Faecal impaction
3 Neuropathic pain
4 Iatrogenic weakness/weakness as side effect
5 Low compliance
6 Hypomania
7 Lack of family network

In front of the emergence of subjectivity, the doctor has three tasks.

The first is related to **management**, i.e. to investigate the patient's agenda and to focus on the presenting problems [9].

The final result is a list of clinical or non-clinical problems, i.e. everything requiring the action of the doctor [11]. This is a list of everything that the patient experiences as a problem, according to Engel's biopsychosocial model [20] (see Table 2.5 and see Box 2.2).

Box 2.2

Problems listed during consultation

Classical clinical symptoms (i.e. sore throat)

Besides diagnosis (i.e. thyroid node in neck scan)

Laboratory test results (i.e. anaemia)

Functional problems (i.e. older patient with walking difficulties)

Risky behaviours (i.e. alcohol intake)

Family problems (i.e. marital tension)

Psychological problems (i.e. anxiety)

Coping problems (i.e. after her daughter's illness, she feels depressed)

Social problems (i.e. older patient left alone)

Administrative problems (certificates, sick notes)

The second task involves **communication**: collecting information by allowing patient expression. The doctor becomes aware of the patient's ideas, concerns and expectations and of the impact of the problems on the patient's life [9], not only of mere physical symptoms.

The third task is related to the starting point of **clinical reasoning**, which means generating early clinical hypotheses, not communicated to the patient, at least not in this phase, which will help the subsequent collection of data and testing work, as stated by Elstein and Schwartz in 2002 [21].

> *The clinical engine starts suddenly and will go along with the doctor throughout the consultation. It functions as the keel of a boat: it helps the doctor to go in the right direction using the subjectivity of the patient in order to reach the diagnosis and the subsequent decision* [3].

The tool to be used to perform these tasks is **attention** [22]: *the doctor receives what can be learned about that person's situation acting as a container for a flow of great value or, with a different image, registering a transmitted radio signal from far away* [22].

It is a non-judgemental acceptance of what the testimony of the sufferer adds to our understanding.

These words aren't trivial. Especially with older people, the point of view of the patient is often different to what the doctor imagines. Younger relatives and younger professionals are not aware of preferences and the thoughts of aged: the cultural distance is high; the different stages of life imply different ideas, for example, about death, that in an older patient are no longer necessarily a concern.

Therefore, the message is to **listen to the older patient** and avoid trying to lock him/her into scientific frames.

Personal experiences of illness are sensitive to a broad range of internal bodily processes [23], micro- and macro-contextual influences, and are highly predictive, not only of prognosis and illness of the patient but also of health-care costs and outcomes [24, 25].

Humans are able to make sense of their personal health state better than sensors and objective biometrics [23].

In Table 2.6 we outline some tips useful in this phase.

2.4 Examination

Examination is a communication and reasoning process emerging on the basis of information gathered through subjectivity, in which the doctor collects information actively, through the interview, the objective examination and the consultation of medical records [8].

Table 2.6 Tips to manage subjectivity

Investigate the patient's agenda and focus on the presenting problems
Collect information by allowing patient expression
Be aware of patient's ideas, concerns and expectations
Don't judge
Be curious
Generate early clinical hypothesis
Personal experiences of illness are sensitive to a broad range of internal bodily processes

The **communication** style of the doctor changes from the conversational model to an interviewing style, from open (ended) question or brief repetition of the patient's words (patient's keywords and key concepts) to the more traditional doctor-centred history–taken and the physical examination.

While in the subjectivity phase the doctor lets the patient lead the dance, in this phase the doctor is the leader [17].

During the examination the **second cognitive routine** starts: the first is inductive reasoning, "forward reasoning", in which data analysis results in hypothesis generation; this second routine is the "backward reasoning" [26], the deductive one, in which the hypothesis is tested.

We also consider a third routine: the "safety routine", implementing cognitive forcing strategies to avoid errors [27]. They are deliberate and based on the reflection of the previous thinking process, providing a recall of what has previously been described as pitfalls in clinical reasoning.

The hypotheses are tested by objective examination, by sending the patient for a laboratory test or scan, but also by a powerful tool: the test of time.

Test of time is descripted by Heneghan [28]: "The course of the disease is used to predict when a person should be better or worse; a "wait and see" strategy allows the diagnosis to become more obvious" [28].

The physical examination is a professional action with a hologrammatic value: it encounters the patient's needs to be examined and reassured by close skin touch of the doctor, but it is also useful to make the patient experiment the symptom or the pain elicited by the manoeuvres of the doctor in a safe environment. Usually, it is used as a test or as a recognition of systems to generate additional hypothesis (see Table 2.7).

The final result of this process is a set of working diagnosis, of different levels of certainty, related to several problems. Other problems which are lacking working diagnosis, whether because they are non-clinical problems or for any other reason, will be managed in the evaluation step.

The **management** task in examination is to consider the doctor's agenda, i.e. problems that are present but not presented by the patient [2, 9].

This is an important task to accomplish with an older patient: the doctor needs a lot of information about patients, which is usually complex, and has to ask for this, during the first visit and, if necessary, in a set of three or four visits, in a span of time of usually over a month. It is sufficient to make a plan to address less important problems in the next consultation.

Table 2.7 The hologrammatic value of the physical examination

The physical examination:
As test
As recognition of systems to generate additional hypothesis
Reassurance by close skin touch of the doctor
Encounter the patient's needs to be examined
Makes the patient experiment the symptom or the pain elicited by the manoeuvres of the doctor in a safe environment

The most relevant issue in older person consultation is medications: the high number of medications taken by the older patients is well known and also the side effects and cumulative effects and unpredictability of these problems [29, 30].

Therefore, it is necessary to check the medications thoroughly and to ask about any over-the-counter medications and alternative treatments, such as dietary supplements, complementary remedies, and so on. It is important to see the pills the patient actually takes, and to ask how many times a day, comencement, and even ask the patient to bring his/her medication in a bag or at least to fill in an information sheet for the doctor.

Another relevant issue is the family structure, useful to assess not only the strength of the social and familiar network but also the reliability of relatives and their interactions with the patient.

But the most interesting issue is **life history** [31]: when the doctor and the patient reach a good confidence and the patient is in a good mood to narrate, the doctor can listen to the patient's narrative. It takes time and perseverance, but the narrative can explain most of ideas of the patient and his/her illnesses. For example, it can explain non-explained symptoms of older patients and their mood and their coping ability. The doctor can discover the losses, griefs, dreams and regrets of an entire life.

To listen to the narrative of an entire life is a special emotional experience [31], and at the end the doctor will see the patient from another point of view, strengthening the relationship with him/her [31].

Another issue, with practical importance, is the functional status: it is worth gathering information about function and disability. You can have a preliminary idea regarding these aspects with five simple questions: "what about eating, bathing and dressing, and what about cooking and shopping", but – more importantly—what about hearing, vision, memory loss and cognitive impairment. The patient may appear cognitively intact during consultation but retain only a little part.

The objective of the GP is to gather information about these issues in 2 months, which allows him to deduce a lot of other information about patient's experience about illness and death and advanced directives and social context and mood (see Table 2.8).

Managing subjectivity and examination are work in which the doctor collects information: according to Simon [32], we can call this work **intelligence gathering.**

Table 2.8 Verbanation examination with older patients

Verbal examination of older patients
ASKED
Medications
Family structure
Life history
Functional status
DEDUCED
Patient's experience regarding illness and death
Advance directives
Social history/networks

2.5   Evaluation

Evaluation is a cognitive process emerging at the end of the information gathering work, made by the doctor [5], in which he or she has three tasks: to give an overall clinical judgement (**clinical task**), to reframe the situation (**management task**) and to inform the patient (**communication task**) [13]. The contents of this phase often include the planning, which will be the next steps for the patient seeking care for a specific reason.

Evaluation is first of all a break in the consultation, a central point of the work of the doctor: he or she divides consultation into two parts; the first part is before the evaluation in which the main task is to gather information, and the second part is after the evaluation, in which he or she has to decide what to do (Fig. 2.1). If the evaluation is correct, also the decision will be correct: the doctor has to stop and evaluate, and only after the evaluation the second part of the consultation, the decision-making part, starts. Usually doctors decide before the evaluation, and evaluation justifies what they have decided, but in complex situations as with older people, this can generate errors.

2.5.1   Evaluation: The Clinical Task

The overall clinical judgement is the awareness of the doctor of the whole situation of the patient, which is the effect of the burden of multimorbidity on the prognosis in terms of physical and mental functioning, quality of life and life expectancy, but also in terms of the capacity of patients for coping with it [3].

This change in perspective enables the doctor to take into account not only the organic failure but also the functional impairment, not only the single and localized

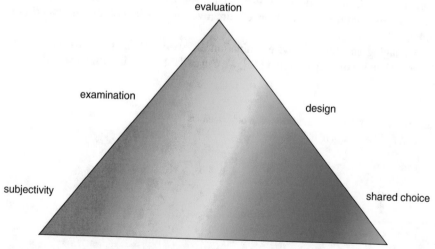

Fig. 2.1 Evaluation: a break in the consultation (*modified from Parisi, Pasolli* [3])

disease but also the person's health. The doctor is not just a follower of protocols but a professional, personalizing medicine and taking care of *that single patient*. And this change in perspective that in general practice is desirable, with older patients it is necessary.

2.5.1.1 Prioritization

To give an overall clinical judgement, the doctor has to start not only from working diagnosis but also from the problems focused on in the first part of the consultation and to prioritize them (see Table 2.5).

Prioritization is not up to the doctor alone but also involves the patient and his/her preferences.

Therefore, the skills needed to an optimized prioritization are shared decision-making skills and the capacity to elicit patient preferences, based on good communication and listening skills. The previous knowledge of the patient helps the doctor in this cooperative work, and confusing and conflicting information are barriers to it. In Table 2.9 we list the facilitators of a good prioritization [33, 34].

Prolonging life is not the unique objective when managing with older patients: while in younger patients it is not questionable with some due exceptions, in older ones it is only one among several objectives, i.e. to guarantee to the patient the best possible quality of life, in accordance with his/her perception, beliefs and personal dignity.

2.5.1.2 Risk and Uncertainty

In medicine, as in every environment of the real world, the professionals have to deal with decisions which have a core of risk—with a known probability of the occurrence of a outcome—embedded in a cloud of uncertainty. The residual uncertainty is always present (Table 2.10) [34].

Table 2.9 Prioritization

Facilitators of a good prioritization
Precision diagnosis
Active involvement of the patient
Eliciting feelings and ideas, concerns and expectations of the patient
Reassure about the effectiveness of the treatment
Assure stable monitoring
Assure a framework to care for the patient
Don't deny but clarify side effects of medication, if it is the case, and reassure the patient about them

Table 2.10 Risk and uncertainty

Certainty if each action is known to lead invariably to a specific outcome
Risk if each action leads to one of a set of possible specific outcomes, each outcome occurring with a known probability. The probabilities are assumed to be known to the decision maker
Uncertainty if either action or both have as its consequence a set of possible specific outcomes, but where the probabilities of these outcomes are completely unknown

Usually, the doctor evaluates the severity of a problem that is life-threatening or disabling. The doctor knows that some problems, such as acute chest pain or fever in an older patient with dementia, pose more risk to life than a sore throat or low back pain in healthy patients, and this is easy to estimate with a known probability, even if there is always a residual uncertainty in diagnosis.

But there is also another aspect of the situation to take into consideration: the "second order uncertainty", about the quality of the evidence itself. If the doctor makes any interventions, he/she has to be confident in the evidence on which his decision is based. The uncertainty is low if the doctor manages a patient with chest pain in a proper way: the risk decreases in a known rate/percentage. The same situation is found in a low-risk disease such as sore throat or low back pain. But the uncertainty is higher in "grey" situations, when no guidelines are available, or in the complex situation where the determinants are multiple or unknown.

The lack of reliability is not always due to incompleteness of scientific knowledge but can also rely on the complex situation of a multiplicity of causal factors and interpretative cues [35].

This last situation is common when the doctor takes care of older patients. For example, the situation of a patient with dementia with the first episode of dysphagia and fever has an unpredictable outcome, but also the effect of a new medication in a polymorbid patient assuming more of four drugs is unpredictable.

It is possible to frame situations with different degrees of severity and uncertainty in different scenarios (see Table 2.11) [36]. In the older patient, we can use a two-scenario framework.

Each scenario implies a different approach of the organization of the service and of the clinical reasoning and communication, and this can affect the final choice.

2.5.1.3 Analytic and "Fast and Frugal" Clinical Reasoning, Values

Once the doctor has established which scenario he has to handle, he is ready to evaluate the problems. This distinction among different kinds of scenarios helps the doctor to use the appropriate tool of reasoning according to the scenario in which the decision is made.

The doctor in the past did not take into account this distinction and used the "rule of thumb" in every situation. Today the opportunities given by clinical prediction rules incorporated in computerized decision support systems linked to electronic health records allow doctors to calculate the **risk** using a statistical and systematic approach, settling pros and cons of each option, weighing every dimension and ultimately choosing the option with the greater number of better dimensions. On the contrary, to face **uncertainty** and complexity, pure statistical inferences are worthless, and the doctor can still use the "rule of thumb". The latter is studied as heuristic. A heuristic is a simple decision making strategy that ignores part of the available information and focuses on a few relevant predictors, and Gigerenzer and Marewsky state that heuristics are better than systematic inferences to predict outcomes in highly uncertain environments [37].

Therefore, the doctor uses an adaptive toolbox, an ecological one (taking into account every determinant of the situation), handling with analytical models—and helped by expert systems if it is necessary—and with fast and frugal heuristics.

Table 2.11 Uncertainty in older patients

Older patient	Complex situation	Mild grey situation
Severity	*Severity of the problem posing a Threat to life and disability* High	*Severity of the problem posing a threat to life and disability* Low
Uncertainty	*Several options—Uncertainty of outcome if you make the intervention* High	*Several options—Uncertainty of outcome if you make the intervention* High
First contact	Dedicated doctor	Receptionist
Timing of the consultation	In a day	In a week
Point of care	Everywhere (surgery or home)	Nurse + doctor's office: Chronic problems
Professionals	Nurse + doctor (chosen)	Nurse + doctor (chosen)
Scheduled consult. Length	Not scheduled	20'
Decision-making focus	Fast and frugal strategies/decision instability/ preferences of patient/values	Management of uncertainty
Shared decision-making	Accurate	Accurate
Information	About options/in order to involve	About options/in order to involve
Consent	In order to involve	In order to involve
Involvement	As opportunity	As opportunity
After intervention	Safety net	Fixed follow up
Competences	Palliative care, geriatric care, psychiatry	General practice: Chronic disease, cardiovascular risk
Classic examples	Patient with dementia who is being taken care of by a foreign caregiver, with the first episode of dysphagia and fever Terminally ill patient	Patient with cardiovascular risk Chronic patient with acute disease

Today a good doctor is one whose decisions rely neither exclusively on the evaluation of risk with analytic models nor exclusively on using fast and frugal heuristics. He is apt to take into account every determinant and, moreover, also the results of the interaction of the determinants among them [38]. The decision, not the uniquely correct but one among several, "emerges" from situated, active integration within an external environment and context, rather than primarily within the internal confines of externally imposed disease criteria, taking into account personal narratives, perceptions, desires and beliefs of the patient.

Furthermore, the doctor has to take into account his values as well as the patient's. Humans decide not only to reach the expected utility but also to reach values in which they trust. The doctor tests the compatibility between his and the patient's principles (technically called "value image" in the theory exposed by Beach [39]) and the "candidate" goals or plans. If the test is positive, he possibly adopts the decision.

Values are a resource but can also be a source of bias. The wrong preconceptions about ageing can impair decision making and the attention to the objectives and values of the patient: for example, the idea that ageing is an illness. In fact, ageing alone doesn't cause illness, and illness is not an inevitable result of ageing. Another preconception is to consider "the older adults" as a uniform category: on the contrary, they have different situations at different ages, and a 65-year-old patient may be more ill and impaired than an 85-year-old individual.

In the complex situation of dealing with an older patient, the doctor has to calculate risk at first, then to evaluate context with fast and frugal heuristics and finally to take into account his values and to elicit those of the patient.

2.5.2 Evaluation: The Management Task

On the base of the overall clinical judgement, the doctor can reframe situation, enlarging the view to the context: the family of the patient, the social network, and so on. The sense and meaning of a problem can change once they have been put in a different situation. The pneumonia of an older patient without any reliable caregiver or social network is quite different from the pneumonia of an older patient who is well cared for: the story of the disease and the outcome will be different, and this also affects the work of the doctor. Having a more ecological view gives more information for good decisions.

2.6 Design

After the evaluation of the present situation, the doctor has to think about the future: what will be the course of action? How many alternatives? What kind of diagnostic or therapeutic action/path? This task is called design: to design is not yet acting or planning. Design needs creativity, a continuing interaction with the patient and to focus reasoning on the alternatives, enduring the anxiety of uncertainty, foreshadowing several scenarios.

Design is the core of professions and makes it possible to distinguish professionals from scientists: "scientists study how the world is, professionals study how the world should be" [32].

To design actually is to map out some plans, in order to decrease a huge amount of possibilities to a limited set of options (which can be counted on the fingers of one hand).

As the final outcome with older patient is often unpredictable, to design several scenarios is always fair; in other words the doctor must always have a "B" plan.

2.7 Shared Choice

Once the doctor has the set of options in mind and the best decision from his point of view, he has to share it with the patient. This is a communicative task.

To share the decision the doctor has to reach three objectives: to inform, to obtain consent and to involve the patient, which aren't visible and codified actions, but embedded in the communication process. The course of action towards these objectives *is* the sharing.

The patient gives, feedback, verbal, paraverbal and non-verbal cues in real time, which modulate the communication with the doctor.

The final result is connected to the interactional process, relying on doctor's and patient's contributions.

Shared decision-making is in some sense a matter of perception [15].

Similar objective states of shared decision-making (if these could be defined) might well be both perceived and valued differently by different patients [15].

2.7.1 The Three Objectives

The first objective is **to inform** the patient.

Doctors have the conviction that information is what they say, no matter if it is expressed in jargon or if it is too difficult for the patient. Information can be evaluated by its impact, thus by the change obtained in the receiver of information. Therefore, doctors should try not to deliver too much information, focusing on that necessary to that peculiar contingency.

First of all, the doctors will have to collect the ideas, concerns, expectations and reason for encounter from the patient, merge and transduce this data into information and then tailor on the patient what to tell. There is not a one-size-fits-all model.

The information has to *fit* the situation.

In a second moment conversely, the doctor will have the additional task of transforming the technical data into narrative ones, which is understandable for the patient.

2.7.1.1 How to Communicate?

In managing an older patient, the first relevant concern is to communicate by following the principle of good communication (see Table 2.12).

2.7.1.2 Who to Inform?

In managing an older patient, the second relevant problem is who to inform.

The first is the patient and, if the patient gives the consent, the caregiver. But this isn't enough: in addition to the caregiver, other relatives, especially in decisions concerning issues of life and death, have the right to be informed, if the patient gives his/her consent.

Table 2.12 Tips for a good communication

- Introduce yourself clearly
- Address the patient with respect
- Do not speak too fast
- Give the patient enough time to process the information
- Do not hurry the patient
- Express yourself clearly
- Allow the patient to read your lips while maintaining eye contact at his/her eye level
- Do not whisper; do not shout
- Avoid jargon
- Give a written plan to take home if necessary (but always if you prescribe something)

If the patient lacks the capacity to understand, the doctor has to inform the caregiver in order to collect the past and present wishes and feelings, beliefs and values that would be likely to influence the decision.

The communication task is to inform the patient about the present situation, check the comprehension of the patient and *after that* inform the patient about the courses of action to implement [9].

The second objective is **to reach a consent**.

We examine the process of obtaining a consent. In Italy and in the rest of Europe, it is requested for every intervention of the doctor [40] (see Box 2.3).

Box 2.3

An intervention in the health field may only be carried out after the person concerned has given free and informed consent to it. This person shall beforehand be given appropriate information as to the purpose and nature of the intervention as well as on its consequences and risks. The person concerned may freely withdraw consent at any time.—*Oviedo 1997* [40].

If the patient lacks the capacity to understand, use and weigh information, retain it in his mind, or to communicate his decision, due to either a permanent or a temporary cognitive impairment (trauma, acute disease), the doctor has to evaluate and record the situation and to share this decision with the patient's caregiver, relatives and advocates, in the patient's best interest.

If the cognitive impairment is permanent and severe, the doctor has to suggest the intervention of an advocate, according to the local law.

The third objective is the **involvement of the patient**.

About half of all patients refuse to be involved in the decision-making process; nevertheless they want to be informed; therefore, the doctor has to ask if the patient or his/her relatives would like to be involved [41].

"Involvement" is not synonymous with "participation". "Involvement" is a relational process, and although it is put into action, we cannot know if it will lead participation or not [41, 42].

Anyway, the involvement of the patient is always an objective to be taken into account, whether it will elicit the participation of the patient or not, for two kinds of reasons. The first reason is ethical: the patient has the right to be involved if he wants, in every situation, while the second one is clinical: in uncertain situations the participation of the patient is often important and gives a contribution to the clinical reasoning.

So, in a situation where the uncertainty is low, the importance of activating a process of involvement of the patient is low, while in a situation with high uncertainty, it has a higher importance. According to the importance of the involvement for the decision, it is possible to apply several strategies of involvement, placed in a continuum, from no involvement to explicit involvement (see Box 2.4).

Box 2.4
Strategies of Involvement.
   Follow these examples:
   "Now I will prescribe a scan!" The doctor is informing the patient and no involvement is elicited.
   "I would prescribe a scan…" The doctor implicitly involves the patient.
   "What about a scan?" The doctor explicitly involves the patient, by keeping open the possibility of refusing involvement.
   "What do you think if I prescribe a scan?" The doctor involves the patient more, by eliciting his thoughts. It is not only the consensus but also the point of view of the patient that is important. In uncertain situations when there is more than one option, the doctor has to declare alternatives. The suggested sentence is:
   "There is more than one reasonable way to deal with this problem", or "there is information about how these two surgical procedures differ that I'd like to encourage you and your family to look at".

2.7.2   Communication in the Two-Scenario Framework

The communication process, directed towards informing the patient, gaining a consent and involving the patient, is strongly modulated, on one hand by the level of severity of the presented problem and on the other hand by the level of uncertainty of the outcome [36].

When facing a mild disease, non-life threatening (e.g. pharyngitis), the doctor can implicitly reach a consent; on the contrary, when facing a life-threatening problem (e.g. acute abdominal pain) or an emergency situation (e.g. dyspnoea), the doctor might inform the patient in a more detailed way and reach a more explicit consensus. The communication process is quite different in the two situations.

2.7.3   Unpredictability

When caring for the older patient, the usual reductionistic medical model is not effective: the doctor faces a complex situation well described by the concept of complex adaptive system [43].

The older patient often has multiple chronic conditions and ageing syndromes, frailty and environmental support needs. The environment mostly has the function of a prosthesis for the older patient, so if the environment changes, it is as if a body function changes as well. Furthermore, a broader use of the concept of frailty in this case can explain the lack of coping, the reduced resilience: even a little change in the environment or in the physical physiological status (individual health states) can modify the homeostasis. The outcome is barely predictable. The doctor cannot rely his/her judgement on mere biological knowledge but on the entire "cloud" of underlying determinants: the classic cardiac or respiratory decompensation is only a simplistic—often untrue—justification that obscures the deep and unknown non-clinical determinants.

To face these complex situations, the doctor first of all has to be aware that the outcome is unpredictable; that unpredictability precludes a "one" right answer approach, because only in a linear reductionist model is there a single answer contemplated. Therefore, it is important to guide the older patient or his/her relatives to consider their options and to be involved in the decision-making process, taking into account values, preferences, ideas and concerns.

In Box 2.5 is an example of a frequent decision process in a complex situation: the hospitalization.

Box 2.5

An example of a frequent decision process in a complex situation: the hospitalization

The story	Observations
Mr. John is 84 years old and he has been affected by dementia for more than 10 years; he is often confused, anxious and mentally disturbed.	**Previous knowledge** of the patient: Serious mental impairment
He is suffering from hypertension, chronic heart failure and type 2 diabetes mellitus NID (not insulin dependent) well controlled; 1 year ago he was catheterized due to benign prostatic hypertrophy, and his nurse changes his catheter every 15 days.	**Opening**: Catch early warnings Multimorbid patient and polypharmacology Risk of urinary tract infections
He is cared for by his wife, who is 78 years old, and by his sons who take turns caring for him every week. They trust me and they usually follow my advice.	Good relationship and high trust in the doctor
They call the doctor for a home visit because Mr. John has been running a temperature of 37.8 degrees Celsius for 2 days; he is also coughing and agitated. The doctor arrives at home.	These symptoms should immediately start running the clinical engine. Early generation of hypothesis: Lower respiratory tract infection
The wife: "Even if he were affected by a severe illness, I wouldn't want to admit him to the hospital"	**Subjectivity** The relative expresses her preference, based on her experiences.

The story	Observations
"In the hospital there is an increased risk of infections: He could get worse than now! I took care of my sister who was admitted to the hospital and died in the end, and she terribly suffered from leg ulcers…"	Information gathering, with particular attention to ideas, concerns and expectations (ICE) of the caregiver, useful to know patient preferences
"After all these years I want him at home. You know the sacrifices I have made to take care of him at home."	The relative reminds the doctor that she is a reliable person
"And my husband always said that he would like to die at home"	Reported patient preferences
"But if you, doctor, decide that he has to go to the hospital I will obey!"	The relative communicates that the choice will be conferred by the doctor: She would like to be involved in the decision-making process but not in the choice
The doctor visits the patient. Respiration rate: 26–28 per min Pulse: 100 per min BP: 115/60 Sp O2: 92%	**Examination/evaluation** The CRB65 risk of mortality in 30 days is intermediate (confusion score 1, resp. score 0, bp score 0 and age score 1)
Thorax: Palpation—Restricted expansion of the lower part of the right thorax Auscultation—Basal crackles heard in the right lung	Hypothesis testing: The probability of having a respiratory tract infection is higher
Abdomen: Normal	Hypothesis testing: The probability of having a abdominal infection is lower
The patient has swollen legs but they are no more swollen than they were in the past Patient is more confused and agitated than the last time the doctor saw him	The confusion is an important element

At this point the doctor puts the instruments in his bag and asks to wash his hands and doesn't say a single word. He is thinking within himself, accomplishing the evaluation task:

"The likelihood of pneumonia is high, and therefore severity is high: unfortunately, I know the high risk of dying from pneumonia in patients admitted to the hospital. At the same time, the uncertainty is also high: there are too many determinants and no guideline for the specific situation of this patient. I have to face the complex scenario: I probably need the help of other professionals, nurses and other colleagues, and I have to take my time to organize the setting. In these situations, the decisions are unstable, whatever decision I make it is neither right nor wrong, it is a chance, and has to take into account the preferences and values of the patient".

The doctor has identified the scenario of decision-making and the typology of the decision. He knows that he needs the help of the patient to decide, because in this situation there is no right or wrong answer. But this doesn't absolve him from the analytic process of decision:

"I have to balance quality of life with the probabilities of survival".

He pictures in his mind a scheme as presented in Table 2.13.

Table 2.13 Analytic process of decision-making

Scenarios	Pros	Cons
1. Intensive care at home	*Higher quality of life* *Respect for advanced will*	*Higher risk of death*
2. Send to the hospital	*Higher safety for the patient* *Less regret for the wife if the patient dies*	*Wife absence, high risk of nosocomial infections, advanced will expressed by the patient and preferences of the caregiver*

Then, the doctor tests compatibility between the course of action and his/her principles and patient's ones: "My value is to respect the autonomy of the patient expressed as an advanced will. What are the values of the patient? A reliable witness, his wife, communicates that quality of life is preferred over prolonging it. The advanced will of the patient and quality of life against life extension".

Principles and values serve to internally generate candidate goals and plans for possible adoption, and they guide decisions about externally generated candidate goals and plans.

In the end the doctor:

"Am I able to take on the responsibility of keeping the patient at home, respecting the value of quality of life and advanced will and not the higher safety for the patient?"

The doctor answers to this question within himself and, drinking the coffee at the kitchen table, informs the wife about severity and uncertainty, about the two options, about pros and cons of each option, about the refusal of the wife to share the decision, but thanking her for speaking out. The wife declares she will obey to the doctor, in whatever decision he will make, and the doctor expresses his choice.

2.8 Summary and Take-Home Messages

2.8.1 Managing the Older Patient

In managing an older patient, the consultation is an opportunity for a unique face-to-face encounter which could strongly affect his/her complex situation. The consultation can be seen as a procedure, composed of discrete elements emerging from "thick" interaction between the doctor's competences and patient's needs. The organization of the service affects the consultation itself: the doctor has to ensure an effective appointment system, enough time for each patient and privacy; older people should have a fast track in acute situations, and follow-up should be booked in advance in consultation for chronic disease. Before starting the consultation, the doctor has to ask the patient if he or she wants somebody else with him during the consultation.

2.8.2 Subjectivity of the Patient

The main aim of the consultation with an older patient is to investigate his/her agenda and to focus on the presenting problems by allowing patient expression, becoming aware of patient's ideas, concerns and expectations and of the impact of the problems on the patient's life.

The point of view of the patient is often different to what the doctor imagines; therefore, listen to older patient and avoid trying to lock him/her into scientific frames.

2.8.3 Examination

The second aim is to select and test previously gathered hypotheses in order to reach the correct diagnosis or to decide how to manage the case ("backward reasoning"). This is made by converting data into an information necessary for the further decisional step. The test of time is the most common test performed in general practice.

Check through all medications thoroughly and ask about the over-the-counter medications and alternative treatments, and assess family structure and the reliability of relatives and relations with the patient. Gather information about functional status. When you have the opportunity, let the patient tell his/her life history.

2.8.4 Overall Clinical Judgement

Be aware of the whole situation of the patient, the effect of the burden of multimorbidity on the prognosis in terms of physical and mental functioning, quality of life and life expectancy, but also in terms of the capacity of patients for coping with it and elicit patient's preferences in order to prioritize problems.

2.8.5 Choice

Map out some plans, in order to decrease a huge number of possibilities to a limited set of options; have a "B" plan anyway.

In order to decide, at first calculate risk, then evaluate context with fast and frugal heuristics, and finally take into account the doctor's values and elicit those of the patient.

2.8.6 Shared Decision-Making

Share the decision with the patient reaching three objectives: to inform, to obtain consent and to involve the patient, through an interactional process, relying on doctor's and patient's contributions. If the patient lacks the capacity to understand, the doctor has to evaluate and record the situation and to share this decision with the patient's caregiver, relatives and advocates, in the patient's best interest.

In a situation with high uncertainty, the involvement of the patient has a higher importance.

References

1. Delvecchio G, Vettore L. Decidere in terapia. Genova: Liberodiscrivere; 2013.
2. Stott N, Davis R. The exceptional potential in each primary care consultation. JR Coll Gen Pract. 1979;29:201–5.
3. Parisi G, Pasolli L. Clinica, relazione, decisione. La consultazione medica nelle cure primarie: La consultazione medica nelle cure primarie. FrancoAngeli, 2016.
4. Geertz C. The interpretation of cultures. Basic books; 1973.
5. Byrne P, Long B. Doctors talking to patients. Department of Health and Social Security. London: HMSO; 1976.
6. Nash A, Fitzpatrick JM. Views and experiences of nurses and health-care assistants in nursing care homes about the Gold Standards Framework. Int J Palliat Nurs. 2015;21:35–41.
7. Neighbour R. The inner consultation: how to develop an effective and intuitive consulting style. Radcliffe Publishing; 2004.
8. Weed LL. Medical records that guide and teach. N Engl J Med. 1968;278:652–7.
9. Pendleton D. The consultation: an approach to learning and teaching. Oxford University Press; 1984.
10. McWhinney I. Family medicine: a textbook. Oxford: Oxford University Press; 1989.
11. Gérvas J. Los problemas de salud en atencion primaria y su clasificacion. Aten Primaria. 1987;4:429–31.
12. Tuckett D et al. Meetings between experts: an approach to sharing medical ideas in medical consultation. London: Tavistock; 1985.
13. Makoul G, Cochran N. Models for teaching shared decision making. In: Elwyn G, Edwards A, Thompson R, editors. Shared decision making in health care: achieving evidence-based patient choice. 3rd ed. Oxford: Oxford University Press; 2016. p. 145–154.
14. Middleton JF. The exceptional potential of the consultation revisited. J R Coll Gen Pract. 1989;39:383–6.
15. Charles C, Gafni A, Whelan T. Shared decision-making in the medical encounter: what does it mean?(or it takes at least two to tango). Soc Sci Med. 1997;44:681–92.
16. Muth C, van den Akker M, Blom JW, Mallen CD, Rochon J, Schellevis FG, Becker A, Beyer M, Gensichen J, Kirchner H. The Ariadne principles: how to handle multimorbidity in primary care consultations. BMC Med. 2014;12:223.
17. Roter D, Hall JA. Doctors talking with patients/patients talking with doctors: improving communication in medical visits. Greenwood Publishing Group; 2006.
18. Karp F. Talking with your doctor: a guide for older people. National Institute on Aging, Public Information Office; 1994.
19. de Wit N. A "time out consultation" in primary care for elderly patients with cancer: better treatment decisions by structural involvement of the general practitioner. Eur J Cancer Care. 2017;26:e12711.
20. Engel GL. The need for a new medical model: a challenge for biomedicine. Science. 1977;196:129–36.
21. Elstein AS, Schwarz A. Clinical problem solving and diagnostic decision making: selective review of the cognitive literature. BMJ. 2002;324:729–32.
22. Charon R. What to do with stories: the sciences of narrative medicine. Can Fam Physician. 2007;53:1265–7.
23. Jylhä M. What is self-rated health and why does it predict mortality? Towards a unified conceptual model. Soc Sci Med. 2009;69:307–16.

24. Nielsen ABS, Siersma V, Kreiner S, Hiort LC, Drivsholm T, Eplov LF, Hollnagel H. The impact of changes in self-rated general health on 28-year mortality among middle-aged Danes. Scand J Prim Health Care. 2009;27:160–6.
25. DeSalvo KB, Jones TM, Peabody J, McDonald J, Fihn S, Fan V, He J, Muntner P. Health care expenditure prediction with a single item, self-rated health measure. Med Care. 2009;47:440–7.
26. Patel VL, Arocha JF, Zhang J. Thinking and reasoning in medicine. The Cambridge handbook of thinking and reasoning. 2005;14:727–50.
27. Croskerry P. Cognitive forcing strategies in clinical decisionmaking. Ann Emerg Med. 2003;41:110–20.
28. Heneghan C, Glasziou P, Thompson M, Rose P, Balla J, Lasserson D, Scott C, Perera R. Diagnostic strategies used in primary care. BMJ. 2009;338:b946.
29. Kozier B. Fundamentals of nursing: concepts, process and practice. Pearson Education; 2008.
30. Veronese N, Stubbs B, Noale M, Solmi M, Pilotto A, Vaona A, Demurtas J, Mueller C, Huntley J, Crepaldi G. Polypharmacy is associated with higher frailty risk in older people: an 8-year longitudinal cohort study. J Am Med Dir Assoc. 2017;18:624–8.
31. Charon R. Narrative medicine: a model for empathy, reflection, profession, and trust. JAMA. 2001;286:1897–902.
32. Simon HA. A behavioral model of rational choice. Q J Econ. 1955;69:99–118.
33. Kastner M, Hayden L, Wong G, Lai Y, Makarski J, Treister V, Chan J, Lee JH, Ivers NM, Holroyd-Leduc J. Underlying mechanisms of complex interventions addressing the care of older adults with multimorbidity: a realist review. BMJ Open. 2019;9:e025009.
34. Han PK, Klein WM, Arora NK. Varieties of uncertainty in health care: a conceptual taxonomy. Med Decis Mak. 2011;31:828–38.
35. Badger F, Plumridge G, Hewison A, Shaw KL, Thomas K, Clifford C. An evaluation of the impact of the Gold Standards Framework on collaboration in end-of-life care in nursing homes. A qualitative and quantitative evaluation. Int J Nurs Stud. 2012;49:586–95.
36. Whitney SN, McGuire AL, McCullough LB. A typology of shared decision making, informed consent, and simple consent. Ann Intern Med. 2004;140:54–9.
37. Marewski JN, Gigerenzer G. Heuristic decision making in medicine. Dialogues Clin Neurosci. 2012;14:77.
38. Woolever D. The art and science of clinical decision making. Fam Pract Manag. 2008;15:31.
39. Beach LR. Image theory: an alternative to normative decision theory. ACR North American Advances; 1993.
40. Europe Co. Convention for the protection of human rights and dignity of the human being with regard to the application of biology and medicine: convention on human rights and biomedicine; Oviedo, 4. 4. 1997. Conseil de l'Europe, Service de l'Édition et de la Documentation, 1997
41. Levinson W, Kao A, Kuby A, Thisted RA. Not all patients want to participate in decision making: a national study of public preferences. J Gen Intern Med. 2005;20:531–5.
42. Gigerenzer G, Gray J. Better doctors, better patients, better decisions: envisioning health care 2020. The MIT Press; 2011.
43. Sturmberg JP, Martin C. Handbook of systems and complexity in health. Springer Science & Business Media; 2013.

Dealing with Older Patients: Health and Disease in Old Age

3

Norma Sartori and Fabrizio Valcanover

Abstract

In this chapter the focus of our attention is on the older person who is not necessarily sick. The key concepts are the subjectivity and personal experiences of the patient. In connection to these perceptions, the patient generates his/her hypotheses of diagnosis and therapy, which he or she then brings to the consultation and that influence his/her relationship with the medical and care staff. We in the medical world must interrogate on ourselves the meaning of healthy elderly person, on how to trace a boundary between the concept of health and sickness in old age, but also the meaning of frailty. The elderly person is immersed in a net of relations, which include those of care, that have been built throughout their whole life and have been moulded through the contact with the health system, doctors and the sanitary consumerism which is typical of our day and age. In this chapter we go further into these ideas with the aid of real stories. The use of these stories allows us to integrate humanities with medical and scientific knowledge. We mention also the educational field and we use stimuli from anthropological and sociological literature.

Keywords

Older patient · Subjectivity · Healthy older patients · Negotiation · Social dimension

N. Sartori · F. Valcanover (✉)
CLIPSLAB-IT, Trento, Italy
e-mail: fabrizio.valcanover@yahoo.it

3.1   Introduction and Aims

The concept of patient-centred is now accepted both at territorial and specialist levels.

The importance of the doctor-patient relation is a topic, along with the debate on incidence and inequality, that occurs when we speak of patient treatment, especially if complex as with older patients. These concepts obviously require a personalization of the steps of the treatment [1, 2].

"People-centred means treating people, patients, their loved ones, careers and other with compassion, dignity and respect ... To deliver the people-centered health systems of tomorrow, we need to change how we provide care and how we measure health system today" [3].

We investigate the subjectivity of the patient as **his or her perception of being healthy or sick. In connection to these perceptions, the patient generates his/her hypotheses of diagnosis and therapy, which he or she then brings to the consultation and that influence his/her relationship with the medical and care staff.**

The perception of health and sickness evolves over time. It is founded on social and cultural elements, on family myths and beliefs, but also on repeated interactions with the health service [4–6].

We can imagine that in an older patient, these experiences are firmly rooted and difficult to change as they are the outcome of an entire lifetime.

Generally, the patient's subjectivity is described by the medical staff, who interprets and deduces it through referred signs and symptoms or through questionnaires or complaints.

Investigating the patient's perception of health and sickness gives us an insight on his/her subjectivity. We find it particularly important when the patient is a senior citizen.

This insight can effectively add to the consultation with the senior patient [7, 8].

Finally, in the teaching field, we find it relevant to insert the analysis of a patient's past experiences of health and sickness as support for a correct diagnosis and therapy.

3.2   Health and Sickness in Old Age (Table 3.1 **Everlasting I. Fraizer)**

Speaking of older patients raises a series of questions.

When does old age begin? Does "pure" ageing exist? Does a physiology of ageing exist?

What is the boundary between health and sickness in old age [9]?

These questions tie in with the concept that illnesses occur in a different form at a young age and that both at a diagnostic and therapeutic level particular caution is necessary [10–12].

John W. Rowe [13, 14] introduced the concepts of successful ageing and usual ageing old person whereby the successful ageing old person is typified by the absence of severe physical impairment, psychological and emotional health and rich social interaction.

Table 3.1 Everlasting by Ian Frazier (New Yorker 2003–10). https://www.newyorker.com/magazine/2003/10/27/everlasting-3

The shock our family experienced at the death of our beloved uncle Simon is beyond my power to describe. You feel so helpless, so bereft… for months afterward we stumbled around in a fog of numbed incomprehension. But then grief naturally began to turn to anger. How could something like this have happened? Simon was a strong, healthy man of 97 years. He had never been sick a single day or suffered any serious injury. In my mind, that profile sent up a red flag right away. Here's a man who has lived without any health problems at all for nearly a hundred years, and suddenly one morning, out of the blue, he dies
Obviously, the facts point to hidden negligence or other underlying causes. A few of our acquaintances, no one close to us, of course, whispered that Simon had brought his death on himself by being "old". That blame-the-victim approach is hardly worth responding to, except to say that "old" is a relative term, and reducing anybody's life to a number seems inaccurate and unfair. One or two other people have been insensitive enough to inform us, witlessly, that we all have to go sometime. As if such platitudes spoke to our sorrow and outrage! Yes, many human beings do go… After a certain number of years. But do we have to? By no means
In Simon's case, there wasn't a reason in the world for this man to die. Simon's blood pressure was at exactly the level posted on the A.M.A.'s web site, and when they lowered the recommendation not long ago Simon's pressure, amazingly, went down just enough to meet it

We will not be tackling these topics.

We want to introduce the concept of "healthy" patient, whereby being healthy is mainly referred to the lifelong experiences of the older patient and the cultural and social environment where he or she lives [15].

With this outlook acute and chronic illnesses take on a new meaning, and, maybe, the concept of frailty is implicitly redefined, even if we do not go into this aspect more deeply.

Therefore, we propose the idea of a healthy elderly person, who does not need treatment and to whom, respecting their age and experience, prevention should be directed in a precise but light manner. The concept of "frailty" however remains a useful tool even if we feel that it is more important for organizing care and therapy paths than for defining a status (and giving a stigma). This, however, is not the specific focus of this chapter.

This division is not so clear in real life. A slightly more thorough way to group people would be the following:

- Healthy people who see themselves as healthy.
- Sick people who see themselves as healthy.
- Healthy people who see themselves as sick.
- Sick people who see themselves as sick.

This point of view should be considered in a social dimension that puts culture and values before patient's inner self.

Whereby, for example, healthy people see themselves as sick shouldn't be dismissed as suffering from somatoform neurosis, or depression, but as offspring of their own history and generation which have passed down to them a particular

Table 3.2 Aurora's story—dying healthy

Aurora died aged 90, having been in full health up to a month before passing. The cause of her death was the flu, first real illness from which she suffered throughout her life. The only thing to bother her had been arthrosis in her knees which, from the age of 85 onwards, kept her from leaving the house autonomously. Since that age her shopping/groceries would be delivered to her. She listened to mass on the radio. She had lost the will to go for walks in the sun. she had no children or husband. Her only niece would visit her regularly and sometimes help her with the housework. A general practitioner, at her niece's insistence, would visit her once a month. Aurora's blood pressure was always normal, her cardio-respiratory system was in excellent condition, and her peripheral arterial and venous circulation undamaged. Her lab exam results are always normal. No sign of any pathologies was ever picked up on during her regular doctor visits. The pain caused by the arthrosis was kept under control with the occasional use of paracetamol. But Aurora felt she was ill and was almost annoyed by the exam results always coming back stating that everything was fine. In the absence of true symptoms, she would complain about the food and how it had lost all taste, about the sun and how it didn't warm her anymore and of dead friends and relatives.

interpretation of health and sickness and the implications of the part healthy or sick person plays in society (Table 3.2 Aurora's story).

A depressive pathology therefore should be investigated only after having a clear general understanding of how the elderly person interprets health and sickness.

In Western society, where the older people makes up an ever-growing percentage of the population, we find ourselves having to redefine their physio-pathological, cultural and social traits, not as singular or exceptional but as a whole which influences the social and political choices of one's country.

To trace a boundary between health and sickness in old age, we think it is necessary to broaden our view.

The immersion in subjectivity (which we will do using histories of healthy older persons) allows us to investigate some aspects of the older patient and particular importance:

- What dying means to the older.
- What health and disease mean to the older persons.
- His/her ability to cope.
- Adapting previous knowledge/experience to new situations.
- New roles and identities (acquired with age) in one's familiar and micro-social environment.
- Ageing as the betterment of certain functions (knowledge, experience) and the worsening of others (memory, attentiveness, speed of thought).
- Stigma: healthy, whiny, diabetic, senile elderly person.
- Demand of financial benefits and the right to healthcare connected with age.

All the points above are important. We are following up just the first and second.

3.2.1 What Dying Means to the Older People

If at a younger age the thought of death is rare and temporary, the passing of years brings about the awareness that life has an end. This awareness has an impact on whether one feels sick or healthy.

The patient's point of view and his/her understanding of health and sickness (and of dying) have been tackled by sociologists, anthropologists, psychiatrists, psycho-analysts, psychotherapists, ethicists and religious figures from different angles and different analysis methods [4–6, 16, 17].

The points of view of the patient about dying and disease are shared with the family and often with the community. In the case of Simon (97 years old) the patient would have probably reacted in the same way as the relatives (Table 3.1).

This literature, interpretive methods aside, suggests that in old age the perception of death, health and sickness is only partly re-elaborated by the physio-pathological status and the medical vocabulary which nowadays passes through the medias and social networks and is best represented by "doctor Google" and that maybe is affected by the economic interests at play.

After all the health service is a business which, despite the economic crises of the last decades, never feels its effects.

3.3 Knowing the Patient, their Relations and Environment

Dealing with older people not only means driving into a patient's subjectivity (concerns, feeling, etc.) but also dealing with a network which is composed of relatives, friends, caregivers, nurses, social workers, specialists and GPs.

The patient is often deaf or blind or demented or with other inabilities: it is not the direct interlocutor; however, it is mandatory to investigate the residual subjectivity.

"Don't tell me this sickness is due to the fact I'm old!" This older person believes their symptoms are due to an illness and not old age.

If this person has a sudden temperature with a cough and discomfort, their observation is fitting. If we encounter other problems such as backache, we need to start digging deeper. Some chronic diseases like COPD or diabetes type 2 can be seen as illnesses or the onset of old age. In this case there is a window for negotiation during the consultation, which makes reaching a mutual agreement possible. The doctor who is awareness of this concept becomes a good professional [18].

3.4 Care Paths and Social Dimension

In the sociological field, the term "care paths" is used to indicate the overall organization of work during the course of an illness and the impact it has on all those involved in such organizing doctor/patients included. The term "disease paths" is used to talk about the course of an illness in strictly clinical terms.

The concept of care paths is useful for looking at (imagine a still frame that captures the evolving dynamic concept of paths at a particular moment) the high number of possible relations when a patient, in most cases an elderly person, is defined as complex.

In this particular context, we do not wish to analyse the organization of a cure path nor its development, implications and characteristics but rather how much this dimension imposes itself in a subconscious and informal way on the doctor, the patient and all the players involved, with particular attention on what are called the "beliefs" of health and sickness [18].

If the analysis can be seen as a pattern of paths, interactions, engagements or separations, organizational critical issues, etc., then surely we can assert that there exists an exchange on a relational and negotiating level that involves the feeling of health or sickness of each player taking part and should focus around the patient's past experiences, in this case, the elderly patient.

Even in the absence of an assistance and care network, multiple interactions with the many figures present in an old person's environment exist (Fig. 3.1). With these players the negotiating interactions concerning the concepts of being healthy and sick are not only found on an explicit and relational level but often are manifested with actions, drive intentions and motivations and interfere with therapy paths and the course of the illnesses.

With this point of view, *the relational dimension* gathers complexity, different shades, implied facts, passions and disappointments that, in the older in particular, have a deep impact on the clinical dimension with the diagnosis and therapies and compliance.

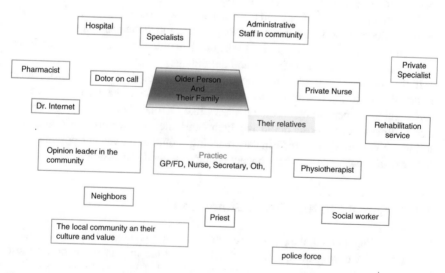

Fig. 3.1 Social dimension: the care paths. F. Valcanover

The care dimension, even in its simple paths, is heavily influenced and can collapse if an important factor is not taken into consideration: older patients see themselves as healthy, sick, old, young and they are constantly trying to make sense of the discomfort and suffering their age is making them live.

This aspect outlines the binds of our intervention and defines possible actions. It also puts forward questions about the "quality of care" and how training, especially when it concerns old age, can create a "re-applicable sensitivity approach" (we will use this term because we are perhaps entering an area where re-applicable is difficult if not impossible) as an embodied work environment amongst professionals [19].

3.5 Anecdotes as a Guide to Therapy

Using true stories as a starting block, we have extracted some "concepts" using a qualitative method [20–22]. This is not a research but a simple tool we have used to investigate our point of view starting with the subjectivity of the older person. Perhaps a detailed study on this point (feeling "healthy") is desirable also to gain further insight into the older person's past, something we consider central in the diagnostic and therapeutic approach.

The choice of telling stories was made to allow us to compare the meaning of health for the patient and for the doctor. The doctor should notice when an older patient thinks he/she is healthy and doesn't realize that something is starting to go wrong. Only in this way can the doctor act in a different way to how she/he would with a young patient.

In particular, Maria tends to deny her health is deteriorating, while Gino and Gina manage to perceive that something is going wrong and the doctor should be consulted, even if they ask to see their GP in an unusual manner (Gino and Gina's story Table 3.3, Maria's story Table 3.4).

The doctor's awareness of the feeling of health of the patient allows him/her to prevent a heart failure (Gino) or to encourage the doctor to send the patient (Maria) to the hospital.

This can happen with patients that consider themselves "healthy".

In the next section, we use three clinical histories to show how the healthy patient variable may influence the clinical approach and therefore the management of the situation and care paths.

3.6 Basic Knowledge and Advanced Knowledge

In the story of Gino and Gina (Table 3.3), the critical point happens to be the decision to visit the doctor the very same evening, even if they arrived in overbooking and the description of the symptom was of little clinical relevance. This makes it possible to reveal a heart failure which could turn into a nocturnal pulmonary oedema.

Table 3.3 Gino and Gina's story

Gino and Gina are a close-knit couple. He is 92; she is 82. They have always had a positive outlook on life with dancing being their biggest passion. To this day they frequent a social club every Saturday evening where they enjoy a lively social life and still dance. Gina has had some health problems: Breast cancer 30 years ago and more recently, 2 years ago to be exact, a gastric cancer, which was dealt with successfully through surgery and has since not resurfaced. Both have dealt with these health issues with optimism and hope. Gino had to undergo urgent cholecystectomy 3 years ago. The operation marked a brief lull for his active dancer lifestyle along with his gardening. Furthermore Gino has been taking warfarin as part of an anticoagulant therapy for the last 4 years to treat an atrial fibrillation. On that occasion he had had a slight cardiac failure so he was prescribed with low doses of beta-bloc and furosemide 25 mg, two pills a day.

One winter evening they show up in the waiting room without an appointment. There are quite a few people already waiting their turn, but they don't give up and patiently wait for their GP to acknowledge them and eventually receive them so they don't have to return the following day. Things don't exactly go to plan. The doctor admits them without enthusiasm; he's tired and was hoping to be on his way home by 8 pm. That said Gino and Gina are neither hypochondriacs nor rude so the doctor resists the temptation to ask them to come back the following day and goes ahead with the examination and to find out what's wrong.

Gino has a "noisy" phlegmy cough which has been gurgling in his chest for 4–5 days. It bothers him mainly at night. He doesn't have a temperature nor other cold symptoms. When he manages to bring up the phlegm, it is clear, almost white. He doesn't show signs of dyspnoea except when climbing stairs, his ankles aren't swollen, but he has put on a couple of kilos since the previous week: "My trousers feel tight... Mind you, I've always liked eating". Gino's statement is refuted by the fact that Gino is tall and slim as a youngster thanks to his regular diet and never overindulging. His TTR of the INR is at 100%.

There are "bubbling sounds" at the base of both lungs with a saturation of 96%, and the irregular cardiac frequency due to the atrial fibrillation is 79.

Well done Gino and Gina for not giving up when the secretary told them they had to wait 3 days for earliest available appointment or when they saw how many people there where in the waiting room.

They didn't want to bother the doctor, who is really busy during this period, with a home visit. Gino got behind the wheel to drive the 2 kilometres to the surgery.

Satisfied they go home with the diuretic therapy doubled and an appointment for a check-up in 3 days.

Also satisfied is the doctor for having averted a possible worsening of the situation one of the following nights

Gino and Gina show up at the doctor in the evening, out of hours. The doctor must make a quick decision: understand if the situation is urgent and needs to be dealt with that same evening or, with no harm to the patient, if it can be dealt with the following day. Despite being tired, the doctor decides to overcome his desire to call it a day and visit the patient the following day, by using, probably

Table 3.4 Maria's story

Maria is 97 years old. I met her shortly after her 70th birthday.

She was an elderly person and was deaf.

Hypertension has never been a serious problem; it has always been kept under control with 20 mg of ACE inhib, without ever showing complications.

Her asthma, however, has at times been a problem for her.

She has always lived on a farm tending to her husband and children. She has never held back on housework or in the fields and a cold has never been seen as a serious issue. However, the colds often turned into bouts of bronchitis, and therefore her asthma would flare up with serious cases of dyspnoeic attacks. Moreover, she has never used foresight. When she would show up at the doctor's, her respiratory situation would often already be serious, and not always would pharmaceutical treatments prevent her from being hospitalized.

Having reached 90 she was an old lady though seemingly not much worse off than when she was 70 – And deaf. The arthrosis in her knees and the ageing of her muscle and bone tissue have forced her to change her rhythm of life; she has relaxed more and has started accepting help from her daughters. She allows them to do housework, cook meals and help her wash. No one comes by the surgery anymore or calls me at home except occasionally about some mild coughing. The asthma has disappeared, and the salbutamol is no longer part of her therapy.

At 97 she still lives alone and is fairly autonomous, thanks to the careful yet relaxed supervision of her daughters, who allow her to decide what time to go to bed (her favoured time is midnight) and get up (around 11–midday) and what to eat; she often prepares her own meals and the shopping is done following her strict orders.

When they call me concerning a persistent cough and a slight temperature, I visit her, and around her thorax there is widespread wheezing as if due to bronchitis; the saturation is good at 95%; the cardiac frequency and blood pressure are also ok. There is a slight swelling around her ankles. She insists she feels fine. "It's just a slight cough, doctor, don't worry!"

She is right; it isn't worrying. An antibiotic and aerosol with salbutamol, Ipratropio bromuro and beclometasone and 25 mg of furosemide once a day for eight days should suffice. (she is no longer able to use inhaling devices). I arrange with the daughter that she will get back in touch in 8 days. She will call me to bring me up to date and, if necessary, fix an appointment for a check-up.

After the 8 days, the daughter, who is very busy with all her engagements, decides to halt her mother's therapy and has not got in touch with me as agreed.

Three days later concerns have arisen: Maybe this cough hasn't totally disappeared, and mother is looking a little pale, even though she's eating, sleeping and going about the house as she always does with her zimmer frame. Maybe I should call the doctor.

This time the visit determines that all bronchial noises have disappeared, but there is still some minimal crackling in the left lung base, which also appears to be hypo-phonetic. Saturation doesn't exceed 86–88%.

Suspicion of pneumonia is now founded, even if the lady keeps claiming she is fine and looks at me with suspicion as if two visits in 11 days are certainly uncalled for. I'm about to prescribe new antibiotics and oxygen.

Then I look around.

(continued)

Table 3.4 (continued)

The daughter has gone out to do the shopping. When she returns, she starts dashing from room to room doing chores while I visit. I take in what is happening and have to make a decision. The big country house with all the cats, open windows and doors and dropping temperatures, a slight draught and the turned off heating probably isn't the ideal place to treat and elderly person with pneumonia. I already know that the daughter doesn't have room or time to keep her mother at home with her. I also know that hospitalization can be potentially dangerous for someone almost 100 years old. But what is more dangerous? Letting her stay alone in this house, though the daughter does drop by once a day, guaranteeing hospitalized with the risk of being bed bound, she takes her medicine? Or after the X-rays, being sores, catheter and benzodiazepine because everyone has to be asleep by 8 pm? It's a tough decision to make.

I take another look around. I used to come here often, and memories of her cardiopathic daughter, who died prematurely, spring to mind.

I realize they are laid back people, if not slightly fatalistic, but certainly not apprehensive and detached from medical consumerism. An illness can manifest itself in one's life but shouldn't be allowed to take up too much of it. Shopping for groceries, decorating the house, taking care of the garden and vegetable patch and looking after the animals remain absolute priorities. The doctor's orders are followed up to the point where they clash with this everyday life full of vitality and energy. They will never ask for instrumental or lab tests let alone to be admitted to hospital.

It is therefore down to me to decide if I send her for X-rays.

Ten days later Maria is back at home. The worse has passed and she can breathe without the need of oxygen, her cough doesn't bother her anymore, and the antibiotic therapy was finished at the hospital. The X-ray, though, is of dubious interpretation: Pleural effusion and lung thickening persist, and geriatrician and radiologist suspect it could be cancer.

Maria has got over her hospitalization without the need of a catheter, without bed sores or disorientation. Her daughter though has realized that her mother cannot be left alone; she has since moved in with her mother and has put in a request for civil invalidity and accompaniment. She is going to look for a career.

subconsciously, his long-time acquaintance with the patient. In particular, the decision is born, in the space of few minutes, of the condensation in the doctor's mind of:

- The type of relationship he/she has with the patient and his wife ("They didn't want to bother the doctor, who is really busy during this period, with a home visit").
- The couple's understanding of the concept health and illness ("neither Gino nor Gina is hypochondriacs").
- Gino and Gina's behaviour when they had got ill in the past ("Both have dealt with these health issues with optimism and hope ... The operation marked a brief lull for his active dancer lifestyle along with his gardening").

– Past acute pathologies and Gino's chronic condition ("Gino has been taking warfarin as part of an anticoagulant therapy for the last 4 years to treat an atrial fibrillation. On that occasion he had had a slight cardiac failure").

We don't know what decision the doctor might have made if his/her relationship with Gino and his wife was not based on mutual respect and good communication, if the patients had had a hypochondriac attitude, or if, when other illnesses had occurred in the past (Gina's neoplasia and Gino's acute cholecystitis), they had reacted in a different manner. If the acute symptom mentioned in the waiting room—the cough—had presented itself in a subject without a chronic cardiac pathology (e.g. Gina), the doctor's decision perhaps would have been different.

It is evident that the doctor cannot base his/her decision only on the symptoms the patient shows or the signs that emerge from the visit. This is particularly evident when the patient is an older person. A young person with a cough in a waiting room without an appointment would have probably not been dealt in the same way by the doctor.

The decision-making of the doctor in Maria's case brings up more aspects along with the ones already examined:

– The partial self-sufficiency of the patient concerning various aspects of her life, in particular taking her medicines, food and hygiene ("has started accepting help from her daughters. She allows them to do housework, cook meals and help her wash").
– The kind of supervision/help given by her daughters ("she still lives alone and is fairly autonomous, thanks to the careful yet relaxed supervision of her daughters, who allow her to decide what time to go to bed (her favoured time is midnight) and get up (around 11–midday)").
– The perception of health and illness by the caregiver (daughter) ("After the 8 days, the daughter, who is very busy with all her engagements, decides to halt her mother's therapy and has not got in touch with me as agreed. Three days later concerns have arisen: maybe this cough hasn't totally disappeared, and mother is looking a little pale, even though she's eating, sleeping and going about the house as she always does with her zimmer frame. Maybe I should call the doctor").
– Myths and family views—health and illness ("I realize they are laid back people, if not slightly fatalistic, but certainly not apprehensive and detached from medical consumerism. An illness can manifest itself in one's life but shouldn't be allowed to take up too much of it"… "They will never ask for instrumental or lab tests let alone to be admitted to hospital" … "The doctor's orders are followed up to the point where they clash with this everyday life full of vitality and energy").
– The relationship between the patient and her daughters.
– The long-time knowledge of the environment in which the patient lives ("I used to come here often and memories of her cardiopathic daughter, who died

prematurely, spring to mind" ..." The big country house with all the cats, open windows and doors and dropping temperatures, a slight draught and the turned off heating probably isn't the ideal place to treat and older person with pneumonia").

– The evaluation of the pros and cons of hospitalization ("I also know that hospitalization can be potentially dangerous for someone almost 100 years old. But what is more dangerous? Letting her stay alone in this house, though the daughter does drop by once a day, guaranteeing hospitalized with the risk of being bed bound; she takes her medicine? Or after the X-rays, being sores, catheter and benzodiazepine because everyone has to be asleep by 8 pm").

In this case also, the decision to send the patient to the hospital was born of all the elements aforementioned together with the objective examination and a suspected pneumonia diagnosis. It is interesting to note how it proved easy for the doctor to propose sending Maria to the hospital, seeing as how she perceives an illness as a small parenthesis of everyday life. She is convinced that full recovery will come soon, and life will go back to as it always was.

3.7   To Negotiate the Meaning of Life

In all these 250 houses down here there's someone who is devoted to Medicine, 250 beds on which 250 bodies lies <u>and testimonies that life has a sense, and that's to me a medical sense</u> (The triumph of medicine, J. Romains 1923) [23].

Early twentieth-century French literature proposes the concept of "medical sense of life". J. Romains is part of the current of playwrights who, from Moliere onwards, were critical of the doctors of the age (Table 3.5). In his play J. Romains proposes, without realising, the concepts of medicalization and medicalization aimed at profit: a "disease mongering" ante litteram. This "medical sense" is born with the "surgery" which sanctions the passage from the practice of medicine as a form of art to the practice of medicine as science. With this passage, which also includes cultural, social and economic aspects, modern medicine stands as candidate not only for a way of easing suffering but also a way to interpret the life and death of human beings. Maybe, without saying it, it starts competing with religions that have always been the guardians of the sense of life and death.

Table 3.5 The triumph of medicine, J Romains 1923 [23]. Summary

A young doctor arrives in a mountain village to take the place of the GP because the old doctor of the village is transferring to a big city. The village was located in countryside, and the inhabitants were living in a simple way, with a very low medicalization. So, the old doctor didn't have a lot of work, and he didn't earn very much, and his work was sometimes boring. When the young doctor, called doctor Knok, came, things changed very rapidly. He started to use a personal method in his work: With the help of the teacher and the pharmacist, he was able to transform all the inhabitants in just 3 months, because they began to feel ill, and a lot of people started to take unnecessary medicine and stayed in bed almost all day, so all the inhabitants became real sick.

Many authors [24–26] have, in different areas, tackled the "sense" concept and its importance in every aspect of human life.

A "medical sense" of life though assumes that every human being harbours within his or her own sense of living (and dying) aspects, concepts and suggestions that come from the medicine world.

In their life plan, older people include a sense of living that therefore also incorporates the sense of being healthy and sick. And each one develops their own, influenced by the social and cultural environment and the relation with the medical world.

Each contact between doctor and patient implies an implicit (and in part explicit) negotiation on the concept of health and sickness which influences how "practice" is carried out and quality of life.

The concept of negotiation has been thoroughly looked into in medical and non-medical spheres [27–30]. It is considered an important relational tool, especially in primary care [30].

Negotiating on what healthy or sick means to an older patient is legitimate and also a very delicate issue because over a certain age even with the lack of insight, perceiving oneself as healthy or sick significantly influences one's life plan, quality of life and conception of death.

The general practitioner/family doctor often interacts with patients (and their families) they have known for many years, during their visits and contacts, at an implicit level regarding the sense of life and therefore what it means to be healthy or sick [31]. It is an implicit concept which has to do with "personalization" of treatment and treating. It is often redefined and renegotiated. It has to do with the relationship being based on trust. In this negotiation the doctor brings his/her "sense of health and sickness" which often, unaware and in an age of high technology, can coincide with a real and true "medical sense" of life.

But this negotiation is even present in occasional contacts, especially if the patient has been hospitalized – there where negotiation has different characteristics.

The doctor's manner towards an older patient in primary care must allow for observation and negotiation that have to do with the sense of living and dying and therefore with the subjective concept of being healthy and sick.

This research is delicate and difficult to trace back to objective criteria.

It can avail itself of what T. Greenhalgh calls intuition [32] (Table 3.6) and of other tools that favour an approach which focuses on the "biological subjectivity" [17, 33–35] of the older patient.

It should be taught at a university to all students of medicine and also for specialists in a personalized form which is adapted to their working context.

Table 3.6 Features of intuition, T. Greenhalgh 2002 [32]

- Rapid, unconscious process
- Context-sensitive
- Comes with practice
- Involves selective attention to small details
- Cannot be reduced to cause-and-effect logic
    (i.e. B happened because of A) addresses, integrates, and make sense of, multiple complex pieces of data

3.8 Teaching Tools for Medical Students, for Post-Grads in General Practice, for Doctors Who Work in the Field

To be a competent GP, you need to be well-read (a true generalist) and have an open, sensible approach to acquiring knowledge that will fill in any gaps. You need to be able to work as part of a team (you will be part of the primary healthcare team, not to mention the doctor-patient aspect), and you need to be open to differing ethical and cultural ideas and beliefs. That's all just for starters [36]!

Handling an older patient is a challenge for any doctor, more so if the patient is "healthy". It is especially the case if the doctor is young and inexperienced or still in their post-grad training. The concepts of prevention and therapy that are applied to young people or older sick people often are not applicable to healthy older subjects. The use of guidelines or literature can come into contrast with the health and/or assistance needs of these subjects [37]. The young doctors undergoing training and students of medicine also need training in general knowledge which should contain philosophical, social and literary thoughts on the sense of life in general and in older people in particular [22, 38].

Using cases that have really happened, writing the story of how they unfolded and discussing it in workgroups or re-enacting it should simulated patients be available can be an effective way of learning [39]. For simulated patient we intend the one with only a minimal level of structure and whose scenario (canvas) must be very lax to leave space for the patient's emotions and feeling that only through this method can emerge. The structured patient who reads from a pre-written and strict script (standard answers to the doctor's questions) is not suitable for this type of in-depth training because it does not allow the simulator to express his past life experiences. Teaching which includes the use of the simulated patient is more suitable for a young professional in training, while for a pre-grad student, it is less suitable because he or she needs basic notions.

Likewise, the use of film in class and the discussion that follows or the reading of literal texts or poems on the subject can broaden a young doctor's point of view. This helps the ability of the doctor to comprehend the older person's past and to start a dialog on subjects that concern their sense of life and death, fears and hopes. It helps in negotiation and, with the difficult task of managing a diagnosis and therapy, the need to send them to specialists or hospitalization.

The most difficult element to grasp and put into practice is the concept of health in old age. University accustoms students and therefore the young doctor to think of older people as a person who inevitably must be sick.

In medical training in general and in particular that of GPs and FDs, as well as focusing on the training of a doctor with clinical knowledge and managing and relational skills, it is appropriate to aim for training that returns a professional who is learned and aware of the environment and values of the community in which he lives and operates and capable to self-assess, listen and think during his actions [40]. Our older cannot but be better off for it.

3.9   Conclusions

In this chapter we began from the subjectivity and the subjective experience of health and sickness in the older patient.

There are some difficulties when we speak about this time of the life. At first it is necessary to re-define the concept of pathology or physiology. Second we must further look into how to establish the boundaries between health and sickness which are usually blurred. One skips rapidly from one condition to another, and not always is the patient, even if conscious, able to grasp this change.

Therefore, we have an ample space of instability that the doctor must know how to grasp.

The subjective approach requires particular attention in the case of older subjects with good resilience and ability to cope. Resilience and ability to cope that are well developed in an older person can change in the person itself the perception of their state of health and underestimate the beginning of an illness or the appearance of alarm bell symptoms.

All these aspects are to be kept in mind in clinical practice and decision-making processes. In general practice an attentive doctor can self-teach these concepts. The young trainee doctors and medical students though must be helped in these teachings through cultural thoughts of literature, philosophy and sociology. Finally let's remind how, from the learning point of view, the simulated patient is a good method for not only fixing clinical knowledge but also training in relations and pondering on what has been presented in a complex environment.

Concepts that are strictly related with what has been affirmed above are consumerism, hyper-medicalization and over-diagnosis.

These aspects are looked into further in another chapter of this book.

In conclusion we remind that the doctor must not only respect the older patient's subjective past of health and sickness but also learn to use them as helpful tools when assessing therapy (Table 3.7, Auden's poetry).

Post. Scriptum July 31, 2020.
The older people in the age of Sars-Cov2.

Table 3.7 Auden's poetry

Give me a doctor partridge plump,
Short in the leg and broad in the rump,
An endomorph with gentle hands,
who'll never make absurd demands
That I abandon all my vices,
Or pull a long face in a crisis,
But with a twinkle in his eye,
Will tell me that I have to die
Wystan Hugh Auden (1907–1973)

We think that even in these tiring first 6 months of 2020 our point of view does not change.

A reflection: the older people all over the world have been considered the historical memory of our civilization, but they have been forgotten: a massacre all over the world.

References

1. Denjoy N, *Why patient-centred approaches are important*, OECD Observer N. 3019 Q1 2017:27.
2. Wenzel M, *Complex patients: how healthcare must adapt to their needs*, OECD Observer N. 3019 Q1 2017:21–22.
3. Guria A, Editorial, *Our health system must put people at the centre*, OECD Observer N. 3019 Q1 2017:3.
4. Kleinman A, Eisenberg L, Good B. Culture, illness, and care: clinical lessons from anthropologic and cross-cultural research. Ann Intern Med. 1978;88(2):251–8.
5. Byron GJ. Medicine, rationality and experience: an anthropological perspective. Cambridge: Cambridge University Press; 1994.
6. Claudine H. The individual, the way of life and the genesis of illness. In: Bury M, Gabe J, editors. The sociology of health and illness. NY: Routledge; 2004. p. 27–35.
7. Middelton J. The exceptional potential of the consultation revisited. J R Coll Gen Pract. 1989;39:383–6.
8. Parisi G, Demurtas J. The consultation with older patient in primary care: communication, management and clinical reasoning. In: J. Demurtas, N. Veronese (eds.), The Role of Family Physicians in Older People Care. Practical Issues in Geriatrics. Springer Nature Switzerland AG. 2022.
9. Fulop T, Larbi A, Khalil A, Cohen AA, Witkowski JM. Are we ill because we age? Front Physiol. 2019;10:1508.
10. Besdine RW. *Quality of life in older people*. Merk Manual Professional version 2019.
11. Bowling A, Dieppe P. What is successful ageing and who should define it? BMJ. 2005;E 331:24–31.
12. American Geriatrics Society. Updated AGS beers criteria® for potentially inappropriate medication use in older adults. JAGS. 2019;67:674–94. By the 2019 American Geriatrics Society Beers Criteria® Update Expert Panel*
13. Rowe JW, Kahn RL. Human aging: usual and successful. Science. 1987;237:143–9.
14. Crowther MR, Parker M, Achenbaum WA, Larimore W, Koenig HG. Rowe and Kahn's *model of successful aging revisited: positive spirituality—the forgotten factor*. The Gerontologist. 2002;42(5):613–20.
15. Parsons T, Turner BS. *The social system, (Preface to the New Edition) First published in England 1951 by Routledge & Kegan Paul Ltd New edition first published 1991 by Routledge 11 New Fetter Lane London EC4P 4EE.*
16. Freidson E. Client control and medical practice. Am J Sociol. 1960;65(4):374–82.
17. Searle JR. Mind, language and society. Philosophy in the real world. Basic Books; 1998.
18. Freidson E. Professionalism. The third logic. UK: Polity Press; 2001.
19. Gherardi S, Strati A. Learning and knowing in practice-based studies. UK: Edward Elgar Publishing inc; 2012.
20. Kleinman A. The illness narratives: suffering, healing, and the human condition. New York, NY: Basic Books; 1988.
21. Anecdotes and empiricism, Editorials, British Journal of General Practice, November 1995: p 571–572.

22. Schön D. The reflective practitioner: how professionals think in action. New York: NY Basic Books; 1983.
23. *Knock; ou, le triomphe de la médecine. J Remains The Triumph of Medicine, J Remains 1923—traduced and acted by Trento's school of general medicine in 2006.*
24. Merleau-Ponty M. Sense et non-sense. Ed. Gallimard 1966.
25. Foucault M. The birth of the clinic. New York: Pantheon Books; 1973.
26. *Quality improvement in practice care: lesson from project in general practice in Improving patient care in primary care in Europe*, editors M. O'Riordan, L. Seuntjes, R. Groll, EQuiP 2004:8–13.
27. Evans DA, Glymour C, Penrose AM. *Evaluation, goals and discourse in clinical decision.* 1985, (Trad. It a S.Bernabè, The Italian Journal of Clinical Pharmacy, 1992 Vol 6, N.2, p 63–75).
28. Bothelo RJ. A negotiation model for the doctor-patient relationship. Family Practice. Oxford University Press; 1992. p. 210–8.
29. Greenhalgh T, Hurwitz B. Narrative based medicine. Dialogue and discourse in clinical practice. BMJ Nooks; 1988.
30. Schelling T. The strategy of conflict. Cambridge: Harvard University Press; 1960.
31. Parisi G, Caimi V, Valcanover F. La continuità relazionale in Medicina Generale—the long-term doctor-patient relationship in general practice. Osp Maggiore. 2002;94(3):275–80.
32. Greenhalgh T. Intuition and evidence—uneasy bedfellows? Br J Gen Pract. 2002;52:395–400.
33. Baron R. *We must learn to hear our patients as well as their breath sounds, after all, what are we listening for?*, an introduction to medical phenomenology. Ann Intern Med. 1985;103:606.
34. Poweley E, Highson R. The arts in medical education. A practical guide. UK: Radcliff Pub. Ltd; 2005.
35. Edelman GM Tononi G. *A universe of consciousness. How matter becomes Imagination.* Basic Books 2000., Reprint edition 2001.
36. Gear S. *The complete nMRCGP study guide*, Radcliffe P. 2008 2008:1.
37. *Determining the harm-benefit balance of in intervention: for each patient*, Prescribe International, Nov 2014/Vol 23 N° 154:274–277.
38. Lee OL, James P, Zevon ES, Kim ES, Trudel-Fitzgerald C, Spiro A 3rd, Grodstein F, Kubzansky LD. Optimism is associated with exceptional longevity in 2 epidemiologic cohorts of men and women. Proc Natl Acad Sci U S A. 2019;116(37):18357–62.
39. Valcanover F, Sartori N, Colorio P. *Simulated patient: a holistic approach like a bridge between theory and practice in medical education.* Poster, Wonca Europe Conference 2009.
40. Weick C. Sensemaking in organization. Sage Publication, Inc; 1995.

Nutritional Issues of Older People in Primary Care

4

Nicola Veronese, Giuliana Ferrari, and Mario Barbagallo

Abstract

Nutritional problems are common in older people. In particular, malnutrition is very frequent and associated with several negative health outcomes. Therefore, the screening of malnutrition through validated tools is mandatory in this population. Weight loss is another common condition in older people and may indicate reversible or not reversible causes: the early diagnosis of weight loss is mandatory for starting the correct diagnostic pathways. The first treatment of weight loss is to treat the cause, if possible. Then, the use of dietary recommendations and nutritional supplementations is of importance. In this chapter, we will discuss how nutritional status should be assessed in older adults, the management of malnutrition, the most common treatments of weight loss, obesity in older individuals, and the role of general practitioners (GPs) in nutritional issues affecting older people.

Keywords

Malnutrition · Weight loss · Older people · Obesity · Nutrition

N. Veronese (✉) · M. Barbagallo
Department of Internal Medicine and Geriatrics, University of Palermo, Palermo, Italy
e-mail: ilmannato@gmail.com

G. Ferrari
Primary Care Department, USL Modena – Emilia Romagna, Modena, Italy

University of Modena and Reggio Emilia, Modena, Italy

4.1   Introduction

Nutritional problems are common in older people. Aging itself, in fact, is characterized by diminished organ system reserves and loss/decrease in homeostatic controls [1]. Indeed, nutritional needs in older people are determined by multiple factors, including specific medical conditions (such as diabetes and dementia), an individuals' level of physical activity, energy expenditure, and caloric requirements, but also the presence of disability and personal food preferences.

In this chapter, we will discuss how nutritional status should be assessed in older adults, the management of malnutrition, the most common treatments of weight loss, obesity in older individuals, and the role of general practitioners (GPs) in nutritional issues affecting older people.

4.2   Malnutrition in Older People

4.2.1   Identification of Malnutrition

To identify malnutrition is of pivotal importance in geriatric medicine. The diagnosis of malnutrition could be made using some validated criteria, as reported in Box 4.1.

> **Box 4.1 Common Criteria for the Diagnosis of Malnutrition**
> *Academy of Nutrition and Dietetics and the American Society for Parenteral and Enteral Nutrition (ASPEN) Criteria* [2]
> *At least two of the following six criteria:*
> 1. Insufficient energy intake
> 2. Weight loss
> 3. Loss of muscle mass
> 4. Loss of subcutaneous fat
> 5. Localized or generalized fluid accumulation that may mask weight loss
> 6. Diminished functional status as measured by handgrip strength
>
> *Global Leadership Initiative on Malnutrition (GLIM)* [3]
> *Combination of at least one phenotype and one etiologic criteria*
> Phenotype criteria—Non-volitional weight loss, low body mass index (BMI), or reduced muscle mass
> Etiologic criteria—Reduced food intake or absorption or underlying inflammation due to acute disease/injury or chronic disease

4.2.2   Screening for Nutritional Status in Older People

Screening of nutritional status is, in our opinion, mandatory in all older people. The most common tools used for this task could be measuring weight, calculating weight loss, and utilizing screening tools.

Weight: Serial measurements of body weight offer the most used and the most obvious screen for nutritional status in older people. However, obtaining periodic body weights may be difficult, particularly in frail and bedridden subjects [1]. For definition, low body weight is defined as <80% of the ideal body weight [1, 2].

Weight loss: Several studies have indicated that weight loss in older adults, especially if unintentional, is a significant predictor of mortality [4–7]. A great debate is still undergoing regarding the amount of weight loss that can increase the risk of mortality and other negative outcomes in older people. In this regard, some studies have reported that a weight loss <5% compared to baseline values is a significant predictor of mortality [7, 8]. Another important topic of discussion is weight loss in overweight/obese older people.

Briefly, weight loss could be considered of clinical importance in the case of [1, 9]:

- ≥2% decrease of baseline body weight in 1 month
- ≥5% decrease in 3 months
- ≥10% in 6 months.

Screening tools: Some screening tools have been developed in order to identify older adults at risk for malnutrition.

- The Nutritional Risk Screening (NRS) 2002 has two parts: a screening assessment for malnutrition and a part for disease severity. Undernutrition is estimated using three parameters: BMI, percent recent weight loss, and change in food intake [10]. Disease severity may range from 0 (for those with chronic illnesses or a hip fracture) to 3 (for those in the intensive care unit with an APACHE score of 10).
- The Simplified Nutrition Assessment Questionnaire (SNAQ), a four-item tool, was tested in community-dwelling older adults and long-term care residents [11]. In those populations, it had a good sensitivity and specificity for the identification of older individuals at risk for 5% or 10% weight loss, respectively.
- SCREEN II (Seniors in the Community: Risk Evaluation for Eating and Nutrition) is a 17-item instrument that evaluates nutritional risk through evaluating food intake, physiological barriers to eating (difficulty with chewing or swallowing), weight change, and social/functional barriers to eating. The tool has excellent sensitivity and specificity, as well as interrater and test/retest reliability [12]. This tool has also an abbreviated version, based on eight questions [12].
- The Malnutrition Universal Screening Tool (MUST) includes BMI, weight loss in 3–6 months, and anorexia for 5 days due to disease. When neither height nor weight is available, the midarm circumference and subjective assessment of physical characteristics, such as very thin, can be used instead. This tool is particularly sensitive for recognition of protein energy undernutrition in hospitalized older patients [13].

- The Malnutrition Screening Tool (MST) was developed for being used in hospitalized patients but also validated in cancer patients [14]. This tool is based on two simple questions: "Have you been eating poorly because of a decreased appetite?" and "Have you lost weight recently without trying?" Even if short, this tool has a good sensitivity and specificity in predicting malnutrition in older people.
- The Mini Nutritional Assessment (MNA) consists of a global assessment and subjective perception of health, as well as questions specific to diet, and a series of body measurements [15]. This tool has been widely validated and translated in several languages and is predictive of poor outcomes [16]. One of the advantage of this tool is that it could be used for the screening and for the diagnosis of malnutrition (also including indicate people at risk of malnutrition) but could be long to do. For this reason, the Mini Nutritional Assessment-Short Form (MNA-SF) uses six questions from the full MNA and can substitute calf circumference if BMI is not available. A validation study demonstrated good sensitivity compared with the full MNA [17].

Using MNA, some authors have proposed some epidemiological data regarding malnutrition in older people. For example, a 2016 meta-analysis on malnutrition in various health-care settings, including data from 240 studies and 110,000 persons, found very different rates of malnutrition: outpatients, 6.0% (95% CI, 4.6–7.5); hospital, 22.0% (95% CI, 18.9–22.5); nursing homes, 17.5% (95% CI, 14.3–20.6); long-term care, 28.7% (95% CI, 21.4–36.0); and rehabilitation/sub-acute care, 29.4% (95% CI, 21.7–36.9) [18].

Box 4.2 Most Common Tools Used for the Screening of Malnutrition in Older People

Tools

Nutritional Risk Screening
Simplified Nutrition Assessment Questionnaire
Seniors in the Community: Risk Evaluation for Eating and Nutrition
Malnutrition Universal Screening Tool
Malnutrition Screening Tool
Mini Nutritional Assessment

4.2.3 Malnutrition and Weight Loss in Older People: From Diagnosis to Management

Poor nutritional status in older people may have a great impact on outcomes, including physical function [19], health-care utilization [20], and length of stay in hospital [21]. A peculiar aspect of older people is the lack of ability to compensate for periods of low food intake (e.g., due to illness) which can result in long-term, persistent weight changes, especially when combined with other factors that can negatively impact body weight.

Involuntary weight loss may be driven by a variety of factors, as follows.

4.2.3.1 Inadequate Dietary Intake

There are multiple causes of weight loss due to inadequate nutrient intake. These include social (e.g., poor economic status, loneliness, social isolation), psychological (in particular depression and dementia), medical (e.g., edentulism, dysphagia), and finally pharmacologic issues.

- Increased likelihood of isolation at mealtimes. About one-third of persons over 65 and one-half over 85 live alone, which typically decreases food enjoyment and calorie intake. In this regard, several studies have reported that older adults who eat in the presence of others consume more than those who eat alone [22].
- Financial limitations affecting food acquisition.
- Cancer is another common cause of unexplained weight loss in older people, particularly when affecting the gastrointestinal tract as well as depression.
- Dysphagia is present in approximately 7–10% of the older adults [23]. Dysphagia is often a consequence of other neurological conditions including stroke and Parkinson disease [1].

When we found an unintentional weight loss in older people, we should also consider the conditions listed in Table 4.1:

4.2.3.2 Physiologic Factors

Physiologic factors associated with weight loss may include age-related decrease in taste and smell sensitivity, delayed gastric emptying, early satiety, and impairment in the regulation of food intake [1].

- Anorexia (of aging): Anorexia, the decrease in appetite, in older adults is influenced by multiple physiological changes. It is known that food intake gradually diminishes with age due to several factors including decreased energy, decreased resting energy expenditure (REE), and/or loss of lean body mass [24]. Changes in taste and smell lead to a decreased desire to eat, and early satiety develops

Table 4.1 Common causes of malnutrition in older people

Apparatus/system/condition	Examples
Endocrine disorders	Hyperthyroidism, new-onset diabetes mellitus
End-organ disease	Congestive heart failure, end-stage kidney disease, chronic obstructive pulmonary disease, hepatic failure
Gastrointestinal disorders	Celiac disease, ischemic bowel, inflammatory bowel disease, pancreatic insufficiency, peptic ulcer disease, gastroesophageal reflux disease
Infections	Tuberculosis
Rheumatologic disorders	Polymyalgia rheumatica, rheumatoid arthritis
Neurologic conditions	Parkinson disease, chronic pain, Alzheimer disease
Medication side effects	Digoxin, opioids, serotonin-reuptake inhibitors, diuretics, and topiramate

with age [25], related to gastrointestinal changes and gastric hormone changes, as discussed above [26]. Moreover, appetite regulation may be affected by some factors cited before such as illness, medications, dementia, and depression [27, 28].

- Cachexia: Cachexia has been defined as a "complex syndrome associated with underlying illness, and characterized by loss of muscle with or without loss of fat mass" [29]. Anorexia, inflammation, insulin resistance, and increased muscle protein breakdown are often associated with the presence of cachexia. Cachexia involves many pathways, leading to a disequilibrium between catabolism and anabolism. Since inflammation and catabolism are present, cachexia often is resistant to nutritional interventions. The cause of cachexia is multifactorial. Therefore, its treatment should be multimodal, including the use of a combination of an appetite stimulant and an agent promoting muscle protein synthesis [30]. Cachexia usually occurs in the setting of underlying illness involving a cytokine-mediated response, such as cancer, renal failure, chronic pulmonary disease, heart failure, rheumatoid arthritis, and acquired immunodeficiency syndrome (AIDS). The role of inflammation in cachexia seems to be pivotal [31], even if anti-inflammatory drugs are not able to modify the course of cachexia itself [30].

4.2.3.3 Evaluation of Weight Loss

Often weight loss is self-reported or based on anamnestic data from the patient and caregivers. Therefore, the first step is to document weight loss during the first visit.

During the first visit, we recommend to estimate body fat and lean muscle mass, through bioelectrical impedance or anthropometric measures, for example. At the same time, in front of an important weight loss, appetite and dietary intake must be assessed using validated tools, such as the MNA. A more formal dietary intake assessment can be obtained with a dietetic consult.

The next step is to perform appropriate laboratory studies, such as metabolic and inflammatory parameters, to include a basic chemistry profile including glucose and electrolytes, thyroid-stimulating hormone (TSH), complete blood count (CBC), and C-reactive protein (CRP) if cachexia is suspected. Chest and plain abdomen radiographs may be considered in the case of suspected cancer or other specific conditions. Order additional studies based on suspicion of underlying disease from the patient's history and examination.

Of importance are older people with no localizing findings and with normal complete blood count, biochemical profile, or chest and plain abdomen radiographs since until one-third of patients were ultimately diagnosed with cancer [32].

4.2.3.4 Tips for Weight Loss Diagnosis

After the diagnosis of weight loss, if it is possible, it is mandatory to treat the condition. The most common causes of weight loss in older people can be described using the acronym "MEALS ON WHEELS" (Table 4.2).

Table 4.2 Causes of weight loss in older adults

Medications
Emotional
Alcoholism, older adult abuse
Late-life paranoia or bereavement
Swallowing problems
Oral factors
Nosocomial infections
Wandering and other dementia-related factors
Hyperthyroidism, hypercalcemia, hypoadrenalism
Enteral problems
Eating problems
Low salt, low cholesterol, and other therapeutic diets

4.2.3.5 Treatment of Weight Loss in Older People

General Recommendations

- Make sure that feeding or shopping assistance is available. Remember that feeding assistance was resource-intensive and required a mean of about 30 minutes and often more [33]. In this regard, social work support may be of importance, if inadequate finances are one of the determinants of poor nutritional status.
- Assure that meals and foods meet individual preferences.
- Increase the nutrient density of food. For example, it could be useful to increase protein content by adding milk powder, whey protein, and egg whites or increase fat content by adding olive oil. If weight does not increase, we suggest daytime snacks between meals.

Nutritional supplements: A meta-analysis included 55 randomized trials of nutritional supplements containing protein and energy to prevent malnutrition in older, high-risk patients [34]. This work resulted in modest improvement in percentage weight change. Moreover, overall mortality was reduced in the groups receiving nutritional supplement, compared with control, but no improvement in disability [34]. In this regard, nutritional supplements seem be able to improve physical performance and muscle strength tests in older people, particularly in frail and sarcopenic subjects [35].

Mirtazapine: Mirtazapine is a common antidepressant leading to more weight gain than selective serotonin reuptake inhibitor (SSRI) antidepressants. For this side effect, it is commonly used for weight loss in older adults due to depression, even if few studies have been specifically performed to evaluate its impact on weight among older adults with weight loss [36].

4.2.4 Obesity in Older People

Even if the prevalence of obesity in people who are 80 years of age is about one-half of that of older adults between the ages of 50 and 59, the fact is that more than 15% of the older American population is obese [37]. However, the epidemiological role of obesity in older people is really debated. It is known that in the general population, obesity is associated with an increased risk of all-cause mortality [38], as well as other disabling conditions including metabolic (e.g., type 2 diabetes) and cardiovascular diseases (e.g., hypertension, coronary heart disease, stroke), but also some types of cancer (e.g., endometrial, breast, prostate, and colon cancers) [39].

However, the association between high BMI values and mortality seems to decline over time, and this seems to be more evident in some special settings such as nursing home in which high BMI seems to be protective for mortality [40]. Other large observational studies observed a decrease in the association of obesity with cardiovascular disease mortality over time [41] and that being overweight does not increase mortality risk for people age 65 years and older [42].

A few studies suggest that being overweight as an older adult is associated with increased mortality:

These findings did not suggest that adiposity per se is protective for mortality but that BMI and weight are not reliable indicators of being overweight or obesity in older people, where normal weight may reflect loss of muscle mass rather than decreased adiposity [1, 43].

This is somewhat demonstrated by the fact that obesity in older adults is associated with new or worsening disability [44], and weight loss can further improve physical function and quality of life in older obese people [45]. Regarding the treatment, recommendations to lose weight must be tailored to the risk profile of particular patients. Those who are experiencing significant adverse effects associated with obesity (the typical example is the patient with pain from osteoarthritis) [46] should be encouraged to have weight loss, but only in the context of regular physical exercise [47].

4.2.5 What's the Role of General Practitioner in Nutritional Issues in Older People?

Older people access very frequently GPs' ambulatories for several reasons [48, 49]. Of curiosity, it is estimated that 10% of the population requiring care from a GP are at risk of malnutrition [50]. Despite the large population at risk of malnutrition and its associated health implications discussed in this chapter, malnutrition is often undiagnosed and untreated by GPs [51]. Many reasons have been suggested for the under-diagnosis of malnutrition in primary care setting, including the absence of nutrition education in medical school curricula and post-graduate training in GPs and the unclear "ownership" of malnutrition care among health-care professionals [52].

However the role of GP in nutritional issues in older people is pivotal. For this reason, we first recommend to assess weight in all older people using the ambulatory, at least one time every 6–12 months. Another important point is to assess, better if through validated screening tools, the presence of malnutrition and start the diagnostic pathway. In this regard, the help of specialists (e.g., geriatrician, gastroenterologist, and others) is recommended as well as the use of laboratory measures.

The use of "MEALS ON WHEELS" could be useful for better and quickly identifying the cause of weight loss. Regarding obesity in older people, it should be noted that the GP was the least likely person to tell a patient to lose weight after partner, family, and friends [53]. Therefore, more is needed to improve the knowledge of GPs regarding obesity in older people.

4.3   Conclusions

Malnutrition is extremely common as condition in older people, but often neglected. In this chapter, we have revised the common tools used for the screening of malnutrition in older people and how to diagnose malnutrition and weight loss. At the same time, obesity is increasing also in older people, probably indicating that it will be a common problem in the next future. The role of the GP is really important, but more knowledge regarding nutritional issues in older people (and their clinical importance) is needed.

References

1. Ritchie C, Yukawa M. Geriatric nutrition: nutritional issues in older adults. UpTo Date. 2009;17.
2. White JV, Guenter P, Jensen G, Malone A, Schofield M, Group AMW, et al. Consensus statement: Academy of Nutrition and Dietetics and American Society for Parenteral and Enteral Nutrition: characteristics recommended for the identification and documentation of adult malnutrition (undernutrition). J Parenter Enter Nutr. 2012;36(3):275–83.
3. Cederholm T, Jensen G, Correia MIT, Gonzalez MC, Fukushima R, Higashiguchi T, et al. GLIM criteria for the diagnosis of malnutrition–a consensus report from the global clinical nutrition community. J Cachexia Sarcopenia Muscle. 2019;10(1):207–17.
4. Wallace JI, Schwartz RS, LaCroix AZ, Uhlmann RF, Pearlman RA. Involuntary weight loss in older outpatients: incidence and clinical significance. J Am Geriatr Soc. 1995;43(4):329–37.
5. Wannamethee SG, Shaper AG, Lennon L. Reasons for intentional weight loss, unintentional weight loss, and mortality in older men. Arch Intern Med. 2005;165(9):1035–40.
6. Gregg EW, Gerzoff RB, Thompson TJ, Williamson DF. Intentional weight loss and death in overweight and obese US adults 35 years of age and older. Ann Intern Med. 2003;138(5):383–9.
7. Pizzato S, Sergi G, Bolzetta F, De Rui M, De Ronch I, Carraro S, et al. Effect of weight loss on mortality in overweight and obese nursing home residents during a 5-year follow-up. Eur J Clin Nutr. 2015;69(10):1113–8.
8. Newman AB, Yanez D, Harris T, Duxbury A, Enright PL, Fried LP, et al. Weight change in old age and its association with mortality. J Am Geriatr Soc. 2001;49(10):1309–18.
9. Zawada ET Jr. Malnutrition in the elderly: is it simply a matter of not eating enough? Postgrad Med. 1996;100(1):207–25.
10. Kondrup J, Rasmussen HH, Hamberg O, STANGA Z, Group AAHEW. Nutritional risk screening (NRS 2002): a new method based on an analysis of controlled clinical trials. Clin Nutr. 2003;22(3):321–36.
11. Wilson M-MG, Thomas DR, Rubenstein LZ, Chibnall JT, Anderson S, Baxi A, et al. Appetite assessment: simple appetite questionnaire predicts weight loss in community-dwelling adults and nursing home residents. Am J Clin Nutr. 2005;82(5):1074–81.
12. Keller H, Goy R, Kane S. Validity and reliability of SCREEN II (seniors in the community: risk evaluation for eating and nutrition, Version II). Eur J Clin Nutr. 2005;59(10):1149–57.

13. Stratton RJ, King CL, Stroud MA, Jackson AA, Elia M. 'Malnutrition Universal Screening Tool' predicts mortality and length of hospital stay in acutely ill elderly. Br J Nutr. 2006;95(2):325–30.

14. Ferguson M, Capra S, Bauer J, Banks M. Development of a valid and reliable malnutrition screening tool for adult acute hospital patients. Nutrition. 1999;15(6):458–64.

15. Vellas B, Guigoz Y, Garry PJ, Nourhashemi F, Bennahum D, Lauque S, et al. The Mini Nutritional Assessment (MNA) and its use in grading the nutritional state of elderly patients. Nutrition. 1999;15(2):116–22.

16. Vellas B, Villars H, Abellan G, Soto M, Rolland Y, Guigoz Y, et al. Overview of the MNA®-its history and challenges. J Nutr Health Aging. 2006;10(6):456.

17. Kaiser MJ, Bauer JM, Ramsch C, Uter W, Guigoz Y, Cederholm T, et al. Validation of the Mini Nutritional Assessment Short-Form (MNA®-SF): a practical tool for identification of nutritional status. JNHA—J Nutr Health Aging. 2009;13(9):782.

18. Cereda E, Pedrolli C, Klersy C, Bonardi C, Quarleri L, Cappello S, et al. Nutritional status in older persons according to healthcare setting: a systematic review and meta-analysis of prevalence data using MNA®. Clin Nutr. 2016;35(6):1282–90.

19. Shen H-C, Chen H-F, Peng L-N, Lin M-H, Chen L-K, Liang C-K, et al. Impact of nutritional status on long-term functional outcomes of post-acute stroke patients in Taiwan. Arch Gerontol Geriatr. 2011;53(2):e149–e52.

20. Baumeister SE, Fischer B, Döring A, Koenig W, Zierer A, John J, et al. The Geriatric Nutritional Risk Index predicts increased healthcare costs and hospitalization in a cohort of community-dwelling older adults: results from the MONICA/KORA Augsburg cohort study, 1994–2005. Nutrition. 2011;27(5):534–42.

21. Lelli D, Calle A, Pérez LM, Onder G, Morandi A, Ortolani E, et al. Nutritional status and functional outcomes in older adults admitted to geriatric rehabilitations: the SAFARI study. J Am Coll Nutr. 2019;38(5):441–6.

22. Locher JL, Robinson CO, Roth DL, Ritchie CS, Burgio KL. The effect of the presence of others on caloric intake in homebound older adults. J Gerontol Ser A Biol Med Sci. 2005;60(11):1475–8.

23. Achem S. Dysphagia in aging. J Clin Gastroenterol. 2005;39:357–71.

24. Morley JE. Anorexia of aging: physiologic and pathologic. Am J Clin Nutr. 1997;66(4):760–73.

25. Toffanello E, Inelmen E, Imoscopi A, Perissinotto E, Coin A, Miotto F, et al. Taste loss in hospitalized multimorbid elderly subjects. Clin Interv Aging. 2013;8:167.

26. Sergi G, Bano G, Pizzato S, Veronese N, Manzato E. Taste loss in the elderly: possible implications for dietary habits. Crit Rev Food Sci Nutr. 2017;57(17):3684–9.

27. Donini LM, Dominguez L, Barbagallo M, Savina C, Castellaneta E, Cucinotta D, et al. Senile anorexia in different geriatric settings in Italy. J Nutr Health Aging. 2011;15(9):775–81.

28. Donini LM, Poggiogalle E, Piredda M, Pinto A, Barbagallo M, Cucinotta D, et al. Anorexia and eating patterns in the elderly. PLoS One. 2013;8:5.

29. Evans WJ, Morley JE, Argilés J, Bales C, Baracos V, Guttridge D, et al. Cachexia: a new definition. Clin Nutr. 2008;27(6):793–9.

30. Ali S, Garcia JM. Sarcopenia, cachexia and aging: diagnosis, mechanisms and therapeutic options-a mini-review. Gerontology. 2014;60(4):294–305.

31. Roubenoff R, Harris TB, Abad LW, Wilson PW, Dallal GE, Dinarello CA. Monocyte cytokine production in an elderly population: effect of age and inflammation. J Gerontol Ser A Biol Med Sci. 1998;53(1):M20–M6.

32. Hernández JL, Riancho JA, Matorras P, González-Macías J. Clinical evaluation for cancer in patients with involuntary weight loss without specific symptoms. Am J Med. 2003;114(8):631–7.

33. Simmons SF, Keeler E, Zhuo X, Hickey KA, Sato HW, Schnelle JF. Prevention of unintentional weight loss in nursing home residents: a controlled trial of feeding assistance. J Am Geriatr Soc. 2008;56(8):1466–73.

34. Milne AC, Avenell A, Potter J. Meta-analysis: protein and energy supplementation in older people. Ann Intern Med. 2006;144(1):37–48.

35. Veronese N, Stubbs B, Punzi L, Soysal P, Incalzi RA, Saller A, et al. Effect of nutritional supplementations on physical performance and muscle strength parameters in older people: a systematic review and meta-analysis. Ageing Res Rev. 2019;51:48.

36. Goldberg RJ. Weight change in depressed nursing home patients on mirtazapine. J Am Geriatr Soc. 2002;50(8):1461.

37. Newman A. Obesity in older adults. Online J Issues Nurs. 2009;14:1.

38. Flegal KM, Kit BK, Orpana H, Graubard BI. Association of all-cause mortality with overweight and obesity using standard body mass index categories: a systematic review and meta-analysis. JAMA. 2013;309(1):71–82.

39. Kyrgiou M, Kalliala I, Markozannes G, Gunter MJ, Paraskevaidis E, Gabra H, et al. Adiposity and cancer at major anatomical sites: umbrella review of the literature. BMJ. 2017;356:j477.

40. Veronese N, Cereda E, Solmi M, Fowler S, Manzato E, Maggi S, et al. Inverse relationship between body mass index and mortality in older nursing home residents: a meta-analysis of 19,538 elderly subjects. Obes Rev. 2015;16(11):1001–15.

41. Flegal KM, Graubard BI, Williamson DF, Gail MH. Cause-specific excess deaths associated with underweight, overweight, and obesity. JAMA. 2007;298(17):2028–37.

42. Diehr P, Bild DE, Harris TB, Duxbury A, Siscovick D, Rossi M. Body mass index and mortality in nonsmoking older adults: the Cardiovascular Health Study. Am J Public Health. 1998;88(4):623–9.

43. Villareal DT, Miller BV III, Banks M, Fontana L, Sinacore DR, Klein S. Effect of lifestyle intervention on metabolic coronary heart disease risk factors in obese older adults. Am J Clin Nutr. 2006;84(6):1317–23.

44. Wee CC, Huskey KW, Ngo LH, Fowler-Brown A, Leveille SG, Mittlemen MA, et al. Obesity, race, and risk for death or functional decline among Medicare beneficiaries: a cohort study. Ann Intern Med. 2011;154(10):645–55.

45. Villareal DT, Apovian CM, Kushner RF, Klein S. Obesity in older adults: technical review and position statement of the American Society for Nutrition and NAASO, the Obesity Society. Obes Res. 2005;13(11):1849–63.

46. Bruyère O, Honvo G, Veronese N, Arden NK, Branco J, Curtis EM, editors. et al., An updated algorithm recommendation for the management of knee osteoarthritis from the European Society for Clinical and Economic Aspects of Osteoporosis, Osteoarthritis and Musculoskeletal Diseases (ESCEO). Seminars in arthritis and rheumatism; 2019.

47. Force UPST. Screening for obesity in adults: recommendations and rationale. Ann Intern Med. 2003;139(11):930.

48. van den Bussche H, Kaduszkiewicz H, Schäfer I, Koller D, Hansen H, Scherer M, et al. Overutilization of ambulatory medical care in the elderly German population?–an empirical study based on national insurance claims data and a review of foreign studies. BMC Health Serv Res. 2016;16(1):129.

49. Frese T, Mahlmeister J, Deutsch T, Sandholzer H. Reasons for elderly patients GP visits: results of a cross-sectional study. Clin Interv Aging. 2016;11:127.

50. Elia M, Russell C. Combating malnutrition: recommendations for action. Nutrition Advisory Group on malnutrition led by BAPEN 2009. 2009.

51. Castro PD, Reynolds CM, Kennelly S, Clyne B, Bury G, Hanlon D, et al. General practitioners' views on malnutrition management and oral nutritional supplementation prescription in the community: a qualitative study. Clin Nutr ESPEN. 2020;36:116.

52. Mogre V, Stevens FC, Aryee PA, Amalba A, Scherpbier AJ. Why nutrition education is inadequate in the medical curriculum: a qualitative study of students' perspectives on barriers and strategies. BMC Med Educ. 2018;18(1):26.

53. Tham M, Young D. The role of the General Practitioner in weight management in primary care–a cross sectional study in General Practice. BMC Fam Pract. 2008;9(1):66.

The Role of Physical Activity in Healthy Ageing: An Overview for the Family Physician

5

Lee Smith, Olivier Bruyere, Kyle Hoedebecke, and Mike Loosemore

Abstract

As individuals age, they are at greater risk of developing non-communicable diseases relating to both physical and mental health. A large body of literature exists to show that regular and sustained participation in physical activity aids in the prevention of many of these conditions. In light of this knowledge, the World Health Organisation has developed physical activity recommendations for older adults to maintain good health; it should also be noted that country-specific recommendations exist. Yet, despite this, global levels of physical activity in older adults are low and tend to decline with age. In recent years interventions to promote physical activity in older adults have been developed, although some have been successful in the promotion of physical activity; it is not known whether these interventions yield long-term behaviour change. Strategies to promote long-term behaviour change in older adults have been identified and should now

L. Smith (✉)
The Cambridge Centre for Sport and Exercise Sciences, Anglia Ruskin University, Cambridge, UK
e-mail: lee.smith@anglia.ac.uk

O. Bruyere
WHO Collaborating Centre for Public Health Aspects of Musculoskeletal Health and Aging, Division of Public Health, Epidemiology and Health Economics, University of Liège, Liège, Belgium

K. Hoedebecke
Department of Family Medicine, The Uniformed Services University of the Health Sciences, Bethesda, USA

M. Loosemore
The Institute of Sport Exercise and Health, University College London, London, UK

© Springer Nature Switzerland AG 2022
J. Demurtas, N. Veronese (eds.), *The Role of Family Physicians in Older People Care*, Practical Issues in Geriatrics, https://doi.org/10.1007/978-3-030-78923-7_5

be woven into interventions to promote physical activity to this population. The role of the family physician in promoting physical activity to older adults is crucial, and this could be achieved by simply promoting physical activity to patients or prescribing physical activity to better health. The following chapter discusses the above topics in detail drawing on the most recent literature and placing an emphasis on findings from systematic reviews and meta-analyses where possible.

Keywords

Older adults · Physical activity · Exercise prescription · Family physician · Non-communicable disease

5.1 Defining and Conceptualising Physical Activity

Physical activity may be defined as any bodily movement caused by contraction of skeletal muscle that requires energy expenditure [1]. Common domains of physical activity in adults and older adults include active travel (e.g. walking and cycling to destinations), occupational physical activity, household chores, gardening, sport, exercise, and play with children or grandchildren. As well as domain specific, physical activity can be conceptualised on its intensity: light, moderate, and vigorous. Light physical activity involves performing tasks at 1.5–3 metabolic equivalents and includes activities such as standing—arts and crafts. Moderate physical activity involves performing tasks at three to six metabolic equivalents and includes activities such as walking and vacuuming. Vigorous physical activity involves performing tasks at 6+ metabolic equivalents and includes activities such as riding a bike or running. These activities sit on a physical activity continuum [2] (see Fig. 5.1).

Of note at the opposite end of the continuum to vigorous physical activity sits sedentary behaviour; these activities involve 0–1.5 metabolic equivalents while in a sitting or lying position. This chapter will only focus on light, moderate, and vigorous physical activity, and the interested reader is referred to the book titled *Sedentary Behaviour Epidemiology* (Leitzmann, Jochem and Schmid 2018) [3] for an overview of the literature surrounding sedentary behaviour and health in adults and older adults.

Sedentary Behaviour	Light Physical Activity	Moderate Physical Activity	Vigorous Physical Activity
0 to 1.5	1.5 to 3	3 to 6	6+

Metabolic Equivalents (1kcal/kg/hour)

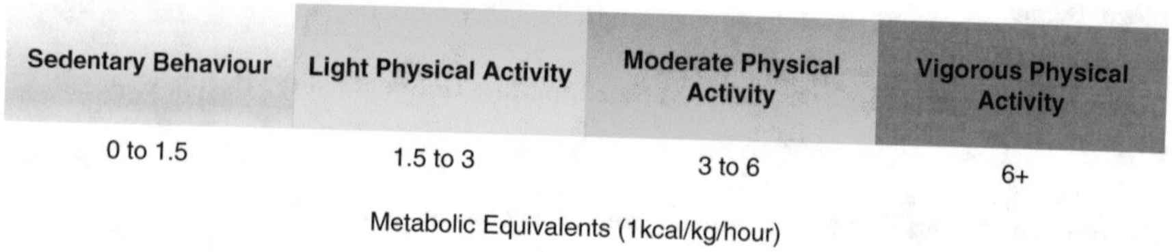

Fig. 5.1 The energy expenditure continuum

5.2 Physical Activity and Health

As individuals age, they are at an increased risk of developing physical non-communicable diseases such as cancer, cardiovascular disease, diabetes, osteoarthritis, and sarcopenia [4–9]. The ageing population are also at increased risk of mild cognitive impairment and dementia [10]. Finally, this group are at increased risk of falls including injurious falls which can lead to morbidity, mortality, and health-care expenditure [11]. Importantly, regular and sustained participation in physical activity, particularly across the lifespan, can aid in the prevention of many of these adverse outcomes [12–16]. Below we provide a summary of this literature drawing on important systematic reviews and meta-analyses in the area.

Regular and sustained participation in physical activity in older adults has been shown to be associated with a plethora of physical and mental health benefits and importantly prolonged survival. In a meta-analysis including nine cohort studies, totalling 122,417 participants, with a mean follow-up of 9.8 ± 2.7 years and 18,122 reported deaths, it was found that a low dose of moderate-to-vigorous physical activity below current recommendations reduced mortality by 22% in older adults. A further increase in physical activity dose improved these benefits in a linear fashion. The meta-analysis concluded that older adults should be encouraged to include even low doses of moderate-to-vigorous physical activity in their daily lives [12]. Moreover, a large body of literature provides empirical evidence that regular participation in physical activity in older adults prevents against diseases of the cardiovascular system, e.g. see [13], and type II diabetes, e.g. see [14].

A recent systematic review of 10 studies integrated and analysed research on physical activity and sarcopenia in the geriatric population. The results of eight studies indicated significant improvement in muscle mass, muscle strength, and physical performance through exercise intervention, as determined by long-term observation. The review concluded that physical activity is an effective protective strategy for sarcopenia [17]. Moreover, other systematic reviews and meta-analyses confirm the beneficial influence of physical activity in general for the prevention of sarcopenia [18, 19].

In a meta-analysis including 11 studies and 1497 participants, it was found that aerobic exercise led to an improvement in global cognitive ability and had a positive effect with a small effect size on memory in people with mild cognitive impairment [15]. Similarly, studies have seen such associations with dementia and Alzheimer's disease [20].

In another meta-analysis of 99 comparisons from 88 trials with 19,478 participants, it was found that participation in exercise (one domain of physical activity) reduced the rate of falls in community-dwelling older people by 21% and thus concluded that exercise as a single intervention can prevent falls in community-dwelling older people [16]. Other meta-analyses on this topic have yielded similar results [21].

One domain of physical activity that has shown significant promise for good mental and physical health in older adults is tai chi [22]. The Compendium of Physical Activities assigned a metabolic equivalent of task score of 4.0 to tai chi, which is classified as moderate-intensity activity [23]. However, and importantly, tai chi is frequently carried out in a gentle and nonstrenuous form (light-intensity physical activity) making it suitable for all ages and fitness levels. Tai chi has shown feasibility and improved physical and psychological outcomes among older adults and also patients with chronic conditions [22, 24]. Moreover, in a meta-analysis of 18 trials with 3824 participants, it was found that tai chi is effective for preventing falls in older adults and the preventive effect is likely to increase with exercise frequency [25]. Other benefits of tai chi identified in multiple meta-analyses include relief of chronic pain [26], relief of fatigue [27], improved self-efficacy [28], improved sleep [29], and enhanced cognitive function in older adults [30]. When recommending physical activity to older adults, the family physician may want to consider suggesting and referring the patient onto a tai chi program.

5.3 Physical Activity Recommendations

In light of these positive health benefits of regular participation in physical activity, the World Health Organisation (WHO) and many nations have developed physical activity recommendations. WHO states that in order to improve cardiorespiratory and muscular fitness and bone and functional health and reduce the risk of noncommunicable disease, depression, and cognitive decline, older adults (65+ years) should do the following [31]:

- Do at least 150 min of moderate-intensity aerobic physical activity throughout the week or at least 75 min of vigorous-intensity aerobic physical activity throughout the week or an equivalent combination of moderate- and vigorous-intensity activity.
- Aerobic activity should be performed in bouts of at least 10-min duration (note: some national guidelines, such as those for people residing in the USA, have now removed this recommendation).
- For additional health benefits, older adults should increase their moderate-intensity aerobic physical activity to 300 min/week or engage in 150 min of vigorous-intensity aerobic physical activity per week or an equivalent combination of moderate- and vigorous-intensity activity.
- Older adults, with poor mobility, should perform physical activity to enhance balance and prevent falls on 3 or more days per week.
- Muscle-strengthening activities, involving major muscle groups, should be done on 2 or more days a week.
- When older adults cannot do the recommended amounts of physical activity due to health conditions, they should be as physically active as their abilities and conditions allow.

There are also several country-specific guidelines that disseminate a similar message; see, for example, UK guidelines [32], American guidelines [33], Australian guidelines [34], and Canadian guidelines [35].

5.4   Levels of Physical Activity

Despite these physical activity recommendations, global population levels of physical activity in older adults are low, and literature shows that physical activity levels decline with age, with the oldest old generally presenting the most unfavourable physical activity profiles. For example, in the oldest old (75+ years) British adults, only 1 in 10 men and 1 in 20 women meet the physical activity guidelines [36]. In America 28% of older adults (50+ years) are inactive, and this low level of physical activity is observed in several other countries, including Australia [37], Canada [38], and across Europe [39]. In addition to low levels of physical activity in older adults, levels also decline as older adults age. For example, Smith et al. (2015) showed in a sample of 5022 participants (mean age 61 years) that over a 10-year period, there was an overall trend for increasing levels of inactivity and a reduction in vigorous activity [40].

5.5   Interventions to Promote Physical Activity in Older Adults

With low and declining levels of physical activity in older adults and the adverse influence this will have on their health, interventions to promote physical activity in older adults are needed. In a systematic review of reviews on physical activity promotion interventions aimed at community-dwelling people over 50 years old, a total of 19 reviews met the inclusion criteria. The study identified that interventions often resulted in sustained improvements in physical activity over the study period, typically at 12 months, and led to improvements in general well-being. Importantly, intervention components associated with increased physical activity include tailoring promotion strategies with a combination of cognitive and behavioural elements and promoting low to moderate physical activity [41]. In a meta-analysis focussing on interventions to increase levels of physical activity in older adults, it was concluded that physical activity interventions significantly improved physical activity behaviour among community-dwelling older adults. Effective physical activity interventions may be efficiently delivered using already available resources and personnel [42]. However, an important limitation of the studies included in both reviews was that they did not shed light on whether or how to sustain increased levels of physical activity past 1 year. Further research is thus required to identify intervention strategies that result in sustained levels of increased physical activity; such strategies will likely yield the greatest results in terms of health benefits and will likely require elements of habit formation [43].

5.6   What's the Role of Family Physicians in the Promotion of Physical Activity for Healthy Ageing

Another important strategy to promote physical activity in older adults is via the family physician. It is feasible that a physical activity recommendation from a health professional could influence behaviour. Receiving physical activity advice in primary care has been shown to increase physical activity levels in sedentary adults [44]. Fisher et al. investigated the association between recalling receiving physical activity advice and physical activity levels in a sample of 15,254 colorectal cancer survivors residing in England [45]. It was found that 31% of participants recalled receiving advice and those who recalled receiving this advice were more likely to participate in brisk physical activity (51% in the advice group vs 42% in the no advice group) and meet the UK physical activity guidelines (25% vs 20%). Other studies of breast cancer survivors have produced similar results [46]. Importantly, colorectal cancer and breast cancer are more prevalent in older adults. It is thus feasible to assume that physical activity advice by a health-care professional in older adults may be an effective route to physical activity behaviour change. It is therefore important to educate medical students on the benefits of physical activity in later life [47] and indeed family physicians on physical activity guidelines and promotion.

Once educated the family physician may then wish to prescribe physical activity in a similar way to which they would prescribe medication. Key components of the prescription should include setting achievable activity goals, identifying barriers and providing potential solutions, and providing specific recommendations on the type, frequency, and intensity of activities. A detailed discussion on how to write an exercise prescription is beyond the scope of this chapter; however, we refer the interested reader to [48] which provides a detailed overview of this topic.

Finally, any attempt to promote physical activity to older adults needs to consider adherence to aid in the prevention of dropout. Indeed, sustained participation in physical activity is likely to have the greatest benefits for both physical and mental health. One way to achieve this is to involve peers. A recent meta-analysis was carried out to evaluate the effectiveness of peers to deliver programs or encourage older people to be physically active. Eighteen articles were included in the review, including a total of 3492 intervention participants with an average age of 66.5 years. The review found that exercise programs involving peers can promote and maintain adherence to exercise programs [49]. Other ways in which exercise adherence may be achieved is through counselling, such as utilising motivational interviewing [50], or through incorporating habit theory into interventions [51].

5.7 Summary

In summary, many of the non-communicable diseases that older adults are at an increased risk of developing can be somewhat negated if the older adult participates in sustained levels of physical activity. In light of this knowledge, physical activity guidelines have been developed specifically for older adults to maintain good health. However, despite this physical activity levels in older adults are low and decline with age. Interventions, to increase physical activity in older adults, have been successful, but it is not known whether this success is sustained over the longer term. The family physician should be encouraged to promote/prescribe physical activity in practice where appropriate by tailoring promotion strategies with a combination of cognitive and behavioural elements, promoting low to moderate physical activity (e.g. tai chi), and utilising strategies to promote adherence.

References

1. Caspersen CJ, Powell KE, Christenson GM. Physical activity, exercise, and physical fitness: definitions and distinctions for health-related research. Public Health Rep. 1985;100(2):126.
2. Smith L, Ekelund U, Hamer M. The potential yield of non-exercise physical activity energy expenditure in public health. Sports Med. 2015;45(4):449–52.
3. Jochem C, Schmid D, Leitzmann MF. Introduction to sedentary behaviour epidemiology. Sedentary behaviour epidemiology. Springer; 2018. p. 3–29.
4. Lear SA, Hu W, Rangarajan S, Gasevic D, Leong D, Iqbal R, et al. The effect of physical activity on mortality and cardiovascular disease in 130 000 people from 17 high-income, middle-income, and low-income countries: the PURE study. Lancet. 2017;390(10113):2643–54.
5. Kalyani RR, Golden SH, Cefalu WT. Diabetes and aging: unique considerations and goals of care. Diabetes Care. 2017;40(4):440–3.
6. Aunan JR, Cho WC, Søreide K. The biology of aging and cancer: a brief overview of shared and divergent molecular hallmarks. Aging Dis. 2017;8(5):628.
7. North BJ, Sinclair DA. The intersection between aging and cardiovascular disease. Circ Res. 2012;110(8):1097–108.
8. Loeser RF. Aging and osteoarthritis. Curr Opin Rheumatol. 2011;23(5):492.
9. World Health Organisation; Yoshida S. A global report on falls prevention epidemiology of falls. 2007.
10. Corrada MM, Brookmeyer R, Paganini-Hill A, Berlau D, Kawas CH. Dementia incidence continues to increase with age in the oldest old: the 90 study. Ann Neurol. 2010;67(1):114–21.
11. Rubenstein LZ. Falls in older people: epidemiology, risk factors and strategies for prevention. Age Ageing. 2006;35(suppl_2):ii41.
12. Hupin D, Roche F, Gremeaux V, Chatard J, Oriol M, Gaspoz J, et al. Even a low-dose of moderate-to-vigorous physical activity reduces mortality by 22% in adults aged≥ 60 years: a systematic review and meta-analysis. Br J Sports Med. 2015;49(19):1262–7.
13. Soares-Miranda L, Siscovick DS, Psaty BM, Longstreth WT Jr, Mozaffarian D. Physical activity and risk of coronary heart disease and stroke in older adults: the cardiovascular health study. Circulation. 2016;133(2):147–55.
14. Colberg SR, Sigal RJ, Yardley JE, Riddell MC, Dunstan DW, Dempsey PC, et al. Physical activity/exercise and diabetes: a position statement of the American Diabetes Association. Diabetes Care. 2016;39(11):2065–79.
15. Zheng G, Xia R, Zhou W, Tao J, Chen L. Aerobic exercise ameliorates cognitive function in older adults with mild cognitive impairment: a systematic review and meta-analysis of randomised controlled trials. Br J Sports Med. 2016;50(23):1443–50.
16. Sherrington C, Michaleff ZA, Fairhall N, Paul SS, Tiedemann A, Whitney J, et al. Exercise to prevent falls in older adults: an updated systematic review and meta-analysis. Br J Sports Med. 2017;51(24):1750–8.
17. Lee S, Tung H, Liu C, Chen L. Physical activity and sarcopenia in the geriatric population: a systematic review. J Am Med Dir Assoc. 2018;19(5):378–83.
18. Steffl M, Bohannon RW, Sontakova L, Tufano JJ, Shiells K, Holmerova I. Relationship between sarcopenia and physical activity in older people: a systematic review and meta-analysis. Clin Interv Aging. 2017;12:835.
19. Beaudart C, Dawson A, Shaw SC, Harvey NC, Kanis JA, Binkley N, et al. Nutrition and physical activity in the prevention and treatment of sarcopenia: systematic review. Osteoporos Int. 2017;28(6):1817–33.
20. Vogel T, Brechat P, Leprêtre P, Kaltenbach G, Berthel M, Lonsdorfer J. Health benefits of physical activity in older patients: a review. Int J Clin Pract. 2009;63(2):303–20.

21. de Souto Barreto P, Rolland Y, Vellas B, Maltais M. Association of long-term exercise training with risk of falls, fractures, hospitalizations, and mortality in older adults: a systematic review and meta-analysis. JAMA Intern Med. 2019;179(3):394–405.
22. Smith L, Gordon D, Scruton A, Yang L. The potential yield of tai chi in cancer survivorship. Future Sci OA. 2016;2(4):FSO152.
23. Ainsworth BE, Haskell WL, Herrmann SD, Meckes N, Bassett DR Jr, Tudor-Locke C, et al. 2011 compendium of physical activities: a second update of codes and MET values. Med Sci Sports Exerc. 2011;43(8):1575–81.
24. Solloway MR, Taylor SL, Shekelle PG, Miake-Lye IM, Beroes JM, Shanman RM, et al. An evidence map of the effect of tai chi on health outcomes. Syst Rev. 2016;5(1):126.
25. Huang Z, Feng Y, Li Y, Lv C. Systematic review and meta-analysis: tai chi for preventing falls in older adults. BMJ Open. 2017;7(2):e013661.
26. Kong LJ, Lauche R, Klose P, Bu JH, Yang XC, Guo CQ, et al. Tai chi for chronic pain conditions: a systematic review and meta-analysis of randomized controlled trials. Sci Rep. 2016;6:25325.
27. Xiang Y, Lu L, Chen X, Wen Z. Does tai chi relieve fatigue? A systematic review and meta-analysis of randomized controlled trials. PLoS One. 2017;12(4):e0174872.
28. Tong Y, Chai L, Lei S, Liu M, Yang L. Effects of tai chi on self-efficacy: a systematic review. Evid Based Complement Alternat Med. 2018.
29. Raman G, Zhang Y, Minichiello VJ, D'Ambrosio CM, Wang C. Tai chi improves sleep quality in healthy adults and patients with chronic conditions: a systematic review and meta-analysis. J Sleep Disord Ther. 2013;2:6.
30. Wayne PM, Walsh JN, Taylor-Piliae RE, Wells RE, Papp KV, Donovan NJ, et al. Effect of tai chi on cognitive performance in older adults: systematic review and meta-analysis. J Am Geriatr Soc. 2014;62(1):25–39.
31. World Health Organization. Global strategy on diet, physical activity and health, physical activity and older adults. 2004.
32. National Health Service. Physical activity guidelines for older adults. 2018.
33. Office of Disease Prevention and Health Promotion. Physical Activity Guidelines for Americans. 2008.
34. Australian Government Department of Health. Recommendations on physical activity for health for older Australians. 2013.
35. Canadian Society for Exercise Physiology. Canadian Physical Activity Guidelines. 2011.
36. Public Health England. Everybody active, every day: An evidence-based approach to physical activity. 2014.
37. Australian Institute of Health and Welfare. Physical activity across the life stages. 2018.
38. Statistics Canada. Directly measured physical activity of adults, 2012 and 2013. 2015.
39. Gomes M, Figueiredo D, Teixeira L, Poveda V, Paúl C, Santos-Silva A, et al. Physical inactivity among older adults across Europe based on the SHARE database. Age Ageing. 2016;46(1):71–7.
40. Smith L, Gardner B, Fisher A, Hamer M. Patterns and correlates of physical activity behaviour over 10 years in older adults: prospective analyses from the English longitudinal study of ageing. BMJ Open. 2015;5(4):e007423.
41. Zubala A, MacGillivray S, Frost H, Kroll T, Skelton DA, Gavine A, et al. Promotion of physical activity interventions for community dwelling older adults: a systematic review of reviews. PLoS One. 2017;12(7):e0180902.
42. Chase JD. Interventions to increase physical activity among older adults: a meta-analysis. Gerontologist. 2014;55(4):706–18.
43. Gardner B, Lally P, Wardle J. Making health habitual: the psychology of 'habit-formation' and general practice. Br J Gen Pract. 2012;62(605):664–6.
44. Calfas KJ, Long BJ, Sallis JF, Wooten WJ, Pratt M, Patrick K. A controlled trial of physician counseling to promote the adoption of physical activity. Prev Med. 1996;25(3):225–33.

45. Fisher A, Williams K, Beeken R, Wardle J. Recall of physical activity advice was associated with higher levels of physical activity in colorectal cancer patients. BMJ Open. 2015;5(4):e006853.
46. Jones LW, Courneya KS, Fairey AS, Mackey JR. Effects of an oncologist's recommendation to exercise on self-reported exercise behavior in newly diagnosed breast cancer survivors: a single-blind, randomized controlled trial. Ann Behav Med. 2004;28(2):105–13.
47. Izquierdo M, Morely J, Lucia A. Exercise in people over 85. BMJ. 2020;368.
48. Lee PG, Jackson EA, Richardson CR. Exercise prescriptions in older adults. Am Fam Physician. 2017;95:7.
49. Burton E, Farrier K, Hill KD, Codde J, Airey P, Hill A. Effectiveness of peers in delivering programs or motivating older people to increase their participation in physical activity: systematic review and meta-analysis. J Sports Sci. 2018;36(6):666–78.
50. Stonerock GL, Blumenthal JA. Role of counseling to promote adherence in healthy lifestyle medicine: strategies to improve exercise adherence and enhance physical activity. Prog Cardiovasc Dis. 2017;59(5):455–62.
51. Kwasnicka D, Dombrowski SU, White M, Sniehotta F. Theoretical explanations for maintenance of behaviour change: a systematic review of behaviour theories. Health Psychol Rev. 2016;10(3):277–96.

Sexual Health in Older People

6

Lee Smith, Daragh McDermott, Sheila Sánchez Castillo, and Igor Grabovac

Abstract

This chapter provides an overview in relation to sexual health and activity in older adults. It discusses declining levels of sexual activity among older populations and the consequent impact such declines may have on their physical and mental health. This chapter discusses barriers to an active sex life in older adults and makes recommendations to overcome such barriers. In addition, no chapter on sexual activity in older adults is complete without a mention of sexual dysfunction. This chapter does not aim to cover sexual dysfunction in detail but rather to provide the reader with an overview and make recommendations for further reading.

Keywords

Sexual activity · Sexual health · Sexual intercourse · Physical health · Mental health

L. Smith (✉)
The Cambridge Centre for Sport and Exercise Sciences, Anglia Ruskin University, Cambridge, UK
e-mail: lee.smith@aru.ac.uk

D. McDermott
Division of Psychology, School of Psychology and Sports Sciences, Anglia Ruskin University, Cambridge, UK

S. Sánchez Castillo
Faculty of Sports Sciences, University of Murcia, Murcia, Spain

I. Grabovac
Department of Social and Preventive Medicine, Centre for Public Health, Medical University of Vienna, Vienna, Austria

© Springer Nature Switzerland AG 2022
J. Demurtas, N. Veronese (eds.), *The Role of Family Physicians in Older People Care*, Practical Issues in Geriatrics, https://doi.org/10.1007/978-3-030-78923-7_6

6.1   Definition

Sexual health is defined by the World Health Organization as "a state of physical, emotional, mental, and social well-being related to sexuality, not merely the absence of disease dysfunction or infirmity" [1].

6.2   Levels and Patterns of Sexual Activity in Older Adults

Sexual activity is a central component of intimate relationships but has been shown to decline with age. In a population-based study of English adults, sexual activity was found to decrease substantially from age 50–59 years to age ≥ 80 years in both men (from 94.1% to 31.1%) and women (from 53.7% to 14.2%) [2]. A similar trend and magnitude of decline were also observed in a US population-based study [3], and such declines have also been shown among Indian older adults [4]. However, it is important to note that although the frequency of sexual activity declines as people age, older adults are not inherently disinterested in sex and that sexual practices do happen in older age [5, 6].

6.3   Physical Health Benefits of Sexual Activity in Older Adults

A decline in sexual activity as people age is of concern as a regular and problem-free sex life has been shown to be positively associated with better physical health. Frequent sexuality in older adults has been shown to be associated with a lower risk of certain cancers and fatal coronary events [7] as well as with a lower annual death rate [8]. Recent work aimed to investigate cross-sectional and longitudinal associations between declines in sexual activity and function and health outcomes in 2577 men and 3195 women aged ≥50 years participating in the English Longitudinal Study of Ageing. The study found that prospectively, men who reported a decline in sexual desire had 1.41 higher odds of incident limiting long-standing illness and 1.63 higher odds of incident cancer than those who maintained their sexual desire. Men who reported a decline in the frequency of sexual activities had 1.47 times higher odds of deterioration in self-rated health and 1.69 higher odds of incident limiting long-standing illness. In women, a decline in frequency of sexual activities was associated with a 1.64 higher odds of deterioration of self-rated health [9]. Taken together the literature suggests that maintaining an active sex life as one ages is likely an important determinant of good physical health and thus healthy ageing.

6.4 Mental Health Benefits of Sexual Activity in Older Adults

In addition to a plethora of physical health benefits, sexual activity has also been found to be associated with good mental health in older adults. Literature utilizing the English Longitudinal Study of Ageing has shown that sexual activity is associated with greater enjoyment of life [10] and greater life satisfaction [11] and may prevent against cognitive decline [12]. These findings support literature from other countries. For example, in a sample of 1879 US adults aged over 80 years, it was found that increased sexual activity was associated with positive emotional health indicators [13]. Similarly, in a sample of 2373 dementia-free older adults from Rotterdam, Netherlands, it was found that positive psychological well-being was associated with more sexual behaviour in partnered, community-dwelling older adults [14]. Taken together the literature suggests that maintaining an active sex life as one ages is likely an important determinant of good mental health and thus healthy ageing.

6.5 Sexual Orientation and Sexual Activity in Older Adults

Given the advances made in terms of sexual minority rights over the course of the twentieth and early parts of the twenty-first century, there is now a significantly larger population of openly lesbian, gay, and bisexual older adults. A key issue facing these populations is heteronormative presumptions made about older adults, particularly those that enter into elderly care [15] where the primary assumption made about older adults is one of heterosexuality. While many of the issues associated with ageing and sexual activity are familiar between heterosexual and sexual minority populations [16], including sexual difficulties in men [17], heterosexist assumptions serve only to augment and exacerbate adverse physical and mental health outcomes for these populations [18].

6.6 Mechanisms Linking Sexual Activity to Healthy Ageing

Several mechanisms may explain the positive effects of sexual activity on physical and mental health. Firstly, during sexual activity or at the time sexual intercourse is at its peak, there is a release of endorphins, endogenous opioid peptides that function as neurotransmitters, which generates a happy or blissful feeling [19]. Importantly, circulating endorphin levels have been shown to be associated with higher natural killer cell activity [20]. A higher natural killer cell activity may be associated with a lower risk of cancer and viruses; they have also been found to prevent against infections of the lungs and play an important role in improving asthma and many other conditions [21, 22] and thus are also likely to be related to limiting long-standing illness and self-rated health. Second, sex can be considered a form of physical activity; one study conducted in a younger population (22.6 ± 2.8 years) showed that energy expenditure during sexual activity was 85 kCal or 3.6 kCal/min and was performed at a moderate intensity (5.8 METS) [23]. Therefore, it is possible that one may acquire health benefits from regular participation in physical activity via sexual activity. Physical activity has been shown to be associated with better self-rated health, lower odds of having a limiting long-standing illness, lower incidence of certain cancers, lower incidence of cardiovascular diseases, and better mental health [24–26]. Third, those who engage in sexual intercourse with their partner are likely to share a closer relationship [27], and indeed closeness to one's partner has been shown to be associated with well-being per se [28]. Finally, it is possible that early symptoms of cancer and long-standing illness may predict a decline in sexual activity and desire before diagnosis of the conditions. For example, fatigue is a reported early warning sign for cancer and is often experienced before a diagnosis is made [29]; it is plausible to assume that fatigue will be associated with a reduction in sexual activity.

6.7 Sexual Dysfunction in Older Adults

Sexual dysfunction refers to a problem occurring during any phase of the sexual response cycle that prevents the individual or couple from experiencing satisfaction from the sexual activity. The sexual response cycle traditionally includes excitement, plateau, orgasm, and resolution [30]. Sexual dysfunction is experienced in both males and females; approximately 43 percent of women and 31 percent of men report some degree of dysfunction [30]. Sexual dysfunction in males tends to refer to any of the following: inability to achieve or maintain an erection suitable for intercourse (erectile dysfunction), absent or delayed ejaculation despite adequate sexual stimulation (retarded ejaculation), and inability to control the timing of ejaculation (early or premature ejaculation). Sexual dysfunction in females includes inability to achieve orgasm, inadequate vaginal lubrication before and during intercourse, and inability to relax the vaginal muscles enough to allow intercourse. Sexual dysfunctions experienced by males and females include lack of interest in or desire for sex, inability to become aroused, and pain during intercourse.

As people reach older age, there is a general increase in the prevalence of sexual dysfunction. Detailed discussion on all sexual dysfunctions experienced by males is beyond the scope of this chapter, and we refer the interested reader to [31]. In males one sexual dysfunction strongly linked to older age is erectile dysfunction. Findings from the Massachusetts Male Aging Study showed that ageing increases the risk of erectile dysfunction from 1.2% per year for men aged between 40 and 49 years to 4.6% for men aged between 60 and 69 years [32]. The key reason behind the rise in erectile dysfunction as one ages is that the prevalence and severity of its physiological risk factors increase with age. These risk factors include hypertension, diabetes, hyperlipidaemia, and coronary artery disease. Moreover, older males have a higher risk for depression which is also associated with erectile dysfunction. Finally, maintaining adequate levels of physical activity as one ages has been shown to be protective against erectile dysfunction. However, as people age, levels of physical activity substantially decline [33, 34].

Detailed discussion on all sexual dysfunctions in females is beyond the scope of this chapter, and we refer the interested reader to [31]. The incidence of sexual dysfunction in postmenopausal women is in excess of 80% [35]. Thus sexual dysfunction in older females is highly prevalent and an important issue for both physical and mental health of this population. Similar to males an increase in sexual dysfunction in older females is at least in part owing to an increase in age-related conditions that are also associated with sexual dysfunction. These conditions include cardiovascular disease, diabetes, lower urinary tract problems, breast cancer, hysterectomy, oophorectomy, endocrinopathies, bariatric surgery, osteoarthritis, and clinical depression [35]. Moreover, physical activity also declines in older women, and higher levels of physical activity are likely to be protective against sexual dysfunction [34].

6.8   What's the Role of Family Physician's in the Promotion of Sexual Health in Older People

In a review of the scientific literature that aimed to examine help-seeking for, and doctor-patient interactions about, sexual problems in the middle and later life age groups, a total of 25 articles were identified, and the following barriers to seeking medical help were identified: (a) psychosocial factors relating to the patient, such as thinking that sexual changes were "normal with ageing"; (b) psychosocial factors to the doctor—for example, assuming that sex was less important to older patients than it was to their younger patients; and (c) inadequate training at medical school for healthcare professionals. People were more likely to seek help if their doctor had asked about sexual function during a routine visit sometime during the previous 3 years [36]. However, the review also identified that doctors tended not to take a proactive approach to sexual health management and indeed often had limited knowledge of later-life sexuality issues. Findings from this review show that there is a strong need to educate both patients and healthcare professionals to highlight the need to acknowledge that older adults are not asexual and that a frequent and problem-free sex life in this population is related to improved health and well-being. Information on and encouragement to try new sexual positions and explore different types of sexual activity are not regularly given to ageing populations. Engaging in discussions regarding sexuality in later life could help redress perceived norms and expectations about sexual activity in older people and help them live more fulfilling lives.

Addressing treatment practices around sexual dysfunction for males and females is beyond the scope of this chapter, but we refer the interested reader to [37] and [31].

6.9 Conclusion

Levels of sexual activity decline and sexual dysfunction increases with age; this is true for both males and females. However, it is important to note that older adults are not inherently disinterested in sex and that sexual practices do happen in older age. A decline in sexual activity with age is of concern as there is a growing body of literature to suggest that sexual activity per se has been shown to be associated with good physical and mental health. However, the majority of existing literature is of an observational nature, and gold standard experimental studies are now required to allow for inferences and more robust recommendations to be made. Sexual dysfunction has been studied in greater detail than declining sexual activity per se; healthcare practitioners tend to be aware of these issues and as a community are well equipped in the treatment of. Despite this the literature suggests that there is a clear need to educate both patients and healthcare professionals to highlight the need to acknowledge that older adults are not asexual and that a frequent and problem-free sex life in this population is related to improved health and well-being.

References

1. World Health Organization (WHO). Defining sexual health. 2006.
2. Lee DM, Nazroo J, O'Connor DB, Blake M, Pendleton N. Sexual health and Well-being among older men and women in England: findings from the English longitudinal study of ageing. Arch Sex Behav. 2016;45(1):133–44.
3. Lindau ST, Schumm LP, Laumann EO, Levinson W, O'Muircheartaigh CA, Waite LJ. A study of sexuality and health among older adults in the United States. N Engl J Med. 2007;357(8):762–74.
4. Kalra G, Subramanyam A, Pinto C. Sexuality: desire, activity and intimacy in the elderly. Indian J Psychiatry. 2011;53(4):300–6.
5. Træen B, Štulhofer A, Janssen E, Carvalheira AA, Hald GM, Lange T, et al. Sexual activity and sexual satisfaction among older adults in four European countries. Arch Sex Behav. 2019;48(3):815–29.
6. Traeen B, Štulhofer A, Jurin T, Hald GM. Seventy-five years old and still going strong: stability and change in sexual interest and sexual enjoyment in elderly men and women across Europe. Int J Sex Health. 2018;30(4):323–36.
7. Ebrahim S, May M, Ben Shlomo Y, McCarron P, Frankel S, Yarnell J, et al. Sexual intercourse and risk of ischaemic stroke and coronary heart disease: the Caerphilly study. J Epidemiol Community Health. 2002;56(2):99–102.
8. Palmore EB. Predictors of the longevity difference: a 25 year follow-up. Gerontologist. 1982;22(6):513–8.
9. Jackson SE, Yang L, Koyanagi A, Stubbs B, Veronese N, Smith L. Declines in sexual activity and function predict incident health problems in older adults: prospective findings from the English longitudinal study of ageing. Arch Sex Behav. 2019.
10. Smith L, Yang L, Veronese N, Soysal P, Stubbs B, Jackson SE. Sexual activity is associated with greater enjoyment of life in older adults. Sex Med. 2019;7(1):11–8.
11. Jackson SE, Firth J, Veronese N, Stubbs B, Koyanagi A, Yang L, et al. Decline in sexuality and wellbeing in older adults: a population-based study. J Affect Disord. 2019;245:912–7.
12. Smith L, Grabovac I, Yang L, López-Sánchez GF, Firth J, Pizzol D, et al. Sexual activity and cognitive decline in older age: a prospective cohort study. Aging Clin Exp Res. 2019;32:85–91.

13. Bach LE, Mortimer JA, VandeWeerd C, Corvin J. The Association of Physical and Mental Health with sexual activity in older adults in a retirement community. J Sex Med. 2013;10(11):2671–8.

14. Freak-Poli R, De Castro LG, Direk N, Jaspers L, Pitts M, Hofman A, et al. Happiness, rather than depression, is associated with sexual behaviour in partnered older adults. Age Ageing. 2016;46(1):101–7.

15. Daley A, MacDonnell JA, Brotman S, St. Pierre M, Aronson J, Gillis L. Providing health and social services to older LGBT adults. In: annual review of gerontology and geriatrics. Springer Publishing Company; 2017. p. 143–60.

16. Hinchliff S, Tetley J, Lee D, Nazroo J. Older adults' experiences of sexual difficulties: qualitative findings from the English longitudinal study on ageing (ELSA). J Sex Res. 2018;55(2):152–63.

17. Jowett A, Peel E, Shaw RL. Sex and diabetes: a thematic analysis of gay and bisexual men's accounts. J Health Psychol. 2012;17(3):409–18.

18. Hoy-Ellis CP, Fredriksen-Goldsen KI. Lesbian, gay, & bisexual older adults: linking internal minority stressors, chronic health conditions, and depression. Aging Ment Health. 2016;20(11):1119–30.

19. Rokade PB. Release of endomorphin hormone and its effects on our body and moods: a review. In: International Conference on Chemical, Biological and Environment Sciences (ICCEBS'2011). Bangkok; 2011. p. 436–8.

20. Darko DF, Irwin MR, Craig Risch S, Christian GJ. Plasma beta-endorphin and natural killer cell activity in major depression: a preliminary study. Psychiatry Res. 1992;43(2):111–9.

21. Mandal A, Viswanathan C. Natural killer cells: in health and disease. Hematol Oncol Stem Cell Ther. 2015;8(2):47–55.

22. Wu J, Lanier LL. Natural killer cells and cancer. Adv Cancer Res. 2003;90:127–56.

23. Frappier J, Toupin I, Levy JJ, Aubertin-Leheudre M, Karelis AD. Energy expenditure during sexual activity in young healthy couples. Earnest CP, editor. PLoS One. 2013;8(10):e79342.

24. Warburton DER, Bredin SSD. Health benefits of physical activity: a systematic review of current systematic reviews. Curr Opin Cardiol. 2017;32(5):541–56.

25. McPhee JS, French DP, Jackson D, Nazroo J, Pendleton N, Degens H. Physical activity in older age: perspectives for healthy ageing and frailty. Biogerontology. 2016;17(3):567–80.

26. Södergren M, Sundquist J, Johansson SE, Sundquist K. Physical activity, exercise and self-rated health: a population-based study from Sweden. BMC Public Health. 2008;8:352.

27. Kontula O, Haavio-Mannila E. The impact of aging on human sexual activity and sexual desire. J Sex Res. 2009;46(1):46–56.

28. Dolan P, Peasgood T, White M. Do we really know what makes us happy? A review of the economic literature on the factors associated with subjective well-being. J Econ Psychol. 2008;29(1):94–122.

29. De Nooijer J, Lechner L, De Vries H. A qualitative study on detecting cancer symptoms and seeking medical help; an application of Andersen's model of total patient delay. Patient Educ Couns. 2001;42(2):145–57.

30. Sexual dysfunction & disorders I Cleveland Clinic.

31. Wincze JP, Weisberg RB. Sexual dysfunction : a guide for assessment and treatment. 3rd ed. New York: Guilford Press; 2015. p. 230.

32. Johannes CB, Araujo AB, Feldman HA, Derby CA, Kleinman KP, McKinlay JB. Incidence of erectile dysfunction in men 40 to 69 years old: longitudinal results from the Massachusetts male aging study. J Urol. 2000;163(2):460–3.

33. Smith L, Gardner B, Fisher A, Hamer M. Patterns and correlates of physical activity behaviour over 10 years in older adults: prospective analyses from the English longitudinal study of ageing. BMJ Open. 2015;5(4):e007423.

34. Smith L, Grabovac I, Yang L, Veronese N, Koyanagi A, Jackson SE. Participation in physical activity is associated with sexual activity in older English adults. Int J Environ Res Public Health. 2019;16(3):489.

35. Ambler DR, Bieber EJ, Diamond MP. Sexual function in elderly women: a review of current literature. Rev Obstet Gynecol. 2012;5(1):16–27.
36. Hinchliff S, Gott M. Seeking medical help for sexual concerns in mid-and later life: a review of the literature. J Sex Res. 2011;48(2-3):106–17.
37. Reddy MS, Starlin VM. Pharmacological advances in the management of sexual dysfunction. Indian J Psychol Med. 2017;39(3):219–22.

Immunizations in Older Adults

7

Elisabetta Alti, Fiona Ecarnot, Stefania Maggi,
Jean-Pierre Michel, Silvestro Scotti, and Tommasa Maio

Abstract

The age-related decline in immunity known as immunosenescence means that older adults are at increased risk of infection, as well as at higher risk of severe forms, complications, and poor outcomes. In parallel, the burden of infectious diseases is highest among older adults, with the inherent risk of hospitalization, aggravation of pre-existing diseases, frailty, increased disability, and ultimately death. Vaccination is the most effective means to prevent against common infectious diseases, yet vaccine uptake in adults remains consistently below target. We discuss here the physiopathological rationale for vaccination in older adults, focusing on the three main diseases that account for the greatest morbidity and/or mortality in this population, namely, seasonal influenza, pneumococcal disease, and herpes zoster. We discuss the burden of each disease and the available vaccines. We also briefly review other vaccines recommended in older adults. The role of the family physician in promoting vaccination among older adults is key

E. Alti · S. Scotti · T. Maio (✉)
Italian Federation of General Practitioners (Federazione Italiana Medici di Medicina Generale, FIMMG), Rome, Italy
e-mail: tommasamaio@gmail.com

F. Ecarnot
Department of Cardiology, University Hospital Jean Minjoz, Besançon, France

University of Burgundy Franche-Comté, Besançon, France

S. Maggi
National Research Council, Neuroscience Institute, Aging Branch, Padova, Italy

J.-P. Michel
Medical University of Geneva (CH), Geneva, Switzerland

© Springer Nature Switzerland AG 2022
J. Demurtas, N. Veronese (eds.), *The Role of Family Physicians in Older People Care*, Practical Issues in Geriatrics, https://doi.org/10.1007/978-3-030-78923-7_7

89

and can actively drive efforts to improve vaccine uptake in this population, thereby reducing the burden of infectious disease and contributing to healthy aging.

Keywords

Older people · Vaccinations · Vaccine-preventable disease · Immunosenescence Vaccine hesitancy

7.1   Background

In older people, the ability to defend against infective agents or malignant and auto-reactive cells declines with increasing age, whereas susceptibility to disease, cancer, and autoimmune disorders increases. This phenomenon is known as immunosenescence, namely, an age-related decline in immunity that occurs with increasing age [1]. It affects both innate and adaptive immunities, although the latter is compromised to a greater degree. Naïve T cells, T regulatory cells, and B cells all decline in number, as does specific antibody production, whereas the functions of memory cells are relatively preserved. Data suggest that memory B and T cells, once elicited by antigens during youth, are quite resilient to the impact of immunosenescence [2], whereas the ability of B and T cells to interact and respond to new infections, tumors, autoimmune response, or vaccinations becomes limited. The clinical consequence of immunosenescence is therefore an increased susceptibility to infection, along with a greater risk of experiencing severe forms of disease, complications of the disease, and poor outcomes. The reasons for the increased susceptibility to disease in older adults, in addition to the aforementioned waning of immune response, include epidemiological factors, malnutrition, and a large number of other age-associated physiological and anatomical alterations, such as increased risk of invasion by pathogenic organisms due to alterations in the barriers represented by the skin, lungs, and gastrointestinal and urological tract (and other mucosal linings). Research into methods for achieving a higher level of protection over a longer duration, with more persistent immune responses, could improve both vaccine impact and coverage, not only preventing disease but increasing healthy lifespan across the board [3].

The burden of infectious diseases is greatest in young children and elderly adults. It is among older adults that the risk of hospitalization, complications, or aggravation of pre-existing diseases, frailty, increased disability, and death is highest. Seasonal influenza (flu), pneumococcal disease, and herpes zoster (HZ) all have their highest mortality rates in older individuals [4]. However, while vaccination prevention campaigns have achieved high coverage rates in children, vaccine uptake levels remain consistently below target in adults, in both healthy and at-risk populations. A century ago, infectious diseases contributed nearly half of all deaths in developed economies like the USA, but while infectious disease has been greatly reduced, the remaining burden of these diseases is now borne disproportionately by older adults [5].

Pneumonia and influenza are among the top ten causes of death, and the risk of nosocomial infections increases in number and clinical severity in individuals aged 65 and older [6, 7]. Even the clinical presentation of infections in older people is quite often different, with fewer symptoms, low grade fever, delirium, anorexia, or generalized weakness [8], possibly leading to delayed diagnosis or untreated conditions and an increase in related complications and hospitalizations. In the elderly, common infections are more frequent and more severe but older adults with chronic diseases (e.g. diabetes, chronic obstructive pulmonary disease or heart failure) have a greater impairment of immune system and a poorer vaccine response with even more susceptibility [9]. Similarly, residents in senior centers, long-term residential facilities, or other social institutions such as daycare programs have been shown to have a significantly increased risk of infections, with worse outcomes (in terms of morbidity and mortality) compared with non-residents [10].

7.2 Prevention Strategies in Older Adults

There are many strategies to counteract the increased risk of infection in older individuals. In addition to the usual lifestyle recommendations, such as adequate nutrition [11], regular physical exercise, smoking cessation, and stress reduction, routine vaccination is one of the most effective interventions in healthy older adults and a key contributor to healthy aging. Immunization against vaccine-preventable diseases (VPDs) has led to significant reductions in mortality and morbidity from infectious causes. Traditionally, most vaccine policies and initiatives are age-based and focus principally on pediatric vaccination, with less emphasis on vaccine policies for older adults. The benefits of vaccination are most obvious in children because childhood vaccination is well-established as a social norm. By way of comparison, compliance with vaccine recommendations in children exceeds 90% in most high-income countries, but compliance is far lower in adults [5]. In older adults, mortality rates due to VPDs such as influenza and pneumococcal disease have only modestly decreased in recent decades, and these persistently low vaccine uptake rates in adults prevent the full benefits of immunization from being reaped.

Therefore, a shift from the childhood vaccination paradigm to a new life-course approach to vaccination is essential to prevent disability, morbidity, and mortality in older subjects and to promote healthy aging [12, 13].

7.3 Factors Influencing Vaccine Uptake

The low vaccine uptake observed among adults is due to multiple factors. For physicians, barriers to vaccination include a constantly changing landscape with frequent updates to vaccination schedules, lack of knowledge among healthcare providers about the clinical and functional implications of aging, and time and logistic constraints in a busy practice setting. Among patients, obstacles to immunization include social influences, disease-related and vaccine-related factors, general attitudes toward health and vaccines, habit, awareness and knowledge, practical barriers and motivators, and vaccine hesitancy [14]. Vaccine hesitancy refers to the delay in acceptance or refusal of vaccines despite availability of vaccination services [15], a phenomenon identified by the WHO as one of the ten major threats to global health in 2019.

The reasons behind vaccine hesitancy are complex and may be either individual or general. They generally fit into three categories: lack of confidence (in effectiveness, safety, the system, or policy-makers), complacency (a perceived low risk of acquiring VPD), and lack of convenience (availability, accessibility, and appeal of immunization services, including time, place, language, and cultural contexts) [15, 16]. To shift individual and community attitudes, beliefs, and, consequently, their decision-making toward greater vaccine acceptance, we need to enhance "awareness of the health threat prevented by the vaccine, maintaining availability through trusted channels, ensuring accessibility to all populations, safeguarding affordability through national program, and ultimately, encouraging acceptability by countering specific vaccine hesitancy beliefs" [17].

7.4　The Role of General Practitioners

The family doctor or general practitioner (GP) usually has a long-standing relationship with the patient and good knowledge of the person, their family, and the context in which they live. As a result, the GP can be very influential in achieving objectives in terms of individual and collective vaccine coverage. The GP's role in preventive medicine is especially determinant for older adults. The GP knows the health status of older patients (i.e., whether they are healthy or suffering from chronic diseases) and usually has a good idea of their lifestyle or risk factors. With a long history of regular follow-up comes the likelihood that the GP knows the patient's vaccine history, which can often be difficult to elicit and may be subject to memory bias. This comprehensive knowledge of the patient enables the GP to adopt a targeted approach to immunization with specific action, where warranted, to address vaccine hesitancy. Indeed, despite the public's widespread use of the Internet to search for information on vaccination, the family doctor remains the most trusted source of information. In Italy, research performed in 2017 by CENSIS attributed a critical role to the family doctor as a source of information about influenza (flu) vaccine. In this study, 62.7% of respondents reported that they asked their family doctor about the need for vaccination, as the most reliable and trustworthy source of information [18].

Their privileged position as a trusted source of information on vaccines means that family physicians play a key role in driving vaccine acceptance. The awareness of vaccination in adult populations is very low. In developed countries, the majority of the general population does not see a high incidence of VPDs in their entourage. This leads to a failure to perceive the risk of VPDs in comparison to the rare adverse events associated with vaccination. The perceived susceptibility and severity of influenza among elderly people weakly correlate with vaccination acceptance, but recommendations from doctors, nurses, or friends/relatives contracting influenza led to a sudden increase in threat perception and subsequent immunization [19].

There are many strategies to enhance vaccine acceptance, most of which come from studies of pediatric immunization. The main features include telling stories, focusing on the benefits of protection, being honest about side effects when asked, not providing only numbers and facts, and building trust with patients [20]. In a study assessing mothers' decision-making regarding vaccination for their children, trust was built when a provider spent time discussing vaccines, did not deride the mother's concerns, was knowledgeable, and provided satisfactory answers, not scientific facts, with tailored information as the main aspects of communication competence [21].

The goal for every family doctor is to seize every opportunity to discuss vaccination with their patients, not only during the flu vaccine campaign but throughout the year, as an integral part of daily practice. With older patients in particular, there are frequent opportunities for medical contact, such as regular check-ups of chronic disease, prescription refills, or during consultations prior to travel, during which it is possible to strengthen the message about vaccination. It is important not only to discuss personal vaccine coverage, but it is also essential to offer the vaccine as soon as possible, preferably in the same session. A study in two major US cities (Houston, Pittsburgh) showed that reducing the number of missed opportunities is associated with a significant increase in coverage rate [22]. Accordingly, vaccine availability and its affordability play a key role in vaccination in older persons. Ease of access, close to home, and at a convenient time, together with affordability of the vaccine are key factors in enhancing the immunization rates and also happen to be the salient characteristics of the local GP practice.

For older persons, it is determinant to receive the vaccine in a convenient place that is easy for them to reach, at the right time, with people they know, and this is all the more true when the person suffers from several chronic diseases or cognitive impairment. Moreover, it is very important to take enough time with each person to discuss the issue, provide information about side effects or efficacy of the vaccine or about the scheduled vaccines recommended for their age group, check their understanding regularly, and answer any new questions that may arise. In a study based in Los Angeles County, USA, the researchers found that the major obstacles to vaccine receipt in adults were logistical and structural challenges, especially lack of time for counseling and patient flow, vaccine storage and space, or lack of support personnel, whereas use of electronic tools (adult immunization registry or electronic medical records) was associated with a higher likelihood of administering vaccination [23]. For family doctors who face logistic or time constraints and who are unable to offer vaccination themselves, they should refer patients to partner provider who can administer the vaccine, and they should review the issue with the patient at the next visit to make sure the referral followed through to vaccination.

Communication is a further key issue in influencing vaccination, not only in awareness or acceptance but also in reminder-recall programs during flu season or for other recommended vaccine schedules. There are many studies based on technological tools such as mobile phone-based applications (apps) or e-mail campaigns, which greatly facilitate outreach, delivering healthcare messages to large numbers with relative ease [24, 25]. There are technological systems that can help doctors to send reminders to patients, or to be proactive (i.e., every time a patient comes to the practice for a prescription or visit, the nurse or doctor receives an alert on the patient's record), or to directly create a list with planned uptake for age group or risk group (chronic diseases, etc.), employer group, or lifestyle group (travelers, etc.). The use of electronic tools for adult immunization registries (at a local or, ideally, national level) can give family doctors the ability to identify gaps in care, track outcomes, and plan recalls for vaccine defaulters.

Creating a national immunization registry for family doctors could achieve more efficient preventive medicine. Immediate availability of up-to-date information on vaccine history, tracking uptake country-wide, in every healthcare context (e.g., emergency room, GP's office, specialist, etc.) would permit more effective and efficient action for older persons. It would help to increase coverage status, reduce possible defaults, and provide the correct schedule to follow, based on age or comorbidity or lifestyle. A vaccine registry can also be used for benchmarking purposes and as an incentive for quality improvement.

In addition to GP practices, the organization of the health system also has a role to play in promoting vaccine acceptance. Smaller practices (1 or 2 doctors) may have more difficulty offering a full array of vaccine products, including maintaining vaccine temperatures and affording rent for space to store vaccines, whereas larger practices (with 11–30 providers or more than 30 providers) and those affiliated with a hospital or large healthcare system are more likely to administer most vaccines [23].

In a recent study in Lazio, Italy, researchers found that flu vaccine uptake was higher in older people assisted by family doctors who got their master's degree more recently, assisted a relatively high proportion of older patients, received influenza vaccination, had a computer assistant, and were associated with other physicians [26]. Working in a team environment allows targeted evidence-based interventions; possibility of facilities (place for storage, cold chain); better knowledge and analysis of vaccine coverage and benchmarks, local and national; reviews and sharing of safety procedures; and reduction of medical errors.

In summary, the role of family physicians in immunization in older people is determinant and includes periodic review of vaccination and counseling about available and recommended vaccines, together with the offer of and administration of the vaccine, as well as control of possible side effects. For GPs who cannot provide vaccination, they should refer patients elsewhere and review the issue at the next visit to check that the vaccine was received. The healthy aging adult needs a proactive approach with integrative interventions for primary prevention (e.g., lifestyle, smoking cessation, etc.), while older individuals or those with comorbidities need more clinical interventions and decisions for immunization.

Almost all countries have established national recommendations for immunization schedules across the lifespan from childhood to older age. Despite some heterogeneity in age thresholds and vaccine recommendations, there are some core vaccines that are widely recommended for older persons and are reviewed below.

7.5 Tetanus, Pertussis, and Diphtheria Vaccine (Tdap)

Administration of the diphtheria-tetanus-acellular pertussis vaccine is routinely recommended in children, with a single booster dose of a vaccine containing tetanus toxoid, reduced diphtheria toxoid, and acellular pertussis (Tdap) in adolescence and a single booster dose of a vaccine containing tetanus toxoid, reduced diphtheria toxoid (Td), or Tdpa every 10 years in adults, according to national recommendations.

Despite these recommendations, immunity to tetanus, diphtheria, and pertussis continues to wane among adults in Europe and the USA [27, 28]. Clinical tetanus, although rare in the USA and Europe, occurs predominantly in unvaccinated or under-immunized older adults, especially older women, who never received the primary series [28, 29].

Although, in Europe, the most severe symptoms of pertussis occur in infants and young children, and most deaths in 2015 occurred in infants too young to be vaccinated, there is nonetheless an increasing incidence of pertussis in adolescents and adults. These age groups are a major source of transmission to infants, especially because mild and asymptomatic cases in adolescents and adults are often not recognized as pertussis [30]. Therefore, in many countries, the National Immunization Advisory Boards suggest immunization with Tdap booster, especially for pregnant women and older individuals [31].

Pockets of diphtheria are reappearing, primarily in resource-limited countries. Approximately 20 to 60 percent of adults become susceptible to diphtheria because of waning vaccine-induced immunity and failure to receive recommended booster immunization. Unvaccinated or inadequately vaccinated travelers to endemic areas are at risk of acquiring this infection [32].

Older adults with and without comorbidities should be reviewed during clinical visits regarding complete primary immunization against tetanus, diphtheria, and pertussis. Those who have not previously been vaccinated against tetanus and diphtheria should receive a series of three vaccines, the first dose and second dose separated by 4 weeks and the third dose given 6–12 months later.

After complete primary immunization, it is recommended to administer a single booster of Td or Tdap every 10 years, according to national recommendations [31, 33, 34]. Studies of the Td vaccine have demonstrated the efficacy and cost-effectiveness of a single booster in producing sustained immunity to both tetanus and diphtheria among older patients (aged 50–70 years) who had received a primary booster series [35].

Older adults should be reviewed every 10 years for the single booster, especially those with grandchildren or living in families with children or pregnant females, in order to receive Tdap for pertussis immunization.

7.6 Influenza Vaccine

The burden of influenza on world health is major, with influenza-related lower respiratory tract infection responsible for an estimated 145,000 deaths among all ages in 2017 according to the Global Burden of Disease study [36]. Influenza mortality rate was highest among adults older than 70 years [36]. Older people are at high risk of developing serious complications from flu, such as hospitalization (57–70%), increased disability, or death, compared with younger, healthy adults. In the USA, more than 75% of influenza-related deaths occurred among people age 65 and over in the 2018–2019 flu season [37]. Recent studies have investigated influenza infection as a potential trigger for cardiovascular conditions, including acute coronary syndromes and atrial fibrillation [38, 39]. Older adults experience significantly increased morbidity and disability from the flu, especially frail adults older than 65 years or those in long-term care, for whom even relatively mild respiratory illness may lead to a catastrophic chain of events, from taking to bed, disorientation, and respiratory illness to falls, fracture, and worsening clinical conditions of preexistent comorbidities. Vaccination is highly effective in preventing adverse outcomes, as shown by an umbrella review and meta-analysis reporting that in community-dwelling older people, influenza vaccination was associated with a lower risk of hospitalization for heart disease and for flu/pneumonia, with evidence of convincing strength [40].

Most countries recommend flu vaccination for older people, usually from age 60 or 65 years and older. Among the available vaccines, two are specifically designed for people aged 65 years and older, namely, a high-dose flu vaccine (brand name Fluzone High-Dose ®) and the adjuvanted flu vaccine.

The Fluzone High-Dose is a three-component (trivalent) inactivated flu vaccine that contains four times the amount of antigen of standard-dose inactivated influenza vaccines. In the USA, Fluzone High-Dose is licensed only for persons aged 65 years and older [41]. A study published in the New England Journal of Medicine [42] reported that the high-dose vaccine was 24.2% more effective in preventing flu in adults 65 years of age and older relative to a standard-dose vaccine. A separate study [43] reported that Fluzone High-Dose was associated with a lower risk of hospital admissions compared with standard-dose Fluzone for people aged 65 years or older, especially those living in long-term care facilities.

The adjuvanted flu vaccine integrates the MF59 squalene oil-in-water adjuvant, which stimulates a stronger immune response to vaccination. It is licensed for people older than 65 years who often have a lower protective immune response after flu vaccination compared to their younger, healthier counterparts. The adjuvanted flu vaccine was found to be associated with a reduced risk of hospitalization for pneumonia and influenza diagnoses [44] and pneumonia, cerebrovascular, or cardiovascular diagnoses relative to the unadjuvanted vaccine in retrospective studies of medical record data [45].

To date, there have been no randomized, head-to-head comparisons of these two vaccines. No preference is expressed for either vaccine type by the American Advisory Committee on Immunization Practices (ACIP), but it is strongly recommended to administer any available age-appropriate formulation [46]. In Italy, the adjuvanted flu vaccine is recommended [34], but Fluzone High-Dose is not currently available.

The recommendations of the American Centers for Disease Control and Prevention (CDC) and the European Centre for Disease Prevention and Control (ECDC) regarding influenza, pneumococcal, and herpes zoster vaccination in older adults are summarized in Table 7.1.

Table 7.1 Summary of the recommendations from the US Centers for Disease Control and Prevention (CDC) and the European Centre for Disease Prevention and Control (ECDC) for the vaccination of older adults against influenza, pneumococcal disease, and herpes zoster

	Influenza	Pneumococcal disease	Herpes zoster
ECDC	**Inactivated tri- or quadrivalent influenza vaccine** recommended **annually** for:	Vaccination with **PCV13, PPSV23, or a combination of both** is recommended in all European Union countries except Bulgaria, Croatia, Estonia, France, Latvia, Liechtenstein, Lithuania, Portugal, and Romania	Vaccination with the **live attenuated herpes zoster vaccine** is recommended for adults:
	• Adults **≥55 years** in Malta and Poland • Adults **≥60 years** in Germany, Greece, Hungary, Iceland, Netherlands, Slovakia • Adults **≥65 years** in Austria, Belgium, Bulgaria, Croatia, Cyprus, Czech Republic, Denmark, Estonia, Finland, France, Ireland, Italy, Latvia, Liechtenstein, Luxembourg, Norway, Portugal, Romania, Slovenia, Spain, and the UK • Specific risk groups only in Lithuania and Sweden		• **Aged 50–60 years** in Austria • **Aged ≥ 50 years** in the Czech Republic • **Aged ≥ 60 years** in Greece • **Aged ≥ 65 years** in Italy • **Aged 65 to 75 years** in France • **Aged 70 years** in the UK Vaccination with the **inactivated herpes zoster subunit vaccine** is recommended **in Germany** for adults **aged ≥ 60 years**

(continued)

Table 7.1 (continued)

	Influenza	Pneumococcal disease	Herpes zoster
US CDC	**1 dose of influenza vaccine** is recommended **annually** with the inactivated influenza vaccine or the recombinant influenza vaccine for all adults **aged ≥ 65 years**	1 dose of PPSV23 is recommended for all adults **aged ≥ 65 years**. If PPSV23 was administered prior to age 65 years, 1 dose of PPSV23 should be administered at least 5 years after previous dose	For adults **aged ≥ 50 years**, vaccination with the **inactivated herpes zoster subunit vaccine** is recommended (2-dose series, 2–6 months apart, minimum interval 4 weeks), regardless of previous herpes zoster infection or vaccination
		1 dose of PCV13 may be considered in immunocompetent adults based on shared decision-making	For adults **aged ≥ 60 years**, vaccination with the **inactivated herpes zoster subunit vaccine** is recommended (2-dose series, 2–6 months apart, minimum interval 4 weeks) or 1 dose of live attenuated zoster vaccine if not previously vaccinated. The subunit vaccine is preferred over the live attenuated vaccine

PCV13 pneumococcal conjugate vaccine 13-valent, *PPSV23* pneumococcal polysaccharide vaccine 23-valent

7.7 Pneumococcal Vaccine

Pneumococcal disease (PD) can be divided into non-invasive disease, including sinusitis, acute otitis media, and community-acquired pneumonia (CAP), and invasive pneumococcal disease (IPD), characterized by the isolation of *Streptococcus pneumoniae* from otherwise sterile sites and mainly comprising pneumococcal meningitis, bacteremic pneumococcal pneumonia, and pneumococcal bacteremia. The burden of invasive and non-invasive diseases remains high, despite wide access to antibiotic therapies. Furthermore, there is an increasing problem of antibiotic resistance, and susceptibility to macrolide antimicrobials, penicillins, and cephalosporins can no longer be presumed in many countries.

Pneumococcal infections affect people of all ages, but children younger than 2 years of age and adults aged 65 years and older are at higher risk. Invasive pneumococcal disease accounted for over 36,000 cases in the USA in 2011 and 11 to 27 cases per 100,000 in Europe, while incidence rates of non-invasive pneumococcal disease, notably CAP, ranged from 1.6 per 1000 in Spain to 11.6 per 1000 in Finland [47–49]. Both the incidence of pneumococcal disease and the mortality rate increase after age 50 and more sharply after age 65.

There are currently two vaccines against pneumococcal infection, namely, the pneumococcal polysaccharide vaccine (PPSV) and pneumococcal conjugate vaccine (PCV). PCV7 vaccination was first approved for children under 2 years of age in 2000 by the US Food and Drug Administration and in 2001 by the European Union. Additional serotypes were introduced with the update to PCV13 in 2010. Widespread implementation of PCV vaccination in children has profoundly modified the epidemiology of pneumococcal disease in the population [47], with in particular large reductions in IPD in the older population [50]. The randomized CAPITA study investigated the efficacy of PCV13 in preventing IPD and CAP in individuals aged 65 years and older and reported significant efficacy for the prevention of vaccine-type pneumococcal, bacteremic, and non-bacteremic CAP and vaccine-type IPD, but not in preventing all-cause CAP [51].

The pneumococcal polysaccharide vaccine (PPSV23) contains polysaccharide antigen from 23 types of pneumococcal bacteria and has been reported to have a statistically significant effect IPD among healthy individuals aged 65 years of age and older [52, 53]. In a systematic review and meta-analysis of the efficacy of PPSV23 in older adults, pooled efficacy of 73% was reported against IPD caused by any serotype [54].

The US Advisory Committee on Immunization Practices (ACIP) recently revised its recommendations for pneumococcal vaccination in adults, notably removing the recommendation for routine PCV13 use among adults aged ≥65 years on the basis that continued childhood immunization with PCV13 has reduce disease burden among adults to historically low levels via reduced carriage and transmission of vaccine serotypes from vaccinated children (i.e., indirect effects) [55]. In parallel, there has been a substantial decrease in antimicrobial resistance [56].

The ACIP now recommends PPSV23 for all adults 65 years or older and for individuals aged 2–64 years with certain medical conditions or for adults aged 19–64 years who smoke cigarettes. PCV13 vaccination is no longer routinely recommended for all adults aged ≥65 years, but adults aged 65 years or older may discuss and decide, in shared decision-making with their clinician, to receive PCV13 based on the patient's individual risk.

In the European Union, almost all countries recommend either PCV13 or PPSV23, or both, in older adults, but recommendations vary from country to country (https://vaccine-schedule.ecdc.europa.eu/).

7.8 Herpes Zoster Vaccine

Herpes zoster is the clinical manifestation of reactivation of the varicella zoster virus (VZV), which remains latent in the dorsal root or cranial nerve sensory ganglia after primary infection (chickenpox). Herpes zoster affects almost one in three adults during their lifetime. Over 95% of the adult population is seropositive to specific anti-VZV antibodies and therefore is potentially at risk of developing HZ in their lifetime.

In Italy, the estimated incidence is 6.3 cases/1000 person-years; and although hospital admissions are less than 2%, the rate is 69% in patients aged over 65 years [57]. The incidence shows a growing rate of herpes zoster infection with increasing age, reaching over 10 cases per 1000 person-years beyond the age of 80 [58].

Herpes zoster is a considerable cause of morbidity, especially in older, immuno-suppressed, or critically ill patients. The illness is associated with significant pain and complications, the most debilitating of which is post-herpetic neuralgia (PHN). PHN is long-lasting pain that persists for some weeks and even months or years after the disappearance of the rash [59], often requiring hospitalization and considerably impairing daily functioning and quality of life. PHN affects one third of all HZ patients [60], and available antiviral and analgesic treatments are relatively unsatisfactory in reducing pain and length of the disease.

Higher relative risks of diagnosis of cardiovascular diseases (tenfold increase), cerebral vasculopathy (fivefold increase) (including acute stroke and transient ischemia), non-arrhythmic myocardiopathy (sevenfold increase), and neuropathy were identified in adults aged 50 years or older with severe herpes zoster requiring hospitalization [61].

There are two available vaccines against herpes zoster: first, a live attenuated unadjuvanted vaccine prepared from the Oka/Merck strain of varicella zoster virus (ZVL) and, second, a recombinant adjuvanted subunit vaccine (HZ/su or RZV).

The ZVL vaccine is indicated for immunization of individuals aged 50 years or older and is effective and safe in subjects with a positive history of HZ. It is given as a single dose injected under the skin or into the muscle. Clinical studies show a reduction of 51% in the incidence of disease, 61% in disease burden, and 67% in PHN in vaccines [57]. The protection afforded by the ZVL vaccine lasts for 5 years. However, lower vaccine efficacy with increasing age is a feature of existing live attenuated herpes zoster vaccines, falling from 69.8% in those aged 50–59 years to 37.6% in those ≥70 years and 18.3% in those aged ≥80 years [62]. The vaccine is not indicated for the prevention of primary varicella infection (chickenpox) and should not be used in children and adolescents. Contraindications include the following:

- A history of hypersensitivity to any of the excipients or trace residuals (e.g., neomycin).
- Primary and acquired immunodeficiency.
- Immunosuppressive therapy (including high-dose corticosteroids).
- Active untreated tuberculosis.
- Pregnancy.

The recombinant zoster vaccine (RZV) is recommended as the preferred herpes zoster vaccine in the USA, but it is not available everywhere in Europe, despite having received approval from the EMEA. It is given in two doses, administered 2–6 months apart for maximum efficacy. Shingrix has been shown to be highly effective at preventing shingles and post-herpetic neuralgia in adults older than 50 years for at least 4 years after vaccination. The vaccine is also effective at protecting adults older than 18 years who are at increased risk of herpes zoster such as the immunosuppresed patient. Pooled analyses of data from participants aged 70 years and older from the ZOE-50 and ZOE-70 trials (totaling 16,596 participants) reported vaccine efficacy against HZ of 91.3% (95% CI, 86.8 to 94.5; $P < 0.001$) and vaccine efficacy against PHN of 88.8% (95% CI, 68.7–97.1; $P < 0.001$) [63, 64]. The protection conferred by RZV has been shown to last up to 9 years [65]. Studies examined the safety of Shingrix vaccination five or more years after Zostavax vaccination. Shorter intervals were not studied, but there are no theoretical or data concerns to indicate that Shingrix would be less safe or effective if administered less than five years after a patient received ZVL. Anyway, it is possible to administer RVZ after ZVL at least 8 weeks later [34]. It can also be administered in people who have previously had HZ infection. RZV can be co-administered with non-adjuvanted inactivated seasonal influenza vaccine, 23-valent pneumococcal polysaccharide (PPV23) vaccine, or antigen-reduced diphtheria, tetanus and pertussis (acellular component) (dTpa) vaccine. Vaccines should be administered at different injection sites.

Contraindications to RZV are:

- A history of severe allergic reaction, such as anaphylaxis, to any component of a vaccine or after a previous dose of the RZV.
- Persons known to be seronegative for varicella virus. It is not necessary to screen (either verbally or via laboratory serology) for a history of varicella. However, if a person is known to be varicella-negative via serologic testing, providers should follow guidelines for varicella immunization.
- Ongoing infection with herpes zoster.
- Although not evaluated in pregnant or lactating women, it is advisable to delay administration of RZV in this population.

7.9 Other Vaccines

While flu, pneumococcal disease, Tdap, and herpes zoster are the most commonly recommended vaccines in older adults, primary care providers should be mindful that some patients may require other vaccines. For example, immunization against hepatitis A or B, meningococcal disease, or measles, mumps, and rubella may be indicated in certain patients depending on their health status, their occupational exposures or risks, and their lifestyle behaviors. Older persons undertaking travel to areas with endemic diseases should also be advised to receive appropriate vaccinations prior to departure. All these considerations should be explored on a case-by-case basis with each individual patient, during regular review of immunization status.

7.10 Conclusions

Older persons are at particularly high risk of influenza, pneumococcal disease, and herpes zoster infection. When infected, they are additionally at higher risk of experiencing severe forms of disease, complications, and poor outcomes. In patients with chronic diseases, which is often the case of elderly people, the risk is also augmented. In parallel, advancing age leads to a decline in immunity known as immunosenescence, whose consequence is an impaired ability to mount and maintain immune response to infection and vaccination. Despite the wide availability, often free-of-charge, of efficacious vaccines against several common infectious diseases, uptake of vaccination is low in older adults and well below recommended target levels, for a variety of patient-, provider- and system-related reasons. Primary care physicians have an influential role in promoting vaccination among older individuals and are key in driving efforts to improve vaccine uptake in this population. No opportunity should be missed to recommend and provide vaccines to older patients, with a view to contributing to healthy aging and preserving functioning and quality of life in older individuals.

References

1. Agarwal S, Busse PJ. Innate and adaptive immunosenescence. Ann Allergy Asthma Immunol. 2010;104:183–90.; quiz 90-2, 210.
2. Stacy S, Krolick KA, Infante AJ, Kraig E. Immunological memory and late onset autoimmunity. Mech Ageing Dev. 2002;123:975–85.
3. Esposito S, Principi N, Rezza G, Bonanni P, Gavazzi G, Beyer I, et al. Vaccination of 50+ adults to promote healthy ageing in Europe: The way forward. Vaccine. 2018;36:5819–24.
4. Maggi S. Vaccination and healthy aging. Expert Rev Vaccines. 2010;9:3–6. Epub 2010/03/17.
5. Bridges CB, Hurley LP, Williams WW, Ramakrishnan A, Dean AK, Groom AV. Meeting the challenges of immunizing adults. Am J Prev Med. 2015;49:S455–64.
6. El Chakhtoura NG, Bonomo RA, Jump RLP. Influence of aging and environment on presentation of infection in older adults. Infect Dis Clin N Am. 2017;31:593–608.
7. Mouton CP, Bazaldua OV, Pierce B, Espino DV. Common infections in older adults. Am Fam Physician. 2001;63:257–68.
8. Norman DC. Fever in the elderly. Clin Infect Dis. 2000;31:148–51.
9. Gavazzi G, Krause KH. Ageing and infection. Lancet Infect Dis. 2002;2:659–66.
10. O'Fallon E, Schreiber R, Kandel R, D'Agata EM. Multidrug-resistant gram-negative bacteria at a long-term care facility: assessment of residents, healthcare workers, and inanimate surfaces. Infect Control Hosp Epidemiol. 2009;30:1172–9.
11. Gibson A, Edgar JD, Neville CE, Gilchrist SE, McKinley MC, Patterson CC, et al. Effect of fruit and vegetable consumption on immune function in older people: a randomized controlled trial. Am J Clin Nutr. 2012;96:1429–36.
12. Gusmano MK, Michel JP. Life course vaccination and healthy aging. Aging Clin Exp Res. 2009;21:258–63.
13. Michel JP, Lang PO. Promoting life course vaccination. Rejuvenation Res. 2011;14:75–81.
14. Ecarnot F, Maggi S, Michel JP. Strategies to improve vaccine uptake throughout adulthood. Interdiscip Top Gerontol Geriatr. 2020;43:234–48.
15. Salmon DA, Dudley MZ, Glanz JM, Omer SB. Vaccine hesitancy: causes, consequences, and a call to action. Vaccine. 2015;33(Suppl 4):D66–71.
16. Jacobson RM, St Sauver JL, Finney Rutten LJ. Vaccine hesitancy. Mayo Clin Proc. 2015;90:1562–8.
17. Piltch-Loeb R, DiClemente R. The vaccine uptake continuum: applying social science theory to shift vaccine hesitancy. Vaccines (Basel). 2020;8.
18. Tabacchi G, Costantino C, Cracchiolo M, Ferro A, Marchese V, Napoli G, et al. Information sources and knowledge on vaccination in a population from southern Italy: the ESCULAPIO project. Hum Vaccin Immunother. 2017;13:339–45.

19. Kan T, Zhang J. Factors influencing seasonal influenza vaccination behaviour among elderly people: a systematic review. Public Health. 2018;156:67–78.
20. Shen SC, Dubey V. Addressing vaccine hesitancy: clinical guidance for primary care physicians working with parents. Can Fam Physician. 2019;65:175–81.
21. Benin AL, Wisler-Scher DJ, Colson E, Shapiro ED, Holmboe ES. Qualitative analysis of mothers' decision-making about vaccines for infants: the importance of trust. Pediatrics. 2006;117:1532–41.
22. Lin CJ, Nowalk MP, Pavlik VN, Brown AE, Zhang S, Raviotta JM, et al. Using the 4 pillars practice transformation program to increase adult influenza vaccination and reduce missed opportunities in a randomized cluster trial. BMC Infect Dis. 2016;16:623.
23. Equils O, Kellogg C, Baden L, Berger W, Connolly S. Logistical and structural challenges are the major obstacles for family medicine physicians' ability to administer adult vaccines. Hum Vaccin Immunother. 2019;15:637–42.
24. Dale LP, White L, Mitchell M, Faulkner G. Smartphone app uses loyalty point incentives and push notifications to encourage influenza vaccine uptake. Vaccine. 2019;37:4594–600.
25. Cutrona SL, Golden JG, Goff SL, Ogarek J, Barton B, Fisher L, et al. Improving rates of outpatient influenza vaccination through EHR portal messages and interactive automated calls: a randomized controlled trial. J Gen Intern Med. 2018;33:659–67.
26. Fabiani M, Volpe E, Faraone M, Bella A, Rizzo C, Marchetti S, et al. Influenza vaccine uptake in the elderly population: Individual and general practitioner's determinants in Central Italy, Lazio region, 2016-2017 season. Vaccine. 2019;37:5314–22.
27. Centers for Disease C, Prevention. Tetanus surveillance—United States, 2001-2008. MMWR Morb Mortal Wkly Rep. 2011;60:365–9.
28. Cook TM, Protheroe RT, Handel JM. Tetanus: a review of the literature. Br J Anaesth. 2001;87:477–87.
29. McQuillan GM, Kruszon-Moran D, Deforest A, Chu SY, Wharton M. Serologic immunity to diphtheria and tetanus in the United States. Ann Intern Med. 2002;136:660–6.
30. Sanstead E, Kenyon C, Rowley S, Enns E, Miller C, Ehresmann K, et al. Understanding trends in pertussis incidence: an agent-based model approach. Am J Public Health. 2015;105:e42–7.
31. European Centre for Disease Prevention and Control. Vaccine schedules in all countries of the European Union.
32. Stefansson M, Askling HH, Rombo L. A single booster dose of diphtheria vaccine is effective for travelers regardless of time interval since previous doses. J Travel Med. 2018;25.
33. Centers for Disease Control and Prevention. Recommended adult immunization schedule for ages 19 years or older, United States, 2019.
34. Italian Government. Piano Nazionale Prevenzione Vaccinale (PNPV) 2017–2019.
35. Solomonova K, Vizev S. Secondary response to boostering by purified aluminium-hydroxide-adsorbed tetanus anatoxin in aging and in aged adults. Immunobiology. 1981;158:312–9.
36. GBD 2017 Influenza Collaborators. Mortality, morbidity, and hospitalisations due to influenza lower respiratory tract infections, 2017: an analysis for the Global Burden of Disease Study 2017. Lancet Respir Med. 2019;7:69–89.
37. Centers for Disease Control and Prevention. Estimated influenza illnesses, medical visits, hospitalizations, and deaths in the United States—2018–2019 influenza season.
38. Warren-Gash C, Smeeth L, Hayward AC. Influenza as a trigger for acute myocardial infarction or death from cardiovascular disease: a systematic review. Lancet Infect Dis. 2009;9:601–10.
39. Barnes M, Heywood AE, Mahimbo A, Rahman B, Newall AT, Macintyre CR. Acute myocardial infarction and influenza: a meta-analysis of case-control studies. Heart. 2015;101:1738–47.
40. Demurtas J, Celotto S, Beaudart C, Sanchez-Rodriguez D, Balci C, Soysal P, et al. The efficacy and safety of influenza vaccination in older people: an umbrella review of evidence from

meta-analyses of both observational and randomized controlled studies. Ageing Res Rev. 2020;62:101118.

41. Centers for Disease Control and Prevention. Fluzone high-dose seasonal influenza vaccine high-dose flu vaccine, brand name Fluzone High-Dose.

42. DiazGranados CA, Dunning AJ, Kimmel M, Kirby D, Treanor J, Collins A, et al. Efficacy of high-dose versus standard-dose influenza vaccine in older adults. N Engl J Med. 2014;371:635–45.

43. Gravenstein S, Davidson HE, Taljaard M, Ogarek J, Gozalo P, Han L, et al. Comparative effectiveness of high-dose versus standard-dose influenza vaccination on numbers of US nursing home residents admitted to hospital: a cluster-randomised trial. Lancet Respir Med. 2017;5:738–46.

44. Mannino S, Villa M, Apolone G, Weiss NS, Groth N, Aquino I, et al. Effectiveness of adjuvanted influenza vaccination in elderly subjects in northern Italy. Am J Epidemiol. 2012;176:527–33.

45. Lapi F, Marconi E, Simonetti M, Baldo V, Rossi A, Sessa A, et al. Adjuvanted versus nonadjuvanted influenza vaccines and risk of hospitalizations for pneumonia and cerebro/cardiovascular events in the elderly. Expert Rev Vaccines. 2019;18:663–70.

46. Ezeanolue E, Harriman K, Hunter P, Kroger A, Pellegrini C. General best practice guidelines for immunization. Best Practices Guidance of the Advisory Committee on Immunization Practices (ACIP).

47. Drijkoningen JJ, Rohde GG. Pneumococcal infection in adults: burden of disease. Clin Microbiol Infect. 2014;20(Suppl 5):45–51.

48. Almirall J, Bolibar I, Vidal J, Sauca G, Coll P, Niklasson B, et al. Epidemiology of community-acquired pneumonia in adults: a population-based study. Eur Respir J. 2000;15:757–63.

49. Jokinen C, Heiskanen L, Juvonen H, Kallinen S, Karkola K, Korppi M, et al. Incidence of community-acquired pneumonia in the population of four municipalities in eastern Finland. Am J Epidemiol. 1993;137:977–88.

50. Pilishvili T, Lexau C, Farley MM, Hadler J, Harrison LH, Bennett NM, et al. Sustained reductions in invasive pneumococcal disease in the era of conjugate vaccine. J Infect Dis. 2010;201:32–41.

51. Bonten MJ, Huijts SM, Bolkenbaas M, Webber C, Patterson S, Gault S, et al. Polysaccharide conjugate vaccine against pneumococcal pneumonia in adults. N Engl J Med. 2015;372:1114–25.

52. Kraicer-Melamed H, O'Donnell S, Quach C. The effectiveness of pneumococcal polysaccharide vaccine 23 (PPV23) in the general population of 50 years of age and older: a systematic review and meta-analysis. Vaccine. 2016;34:1540–50.

53. Moberley S, Holden J, Tatham DP, Andrews RM. Vaccines for preventing pneumococcal infection in adults. Cochrane Database Syst Rev. 2013:CD000422.

54. Falkenhorst G, Remschmidt C, Harder T, Hummers-Pradier E, Wichmann O, Bogdan C. Effectiveness of the 23-Valent Pneumococcal Polysaccharide Vaccine (PPV23) against pneumococcal disease in the elderly: systematic review and meta-analysis. PLoS One. 2017;12:e0169368.

55. Matanock A, Lee G, Gierke R, Kobayashi M, Leidner A, Pilishvili T. Use of 13-valent pneumococcal conjugate vaccine and 23-valent pneumococcal polysaccharide vaccine among adults aged >/=65 years: updated recommendations of the advisory committee on immunization practices. MMWR Morb Mortal Wkly Rep. 2019;68:1069–75. Journal Editors form for disclosure of potential conflicts of interest. No potential conflicts of interest were disclosed

56. Jansen KU, Anderson AS. The role of vaccines in fighting antimicrobial resistance (AMR). Hum Vaccin Immunother. 2018;14:2142–9.

57. Gabutti G, Franco E, Bonanni P, Conversano M, Ferro A, Lazzari M, et al. Reducing the burden of Herpes Zoster in Italy. Hum Vaccin Immunother. 2015;11:101–7.

58. Alicino C, Trucchi C, Paganino C, Barberis I, Boccalini S, Martinelli D, et al. Incidence of herpes zoster and post-herpetic neuralgia in Italy: Results from a 3-years population-based study. Hum Vaccin Immunother. 2017;13:399–404.

59. Le P, Rothberg M. Herpes zoster infection. BMJ. 2019;364:k5095.

60. Mallick-Searle T, Snodgrass B, Brant JM. Postherpetic neuralgia: epidemiology, pathophysiology, and pain management pharmacology. J Multidiscip Healthc. 2016;9:447–54.
61. Piazza MF, Paganino C, Amicizia D, Trucchi C, Orsi A, Astengo M, et al. The unknown health burden of Herpes Zoster Hospitalizations: the effect on chronic disease course in adult patients >/=50 years. Vaccines (Basel). 2020;8.
62. Schmader KE, Levin MJ, Gnann JW Jr, McNeil SA, Vesikari T, Betts RF, et al. Efficacy, safety, and tolerability of herpes zoster vaccine in persons aged 50-59 years. Clin Infect Dis. 2012;54:922–8.
63. Cunningham AL, Lal H, Kovac M, Chlibek R, Hwang SJ, Diez-Domingo J, et al. Efficacy of the Herpes Zoster subunit vaccine in adults 70 years of age or older. N Engl J Med. 2016;375:1019–32.
64. Cunningham AL, Heineman TC, Lal H, Godeaux O, Chlibek R, Hwang SJ, et al. Immune responses to a recombinant glycoprotein E Herpes Zoster vaccine in adults aged 50 years or older. J Infect Dis. 2018;217:1750–60.
65. Schwarz TF, Volpe S, Catteau G, Chlibek R, David MP, Richardus JH, et al. Persistence of immune response to an adjuvanted varicella-zoster virus subunit vaccine for up to year nine in older adults. Hum Vaccin Immunother. 2018;14:1370–7.

Digital Health in an Ageing World

8

Ana Luísa Neves, Charilaos Lygidakis, Kyle Hoedebecke, Luís de Pinho-Costa, and Alberto Pilotto

Abstract

Population ageing and the technological revolution will impact almost all aspects of society, notably healthcare. There are several key examples in which technology can assist older adults in ageing healthily: digital applications and telemedicine, wearables, ambient assisted living, and digital coaching/teaching. Digital health solutions must be tailored to the motor skills, visual and hearing capacity of older persons, and, importantly, to target their actual needs. To that end, it is critical to partner with patients and to capitalize in user-centred design methods. The use of digital technologies by older persons also poses specific challenges,

A. L. Neves (✉)
Institute of Global Health Innovation, Imperial College London, London, UK

Center for Health Technology and Services Research/Department of Community Medicine, Health Information and Decision, Faculty of Medicine, University of Porto, Porto, Portugal
e-mail: ana.luisa.neves14@imperial.ac.uk

C. Lygidakis
Department of Behavioural and Cognitive Sciences, University of Luxembourg, Esch-sur-Alzette, Luxembourg

K. Hoedebecke
Department of Utilization Management, Oscar Health, Dallas, TX, USA

L. de Pinho-Costa
Department of Community Medicine, Health Information and Decision, Faculty of Medicine, University of Porto, Porto, Portugal

A. Pilotto
Department Geriatric Care, Orthogeriatrics and Rehabilitation, Galliera Hospital, Genoa, Italy

Department of Interdisciplinary Medicine, University of Bari, Bari, Italy

© Springer Nature Switzerland AG 2022
J. Demurtas, N. Veronese (eds.), *The Role of Family Physicians in Older People Care*, Practical Issues in Geriatrics, https://doi.org/10.1007/978-3-030-78923-7_8

including lack of access to technology and digital literacy skills; inadequate medical reimbursement schemes; lack of legal and regulatory frameworks; and concerns about data security. Policy frameworks call for increased access to digital technologies, universal and affordable access to the Internet, and investments in expanding the infrastructure needed. It is thus becoming critical that family doctors develop digital skills to support and best advise their patients on the use of these innovative tools, notably the older persons.

Keywords

Digital health · Older persons · Primary care

8.1 Introduction: The Potential of Digital Health Use by Older Persons

Important demographic and epidemiologic changes affect the demand for health-care services. A declining birth rate and a higher life expectancy, a rise of the old-age dependency ratio, an increase of mobility and urbanization, and a shift towards non-communicable diseases are among the noteworthy factors that are bound to change healthcare. In less developed countries, the population aged 60 years and older is estimated to triple by 2050 [1].

As populations and societies age, digital health promises to play a major role in transforming healthcare services and how they are resourced, organized, and delivered. This is possible thanks to immense computing power, persistent connectivity, decrease in power consumption, and dramatically lower costs. Concomitantly, emerging technologies are promising revolutionary solutions:

- The fifth generation of cellular wireless networks (5G) promises a substantial increase in bandwidth and speed compared to the previous one; offers a drastic decrease in latency (and hence an increase in responsiveness); allows one million connected devices per square kilometre; and supports network slicing, i.e. the establishment of multiple customizable subnetworks that meet specific requirements for different applications [2–4].
- The Internet of Things (IoT) is a system of physical and virtual objects, such as sensors, devices, actuators, and software, which are interconnected, exchange data with each other, and interact with other devices and humans [4–6].
- Edge and fog computing redistributes processing capability and storage capacity closer to the origin of data (i.e. data captured from IoT devices), adding flexibility, reliability, security, while leaving intense processes to cloud computing [6–8].
- Artificial intelligence (AI), with its most common approaches of machine learning and deep learning, is advancing through the leaps in computational performance and the availability and integration of big data sets (deriving from resources such as electronic health records, medical imaging, sensors and patient-generated data, and multi-omics measurements) [9, 10].

8.2   Examples and Uses of Digital Tools in Older Persons

There are many areas in which technology can assist older adults in ageing health-ily, living independently, improving their quality of life, and preventing hospitaliza-tions. Digital technologies are a promising solution to enhance patients' access to centralized medical information, increase access to health information, improve health literacy, and engage with patients as active stakeholders in the management of their health and disease. Digital solutions support self-care and multimorbidity management and facilitate self-management of diseases. Behavioural change tech-niques, such as social support, feedback and monitoring, and goal setting, have been employed in interventions delivered over the Internet, on mobile phones, or with text messages, with mixed effects [11–14]. Given their omnipresence in people's daily lives, digital technologies offer a smooth mode of delivery for health behav-iour change, reaching individuals anywhere and at any time. In this section, we will discuss some key examples.

8.2.1   Digital Applications and Telemedicine

The most widespread use of medical technology is through digital applications (apps) and telemedicine. These software packages show real promise in terms of improving patient outcomes and decreasing medical costs as digital encounters increase healthcare efficiency by reducing the amount of travel and preparation needed for patient care. This, in turn, also improves a community's access to health-care as less urgent medical concerns are addressed digitally—opening appointment availability for in-person care for those with more severe clinical issues.

For example, WellDoc has implemented an app called BlueStar that allows for digital patient monitoring from anywhere. Specific pathology-related parameters—such as blood glucose levels, pulse, or numerous others—are maintained within specific guidelines. BlueStar notifies the patient's medical team so that a digital clinical encounter can occur to address abnormalities. This technology has been associated with a 58% reduction in emergency department visits and hospitaliza-tions in a studied group of patients with type 2 diabetes [15]. Furthermore, another year-long follow-up period reduced the total average number of hospital visits from five to zero and their emergency department visits from 21 to 11 in a trial of 32 patients [15].

Other medical companies take a slightly different approach where patients' vitals and metrics are remotely monitored by a team of nurses. Any abnormal results are brought to their attention where they can then call the patient and set up a plan to solve the issue or schedule an in-person medical evaluation as clinically indicated. When tested with geriatric patients in several different locations, patients experi-enced amazing results including clinically significant reductions in admissions, inpatient hospital days, and fewer medical expenditures [16–18].

8.2.2 Wearables

Wearable medical devices consist of a plethora of autonomous devices designed to be worn with the goal of providing prolonged periods of support and/or monitoring for the user. These accessories incorporate various physiological sensors, allow for data processing, and provide wireless transmission of information. One such example is that of QardioCore—a medical-grade monitor that allows for the monitoring of a patient's heart health. This is accomplished through sensors that record more than 20 million data points that link to a smartphone app [19]. Key clinical details include ECG, heart rate, heart rate variability, respiratory rate, temperature, and physical activity levels. This information can then be shared with the patient's medical team.

Wearable technology offers great potential in dementia research and care management. New digital-based biomarkers from wearables may aid dementia research and provide actionable insights for a timely diagnosis and early/targeted intervention, allowing the delivery of preventive and therapeutic care before full escalation or even on real time—when and where it is most needed—while improving engagement and compliance with the plan of care [20–24].

A magnificent example comes from the UK National Health System, where the Technology Integrated Health Management (TIHM) deploying wearables and other devices/IoT technologies to support people with dementia living at home has been put into trial [20]. Such a system continuously monitors the individuals and their surrounding environment, enabling a team of health professionals to remotely monitor their health and safety, 24/7. While it may raise significant ethical concerns, the potential challenges on personal liberty and data ownership may well be offset by the potential benefits: keeping people with dementia safe(r) and well in their own homes, for much longer, allowing it to be a supportive and reassuring environment, thus reducing carer burnout and unnecessary use of other health resources/interventions—like hospital admissions—while allowing them to be redeployed when/where they are needed. Still, there are technical challenges and financial constraints that also need to be addressed to ensure scalability in addition to effectiveness of these devices/strategies [21–24].

8.2.3 Ambient Assisted Living

Ambient assisted living (AAL) encompasses products and services which combine information and communication technologies enabling people to live independently, in the environment of their choice, stay connected, and improve their quality of life [25, 26]. AAL systems comprise IoT objects, including wireless sensors, actuators, software, and databases, which are all connected and exchange information [25, 27]. AAL applications span from automation (e.g., temperature control, provision of food) and health monitoring (e.g., sensors monitoring vital signs) to safety and security (e.g., reminders, fall detection, and prevention) and social interaction, and they have been employed in various conditions, including congestive heart failure, depression, and chronic obstructive pulmonary disease [28–33].

At the same time, remote monitoring by multidisciplinary care teams, including physicians and nurses, will allow intervening timely and managing patients effectively [34]. Health information systems, video conferencing with patients and within care teams, and high-speed data transfer, including medical imagery, will be key to clinical decision-making [35].

Older adults with sensory impairments will benefit more from voice recognition and haptic systems [26]. Virtual voice assistants offer a simpler way to interact, addressing limitations linked to visual impairments, lack of digital skills, and the complexity of user interfaces, while their combination with robotics will provide a more physical, human-like presence [36, 37]. Virtual reality has shown potential in older adults with mental illnesses and for those in stroke rehabilitation [38, 39].

8.2.4   Digital Coaching/Teaching

Many healthcare services are only available in the clinical setting as this is where specialists and ancillary staff members like dieticians and physical therapists work. This is further complicated by comorbidities, difficulties with ambulation, and socioeconomic limitations. However, digital solutions now allow these treatments to occur in the comfort of one's home. Home physical therapy (PT) makes it possible for patients to meet with a physical therapist digitally for guidance and then access a complete library of exercises with high-quality images and videos for referencing [40].

Similarly, digital coaching is effective for respiratory illnesses. One study working with 51 adults with uncontrolled asthma evaluated a 12-week patient-centred digital coaching program that combined educational pamphlets, symptom trackers, peak flow monitoring, physical activity, and additional services. The continuous support provided an increased level of motivation for self-management of this disease process. Furthermore, there was a statistically significant improvement in mental status, outpatient exacerbation reductions, and body weight—among other key clinical markers. Similar programs are now being tested for other chronic pathologies with the goal of attaining similar results [41].

8.2.5   A Synergistic Technological Focus

All of the above options must work together to make the greatest strides in fighting chronic diseases such as diabetes and its related complications. One scholarly source notes that every 30 seconds somewhere in the world a limb is amputated as a result of diabetic foot ulcers [42]. These ailments collectively cost $17,000 USD per ulceration. This metric rises to $40,000 USD should there be a resultant amputation [42]. Still, there are tech options aimed at diabetic complications. Various products such as Podimetrics mats, TempTouch handheld devices, and Bluedrop scales employ AI and telemedicine to prevent up to 70% of diabetic foot ulcers [43, 44]. Though these products have received FDA approval and millions of dollars in investments, technological solutions in diabetes and countless other disease processes have barely scratched the surface.

8.3   Concerns and Limitations

Despite all the above, the use of digital technologies by older persons also poses specific challenges. Patients' willingness and ability to engage, adopt, and maintain the use of digital technologies are deeply influenced by individual factors (e.g. age, ethnicity, education level, health literacy, and health status), as well as by healthcare delivery (e.g. provider endorsement) [45, 46]. Previous research on the "digital divide" revealed the existence of categorical inequalities between young and old people [47]. Age is, per se, associated with lower adoption rates: older persons have less access to digital tools and less experience performing a variety of online tasks and are less likely to believe that they would be capable of going online for health information and advice [47]. In older subjects, the magnitude of the challenge results not only of increased age as a risk factor for lower engagement but also of the complex and cumulative interplay of other risk factors. Global chronological trends of progressively increased education and health literacy levels also contribute to the digital exclusion of older persons. Furthermore, these patients typically have a lower health status due to an increased prevalence of multimorbidity and use of polypharmacy, which represent additional risk factors for a lower engagement with digital tools, contributing to the digital exclusion of this segment. Although a digital divide does exist, we find that some sub-groups of seniors utilize a plethora of different technologies similar to their younger counterparts. Specifically, the younger geriatric patients (65–70 years old), those with greater economic means, and the highly educated show more affinity towards the use of tablets, smartphones, and high-speed Internet [48].

It is also important to note that, in order to engage with digital technologies, older persons require access to technology and basic digital literacy skills. Access to technology has steadily increased in the last decades, with smartphone ownership surpassing three fourths of the population in several advanced economies [49]. In 2015, it was estimated that 3.2 billion people, representing almost half of the world's population, would be online by the end of the year [50], but usage varies significantly between age groups. In the UK, while 97% of adults aged 35–44 years old use the Internet daily or almost every day, this frequency drops to 55% in those aged over 65 years old [51]. Both digital literacy and digital access have become increasingly important competitive differentiators for individuals using the digital tools meaningfully. Therefore, increasing digital literacy and access to technology for people who may have been left out of the information revolution are a common concern. Older patients emerge, in this aspect, as a particularly vulnerable group.

Lower access to technology in older persons has, on its own, a negative impact on digital literacy. In brief, digital literacy can be described as an individual's ability to find, evaluate, and compose clear information on digital platforms. Lack of access and/or familiarity with digital tools contributes to resistance and anxiety towards its use. Additionally, current technologies are often designed without customization to the circumstances of older persons, therefore limiting its intended effectiveness and beneficial effects in other dimensions of quality and safety of care. Although there is a plethora of services available that can serve some of the user requirements, there is a clear shortage of integrated solutions focusing on older persons [52]. This segment of the population expresses a range of concerns around several themes, including difficulty in identifying credible and relevant sources of information on the web; ownership, access, and responsibility for medical information; and privacy concerns [53].

We must also consider additional barriers. Because technologies are relatively new, medical reimbursement schemes are slow to pay for services such as telemedicine. Furthermore, there is a lack of legal and regulatory framework that ensures high-quality medical encounters with optimal outcomes. Lastly legitimate security concerns exist due to potential hacking of sensitive personal information. While this does not exhaust all of the potential concerns, we see that much more must be done before society can take full advantage of medical technology advancements.

8.4 Partnering with Older Persons to Develop Patient-Centred Digital Solutions

In order to foster acceptance of digital technologies by older persons, digital technologies will need to provide personal and general information that is secure, readily accessible, and easily understood [53]. The importance of better understanding which individual characteristics shape older persons' perceptions and behaviour in using digital tools emerges therefore as a key to design and deliver tools that are better tailored to patient's needs and, therefore, have higher adoption rates and overall impact [54].

As advocated by 2020health, a social enterprise think tank, employing user-centred design methods enables true community engagement, rapid prototyping of products, and early feedback and buy-in from consumers/patients [55]. Partnering with patients creates conditions for digital health solutions to provide better, jargon-free guidance on setup and to become more appealing and intuitive for use by older persons (i.e. more tailored to their motor skills, visual and hearing capacity), thus targeting their actual needs and setting up goals that are perceived by users as realistic.

8.5 New Opportunities and the Way Forward

Population ageing and the technological revolution are key global trends for the coming decades [56]. Such demographic transition and technological advance will impact on almost all aspects of society, notably healthcare [56]. Meanwhile, the debate has moved beyond discussing the challenges such trends pose to highlighting the many they can help solve [56]. Consequently, innovation is not only being embraced but fostered, and the twentieth-century social construct of seeing older persons as an economic burden, dependent and in need of care and services, is slowly but steadily shifting to a new paradigm where elders are seen through an opportunity lens and as a valuable resource.

Policy wise, such transformations have been engraved in the United Nations (UN) 2030 Agenda (2015) and in the Global Strategy and Action Plan on Ageing and Health, adopted by the World Health Organization (WHO) (2016). By pledging to leave no one behind, the UN Assembly called for ensuring the Sustainable Development Goals (SDGs) are met for all segments of society and across the life course, recognizing that older persons must take an active role in social change if inclusive and sustainable development is to be achieved. According to SGD goals, it is essential to ensure healthy lives and promote well-being at all ages, as well as to invest in infrastructure, namely, information and communication technology, as improvements in health outcomes require investment in such infrastructure. WHO, in turn, has furthered the global response to population ageing by building on the UN 2030 Development Agenda, considering that the SDGs reaffirm and support WHO's Healthy Ageing principles.

Such policy frameworks pave the way forward for digital health in the ageing world, as it calls for increased access to information and communications technology, universal and affordable access to the Internet, and much needed investments in expanding and upgrading the infrastructure needed to further develop and implement digital health solutions that can support the well-being and health needs of the ever-increasing numbers of older persons: from optic fibre to 4/5G networks, including augmented and virtual reality technologies, 3D/4D printers and robots, or even artificial intelligence and big data technologies, cloud and quantum computing, brain-machine interfaces, and sensors.

In addition, as the implementation of digital interventions scales up worldwide, there is an increased need to evaluate their impact and, particularly, to investigate their effect in different segments of the population. To ensure the quality and minimize safety risks, reliable mechanisms should also be in place so that users can easily identify the digital health solutions that provide real value, among the many available. In this regard, a proposal has been published by Mathews et al. [57], calling for triple validation of digital health solutions: (1) on the accuracy of any claimed measurements; (2) on the evidence supporting a positive impact on user-centred health outcomes; and (3) on the integration into patients' lives, provider workflows, and healthcare systems. The latter directly addresses the known lack of interoperability that currently hinders digital health, both across digital health solutions (technical interoperability) and across health and social care organizations (service interoperability) [57]. In addition, considering the massive increase of personal data produced by digital technologies, the data protection regulatory landscape will need to continue evolving to discourage the manipulation and misuse of data as well as to diminish the growing concerns over privacy that could result in a climate of distrust and bring technological innovation to a halt [56].

8.6   The Role of the Family Physician

Not only does technology enhance current practices in care, but it can also be a catalyst for rethinking the way services are delivered and the roles of the stakeholders. New tools offer the opportunity to model consultations differently. Many tasks carried out by primary care professionals, such as family physicians and nurses, can be automated, freeing up time and potentially benefiting the relationship with patients if allocated suitably. The relationship of trust between the family doctor—and other primary care professionals—and the patient can become a strong asset in assisting older people in navigating the panorama of digital services and tools. The constellation of applications, however, renders critical the development of competences and skills, including basic artificial intelligence literacy, which will enable primary care professionals, to use digital technologies appropriately and proficiently [55, 58]. A transformation of undergraduate, postgraduate, and continuing professional development curricula is urgently needed in this respect, as well as more co-creation through increased active participation of health workers in the phases of design, development, implementation, and maintenance of technological solutions.

References

1. Chatterji S, Byles J, Cutler D, Seeman T, Verdes E. Health, functioning, and disability in older adults—present status and future implications. Lancet. 2015;385:563–75.
2. International Telecommunication Union (ITU). Minimum requirements related to technical performance for IMT-2020 radio interface(s). 2017.
3. Morgado A, Huq KMS, Mumtaz S, Rodriguez J. A survey of 5G technologies: regulatory, standardization and industrial perspectives. Digit Commun Networks. 2018;4:87–97.
4. Bhatt CM, Dey N, Ashour A. Internet of things and big data technologies for next generation healthcare. Springer International Publishing; 2017.
5. European Commission—Directorate General for Communications Networks: Content and Technology. Commission Staff Working Document: Advancing the Internet of Things in Europe. Digital Single Market. 2016.
6. Thuemmler C, Bai C, editors. Health 4.0: how virtualization and big data are revolutionizing healthcare. New York, NY: Springer; 2017.
7. Oueida S, Kotb Y, Aloqaily M, Jararweh Y, Baker T. An edge computing based smart healthcare framework for resource management. Sensors. 2018;18:4307.
8. Klonoff DC. Fog computing and edge computing architectures for processing data from diabetes devices connected to the medical internet of things. J Diabetes Sci Technol. 2017;11:647–52.
9. Perakakis N, Yazdani A, Karniadakis GE, Mantzoros C. Omics. Big data and machine learning as tools to propel understanding of biological mechanisms and to discover novel diagnostics and therapeutics. Metab Clin Exp. 2018;87:A1–9.
10. Topol EJ. High-performance medicine: the convergence of human and artificial intelligence. Nat Med. 2019;25:44–56.
11. Webb T, Joseph J, Yardley L, Michie S. Using the internet to promote health behavior change: a systematic review and meta-analysis of the impact of theoretical basis, use of behavior change techniques, and mode of delivery on efficacy. J Med Int Res. 2010;12:e4.
12. Michie S, Richardson M, Johnston M, Abraham C, Francis J, Hardeman W, et al. The behavior change technique taxonomy (v1) of 93 hierarchically clustered techniques: building an

international consensus for the reporting of behavior change interventions. Ann Behav Med. 2013;46:81–95.

13. Zhao J, Freeman B, Li M. Can mobile phone apps influence people's health behavior change? An evidence review. J Med Internet Res. 2016;18:e287.

14. Nundy S, Mishra A, Hogan P, Lee SM, Solomon MC, Peek ME. How do Mobile phone diabetes programs drive behavior change?: evidence from a mixed methods observational cohort study. Diabetes Educ. 2014;40(6):806–19.

15. Iyengar V, Wolf A, Brown A, Close K. Challenges in diabetes care: can digital health help address them? Clin Diabetes. 2016;34:133–41.

16. Aranda S. The patient remote intervention and symptom management system (PRISMS)–a telehealth-mediated intervention enabling real-time monitoring of chemotherapy side-effects in patients with haematological malignancies: study protocol for a randomised controlled trial. Trials. 2015;16:472.

17. Evans J, Papadopoulos A, Silvers CT, Charness N, Boot WR, Schlachta-Fairchild L, Crump C, Martinez M, Ent CB. Remote health monitoring for older adults and those with heart failure: adherence and system usability. Telemed e-Health. 2016;22:480–8.

18. Walker AL, Muhlestein JB. Smartphone electrocardiogram monitoring: current perspectives. Advanced Health Care Technologies. 2018;4:15–24.

19. de Vries NM, Staal JB, van der Wees PJ, Adang EM, Akkermans R, Olde Rikkert MG, Nijhuis-van der Sanden MW. Patient-centred physical therapy is (cost-) effective in increasing physical activity and reducing frailty in older adults with mobility problems: a randomized controlled trial with 6 months follow-up. J Cachexia Sarcopenia Muscle. 2016;7:422–35.

20. Rostill H, Nilforooshan R, Morgan A, Barnaghi P, Ream E, Chrysanthaki T. Technology integrated health management for dementia. Br J Community Nurs. 2018;23:502–8.

21. Godfrey A, Brodie M, van Schooten KS, Nouredanesh M, Stuart S, Robinson L. Inertial wearables as pragmatic tools in dementia. Maturitas. 2019;127:12–7.

22. Koumakis L, Chatzaki C, Kazantzaki E, Maniadi E, Tsiknakis M. Dementia care frameworks and assistive technologies for their implementation: a review. IEEE Rev Biomed Eng. 2019;12:4–18.

23. Neubauer NA, Lapierre N, Ríos-Rincón A, Miguel-Cruz A, Rousseau J, Liu L. What do we know about technologies for dementia-related wandering? A scoping review. Can J Occup Ther. 2018;85:196–208.

24. Mangini L, Wick JY. Wandering: unearthing new tracking devices. Consult Pharm. 2017;32:324–31.

25. Memon M, Wagner S, Pedersen C, Beevi F, Hansen F. Ambient assisted living healthcare frameworks, platforms, standards, and quality attributes. Sensors. 2014;14:4312–41.

26. Wang S, Bolling K, Mao W, Reichstadt J, Jeste D, Kim H-C, et al. Technology to support aging in place: older adults' perspectives. Healthcare. 2019;7:60.

27. Tsirmpas C, Kouris I, Anastasiou A, Giokas K, Iliopoulou D, Koutsouris D. An internet of things platform architecture for supporting ambient assisted living environments. Technol Healthcare. 2017;25:391–401.

28. Dohr A, Modre-Osprian R, Drobics M, Hayn D, Schreier G. The internet of things for ambient assisted living. In: Information Technology: New Generations, Third International Conference on Smart Homes and Health Telematics. 2010:804–9.

29. Baig MM, Afifi S, GholamHosseini H, Mirza F. A systematic review of wearable sensors and IoT-based monitoring applications for older adults—a focus on ageing population and independent living. J Med Syst. 2019;43:233.

30. Nguyen H, Mirza F, Naeem MA, Baig MM. Falls management framework for supporting an independent lifestyle for older adults: a systematic review. Aging Clin Exp Res. 2018;30:1275–86.

31. Liu L, Stroulia E, Nikolaidis I, Miguel-Cruz A, Rincon AR. Smart homes and home health monitoring technologies for older adults: a systematic review. Int J Med Inform. 2016;91:44–59.

32. Gellis ZD, Kenaley BL, Ten Have T. Integrated telehealth care for chronic illness and depression in geriatric home care patients: the integrated telehealth education and activation of mood (I-TEAM) study. J Am Geriatr Soc. 2014;62:889–95.
33. Bauce K, Fahs DB, Batten J, Whittemore R. Videoconferencing for management of heart failure: an integrative review. J Gerontol Nurs. 2018;44:45–52.
34. Nakamura N, Koga T, Iseki H. A meta-analysis of remote patient monitoring for chronic heart failure patients. J Telemed Telecare. 2014;20:11–7.
35. Janssen A, Robinson T, Brunner M, Harnett P, Museth KE, Shaw T. Multidisciplinary teams and ICT: a qualitative study exploring the use of technology and its impact on multidisciplinary team meetings. BMC Health Serv Res. 2018;18:444.
36. Ho DK. Voice-controlled virtual assistants for the older people with visual impairment. Eye. 2018;32:53–4.
37. Rieland R. How will artificial intelligence help the aging? In: Smithsonian. 2017.
38. Cho KH, Lee WH. Effect of treadmill training based real-world video recording on balance and gait in chronic stroke patients: a randomized controlled trial. Gait Posture. 2014;39:523–8.
39. Chan CL, Ngai EK, Leung PK, Wong S. Effect of the adapted virtual reality cognitive training program among Chinese older adults with chronic schizophrenia: a pilot study. Int J Geriatr Psychiatry. 2010;25:643–9.
40. Rasulnia M, Ginter R, Wang T, Burton S, Pleasants R, Lugogo N. Assessing the impact of a remote digital coaching engagement program on patient reported outcomes in asthma. Novel Epidemiol Manage Outcomes Asthma. 2017;A2999:795.
41. Boulton AJ, Vileikyte L, Ragnarson-Tennvall G, Apelqvist J. The global burden of diabetic foot disease. Lancet. 2005;366:1719–24.
42. Bloom JD, Linders DR, Engler JM, Petersen BJ, Geboff A, Kale DC, inventors; PODIMETRICS Inc, assignee. Method and apparatus for indicating the risk of an emerging ulcer. United States patent US 9,259,178. 2016.
43. Sousa P, Felizardo V, Oliveira D, Couto R, Garcia NM. A review of thermal methods and technologies for diabetic foot assessment. Exp Rev Med Dev. 2015;12:439–48.
44. Murphy C, Corley G, Kiersey S, inventors; Bluedrop Medical Ltd, assignee. Skin Inspection Device for Identifying Abnormalities. United States patent application US 16/303,296. 2019.
45. Irizarry T, DeVito DA, Curran CR. Patient portals and patient engagement: a state of the science review. J Med Internet Res. 2015;17:e148.
46. Goldzweig CL, Orshansky G, Paige NM, et al. Electronic patient portals: evidence on health outcomes, satisfaction, efficiency, and attitudes: a systematic review. Ann Intern Med. 2013;159:677–87.
47. Gordon NP, Hornbrook MC. Older adults' readiness to engage with eHealth patient education and self-care resources: a cross-sectional survey. BMC Health Serv Res. 2018;18:220.
48. Anderson MO, Perrin AN. Technology use among seniors. Washington, DC: Pew Research Center for Internet & Technology; 2017.
49. Taylor KSL Smartphone ownership is growing rapidly around the world, but not always equally: Pew Research Center. 2019.
50. DataReportal. Digital 2019: Global Digital Overview.
51. Office for National Statistics. Home internet and social media usage: Frequency of internet use, by age group and by income.
52. Kyriazakos S, Prasad N. Delivery of eHealth and eInclusion services for elderly people with mild dementia. In: 2nd International Conference on Wireless Communication, Vehicular Technology, Information Theory and Aerospace & Electronic Systems Technology (Wireless VITAE), 2011.
53. Ware P, Bartlett SJ, Paré G, Symeonidis I, Tannenbaum C, Bartlett G, Poissant L, Ahmed S. Using eHealth technologies: interests, preferences, and concerns of older adults. Interact J Med Res. 2017;6:e3.
54. Rockmann R, Gewald H. Elderly people in eHealth: who are they? Procedia Comput Sci. 2015;63:505–10.

55. Mason K. Health technologies: are older people interested? Discussion Paper. 2020 health. 2016:1–8.
56. European Strategy and Policy Analysis Systems. Global trends to 2030: Can the EU meet the challenges ahead?
57. Mathews SC, McShea MJ, Hanley CL, Ravitz A, Labrique AB, Cohen AB. Digital health: a path to validation. NPJ Digit Med. 2019;2:38.
58. World Health Organization. Digital technologies: shaping the future of primary health care. Technical series on Primary Health Care.

Part II

Tools and Scores for Geriatric Assessment (with Tables and Synopsis)

Scales and Scores for Comprehensive Geriatric Assessment in Primary Care

9

Anna Maria Meyer, Stefano Celotto, Daniele Angioni, and M. Cristina Polidori

Abstract

Older patients' health problems in general practice (GP) are often complex and cannot be assigned to a specific disease. This requires a paradigm shift to goal-oriented, personalized care for clinical decision-making. Geriatric diagnostics is the key to prevent the loss of function with older adults at risk for adverse outcomes by a preventive approach in GP—therefore the role of a general practitioner is highly important in the geriatric care of older adults. Geriatric diagnostics includes geriatric screening, which should be performed in all older adults to identify those in need for further diagnostics. If a patient is screened positive, a comprehensive geriatric assessment (CGA) should be performed to assess the domain or function where the patient displays the risk of adverse outcomes in order to intervene. Approaching single geriatric syndromes might be needed to develop a specific, goal-oriented care plan. Ideally, the CGA should be

A. M. Meyer
Ageing Clinical Research, Dpt. II of Internal Medicine and Centre of Molecular Medicine, University Hospital of Cologne Medical Faculty, Cologne, Germany

S. Celotto
Primary Care Department, Azienda Sanitaria Universitaria Friuli Centrale, Udine, Italy

D. Angioni
Primary Care Clinic, Eastern Piedmont, Novara, South-District, Italy

Diagnostic Medical Sonographer in Vercelli, Vercelli, Italy

M. C. Polidori (✉)
Ageing Clinical Research, Dpt. II of Internal Medicine and Centre of Molecular Medicine, University Hospital of Cologne Medical Faculty, Cologne, Germany

Cologne Excellence Cluster CECAD, University of Cologne, Cologne, Germany
e-mail: maria.polidori-nelles@uk-koeln.de

© Springer Nature Switzerland AG 2022
J. Demurtas, N. Veronese (eds.), *The Role of Family Physicians in Older People Care*, Practical Issues in Geriatrics, https://doi.org/10.1007/978-3-030-78923-7_9

121

performed together with a multidisciplinary geriatric team. Problems in the implementation of CGA in primary care include lack of awareness due to poor access to current scientific evidence, lack of time, sceptical physicians' attitudes and the missing opportunity of a geriatric team in an outpatient setting. However, there is growing evidence that the goal-oriented, systematic implementation of CGA in GP settings is realistic and feasible when mediated by authentic comanagement and intersectoral cooperation of geriatricians and GP physicians.

Keywords

Comprehensive geriatric assessment · General practice · Family physicians Frailty · Ageing

9.1 The Comprehensive Geriatric Assessment: More than Numbers

Older adults are frequent users of general practice (GP), with at least 10% of the people over 60 years visiting their GP over ten times per year, higher percentages for persons older than 70 years [1, 2] and percentages reaching up to 24% for persons aged 85 years and older [3]. Despite this high frequency, the identification of older patients at risk for adverse outcomes is not performed on a regular basis, and they often remain underdiagnosed. Possible reasons are the curtain of multimorbidity, acute diseases and age-related changes affecting older people, making it challenging to uncover leading geriatric syndromes [4]. The frequent underreporting of complaints by older patients is also a main problem in general practice, as some frailty-related symptoms are considered part of "normal ageing" [5]—very often the loss of function occurs in a subtle progression [6], and ageing occurs in the form of many heterogeneous phenotypes [7–9].

However, it is of high importance to promptly identify vulnerability of the systems, i.e. frailty, as well as all those processes which are not part of the physiological, inevitable ageing process—i.e. the so-called geriatric syndromes. Frailty predisposes to geriatric syndromes, and the latter pave the way to a complex geriatric multimorbidity which leads to higher use of healthcare resources, high treatment burden and psychological distress [10], which may in turn result in more comorbidities. By detecting geriatric syndromes, and even more so frailty and prefrailty, a vicious cycle of disability and adverse outcomes can be stopped—therefore an early identification is necessary before the cycle begins. Based on this scheme, showing the importance of risk identification prior to disease onset brings us directly to the importance of the work of general practitioners in this sense. General practice (GP) settings, in fact, are the structures in which older, apparently healthy, patients can be seen due to minor health problems or for an adequate management of their chronic disease. These patients may enormously benefit from the identification of risk conditions before a hospitalization occurs—in this sense, general practitioners are the gatekeepers and the "player managers" of the patients.

The diagnostic approach to older persons should objectively define their needs and identify supportive care approaches for maintaining or achieving an acceptable level of intrinsic capacity, quality of life, independence [11] and self-efficiency [12].

The so-called *comprehensive geriatric assessment* (CGA) is a substantial help, being promoted to be the heart and the soul of geriatrics [13] which can be easily learned in teaching settings at a pre-graduate, post-graduate or multiprofessional level [5].

The history of the CGA began 50 years ago by the work of Lawrence Rubenstein [14]. Since then, it has been used as a diagnostic tool in several clinical settings all over the world [15]. It is defined as a "multidimensional interdisciplinary diagnostic process focused on determining a frail elderly person's medical, psychological and functional capability in order to develop a coordinated and integrated plan for treatment and long-term follow-up" [16]. It has the aim to identifying patient's deficits and problems highlighting the level of functioning of the patient at different dimensions.

The CGA must be strictly separated from *geriatric screening*, which just roughly identifies risk constellations mainly through yes-and-no questions, in order to plan further diagnostic procedures, such as a targeted CGA, on this basis [17, 18].

Generally, the CGA is also kept separated from frailty assessments, which are considered as necessary and targeted when frailty is suspected. However, and within the frame of the new evidence characterizing frailty as a dynamic concept—i.e. reversible to prefrailty and robustness [19]—therefore to be diagnosed as soon as possible, as well as a multidimensional condition [20, 21], frailty is suggested to be captured at best by multidimensional tools. In this sense, frailty can be seen as a surrogate marker of biological age, and its multifactoriality explains its complexity and therefore difficulty in diagnosis on one hand, and on the other hand it underlines the necessity to introduce its assessment in clinical practice [22]. Indeed, frailty identification in the general population through feasible multidimensional tools like the CGA and derivatives might be key for adequate, not futile resource allocation, as we see during the SARS-CoV-2 pandemic [23].

The several existing assessments to identify frailty in older patients focus mainly on physical frailty. The overall frailty, however, might be accurately caught in real life by the GP by means of appropriate tools, and the comanagement with geriatric expertise might enable highly effective interventions and integrated care on different domains of the patient: physiological, cognitive, nutritional, functional and psychosocial [24]. Assessments range from simple tools to very extensive forms to instruments that additionally calculate the patients' prognosis. Since one of the main aims of the CGA is to assess "frailty" and there is no coherent definition of that term, there is accordingly no consensus about which instruments are most appropriate to identify frail older people [25–29]. Some of the most popular frailty indexes that need to be mentioned are the *Fried's frailty phenotype (Cardiovascular Health Study, CHS)* [30]; the *Edmonton Frailty Scale* (EFS) [31]; the *Fatigue, Resistance, Ambulation, Illness and Loss of Weight* (FRAIL) *Index* [32]; the Rockwood *Clinical Frailty Scale* [33]; and the *Clinical Frailty Scale* (CFS) [33]. Despite ongoing debate about frailty definition and frailty assessment in GP settings, all determine a predictive value for the patients' outcomes and to focus on early intervention and preventive measures [34].

When taking a closer look to all these scales, an experienced general practitioner will see that most information is performed "involuntarily" by a normal history collection by addressing the emotional, physical, psychic, functional and social domains of the patient. Every good general practitioner performs multidimensional examination and takes decisions consequently even if not using numbers as in a structured assessment. Therefore, the CGA is equal to a general practitioner's approach of personalized medicine, and the scales are just a structured way to make sure that the doctors are asking for all the information and that not one part is missing. Additionally, it helps to communicate information to other specialties or other physicians, if needed, because this information is objective.

However, all these CGA-delivered numbers need general practitioners with expertise, because numbers, i.e. scores and scales, are not useful (and sometimes even counterproductive) if they are not used with a target-oriented, tailored interpretation taking into account the values, the well-being and the intrinsic capacity of each individual patient.

At the end—despite all numbers and scales—what the health systems want to achieve is the early recognition of frailty and the prevention of repeated negative outcomes like rehospitalizations. Some systems (like the German one, where the geriatric intervention goes through a very special remuneration and therefore insurance algorithm) struggle to find appropriate instruments to triage "geriatric" patients to the respective "geriatric" intervention. But in truth, what medicine needs to recognize is frailty, which is the very substance of geriatric medicine, and leads to the conditions usually encountered in what we call *the geriatric patient* [35]. While screenings per nature cannot identify frailty (they can just identify the probable presence of risk factors), an assessment like the CGA is needed. Indeed, the benefit of CGA-based geriatric interventions is recognized and has been well described in several systematic reviews [15, 36]. While a further description of these benefits goes beyond the scope of this chapter, it is urgent time that all possible efforts are put in action to keep older community-dwellers in their usual environment, i.e. at home, as long as possible. GP physicians, familiar with the measurement of function [37], may constitute a critical role to feasibly implement the CGA [38–40].

9.2 The Unreplaceable Meaning of the Patient-GP-Specialist Triad

As new care systems allow older people to live at home longer, it is likely that more and more GP physicians will be the main medical contact for the treatment of geriatric patients [41]. With the ageing of the population and the rising of multimorbidity, requests for GP consultations and home visits increase exponentially, and it becomes hard to fulfil all of them in a reasonable amount of time; this results in extended waiting times for appointments and a higher rate for referrals. The large spectrum of chronic diseases in these patients as well as unspecific symptoms—such as pain, dizziness, dyspnoea or any weakness—complicates diagnostic and therapeutic processes in older patients in GP [42].

If we want older people to stay healthy, their living conditions should be supported, and therefore prevention is incredibly important in any healthcare system. When it comes to prevention, general practitioners play a central role, because prevention is known to be a core issue in GP. The European definition of GP says that general practitioners "should promote health and wellbeing by applying health promotion and disease prevention, cure, care, palliation and rehabilitation" [43]. The definition implies a continuous flux of information between GP physicians and other healthcare professionals caring for the patient across the long way of chronic conditions. In this sense, the GP physician, who experiences the patient's trajectories for several years, is a central figure in the maintenance of her intrinsic capacity. As the GP doctor possesses unreplaceable information for the adequate management of older patients, the shared approach sketched above as well as a well planned distribution of tasks is highly important for integrated care [44].

A targeted intervention in the management of older patients needs a multidisciplinary treatment of frailty with clinical treatment through the GP physician [29, 45, 46] and, if needed, together with targeted approaches in the fields of physiotherapy, nutrition, neuropsychology, occupational therapy, pharmacy and speech therapy [39, 47], as well as other specialties. As the psychosocial aspect of patient care becomes more important, the intensive cooperation with social services and the full utilization of outpatient rehabilitation options also gain importance [42].

The GP practitioner acts like a "player-manager" for the team of the patient—someone making sense of all the information, explaining medical findings and supporting the patient [48]. In doing so, the GP physician plays a decisive role as a referrer in outpatient management because he makes decisions about further examinations, medical contact and prescriptions [49]. In this sense, the GP doctor-specialist triad is completed by the patient himself, who needs to be an active player in his own treatment. Evidence shows the importance of enabling the patient to collaborate, discuss and share openly what is important to him and his own health [12, 46, 50]. This so called "value-based" patient care is not implemented systematically, even though physicians often know what is good for the patient's health [51, 52]. This can be exemplified by a case study: a patient comes to the physician because he can no longer go up the two stairs to his apartment due to pain in the knee and shortness of breath. In the hospital significant aortic valve stenosis is found and interventional treated. The doctor is satisfied because the ejection volume is increasing and the shortness of breath is significantly reduced. However, even if the patient is now objectively considered to be in a better health condition, the pain in the knee remains, and his initial problem of no longer being able to reach his apartment on the second floor is not resolved. This case example shows that the approach of shared decision-making is highly important because it identifies the patient as an expert on his own condition and the doctor as an expert on the medical findings [52]. For a good doctor-patient relationship, furthermore, the patient needs to be provided with enough medical information [53, 54]. This gives the patient health literacy, which can lead to more health-promoting activities and lifestyle enhancements [55] and also to an increase in compliance, which in turn results in cost savings. Besides the previous external improvement strategies, in fact, patients also have geriatric resources [56] that are worth of consideration. Geriatric resources are characteristics that a patient brings with them, which can protect them against long-term care, dependency and complications in the event of a long course of the disease. Examples are emotional, physical, motivational or financial resources [56].

The general practitioner as a team member of other medical specialities and hospitals is still underrepresented. Especially studies with older patients in GPs can be rarely found although previous studies showed that the use of a CGA in GP is possible and that a worse outcome is associated with a higher number of GP visits [9]. Especially research of the transitional care from inpatient to outpatient setting, to show how a good communication can work, must be enforced [57].

9.3 Through the Jungle of Scales, Scores, Screenings and Assessments: What's What

Although the body of geriatric care is performed in the primary healthcare setting, most CGAs are created for the hospital setting. Previous studies showed the bunch of geriatric problems of older patients in outpatient settings; geriatric syndromes are very common and very often underrecognized. Therefore, they remain untreated [58, 59]. Similarly, and probably most importantly, the identification of (pre)frailty before hospitalization should be considered mandatory as it paves the way to positive trajectories and outcomes upon identification and treatment by prevention of geriatric syndromes [60].

The current German Primary Care Guideline of the Geriatric Assessment has the goal of enabling general practitioners to recognize vulnerable patients with preventive, therapeutic and rehabilitation needs in everyday practice with reasonable financial effort by performing CGAs [6].

Although the working frame of a GP is usually very stressful, GP physicians mentioned in previous studies that the implementation of a geriatric screening in the waiting area could be easily integrated into the practice and that patients were motivated to take part in the test without acceptance problems [6].

9.3.1 Geriatric Screenings: Little Expenditure of Time but Also Not Specific

Geriatric Screening I [6]
(1) **Do you feel full of energy?**
(2) **Do you have difficulty walking a distance of 400 m?**
If one or two questions are positive (question 1 „no", question 2 „yes", there is a need of a further testing by a complete CGA.

Geriatric screening can detect unidentified problems in general practice. In a first step, GPs need a simple screening instrument enabling them to detect older patients at need for a more complete geriatric assessment which can be followed by targeted interventions [61]. A screening tool recommends the use of two signal questions for a pre-selection [6]. Another screening tool recommends a set of five components [62].

> **Geriatric Screening II** [62]
> (1) Fatigue reported by the patient
> (2) **Physical performance**
> (3) **Walking**
> (4) **Number of comorbidities**
> (5) **Nutritional status**

This approach should help increase the benefit of an assessment method and lower labour costs, as a CGA for every citizen over 70 years old would affect too many people and, therefore, would not be logistically manageable. Despite debate on frailty definition, positively screened patients are to be considered frail and need a comprehensive assessment to identify specific geriatric syndromes and resources to target [6].

9.3.2 A Single Geriatric Syndrome Approach: Specific but Not Comprehensive

When there is the wish to assess age-associated problems, it is possible to ask for specific conditions of the older patient like urine incontinence or hearing loss point by point. By assessing these geriatric syndromes, there is the advantage of gaining specific target points for a following intervention [56]. There are many screening instruments which have been developed for the individual syndromes [56, 58]. Similarly to some very detailed scales for the identification of frailty [20], a long-lasting knowledge of the patient and the amount of items to take into account make the identification of single geriatric syndromes time-consuming. Table 9.1 gives an overview of some of the most common evaluation tools.

9.3.3 The CGA: The Problem of Gaining Comprehensive Information in a Timely Frame

In contrast to the single approach, it is possible to carry out a comprehensive assessment, in which one does not test individual syndromes, but rather global functions of the older patient. This procedure has the advantage that the general functional status of an older person can be recorded in a manageable amount of time. In the

Table 9.1 Selection of evaluation tools of single geriatric syndromes, domain functions of the person and frailty

How to test geriatric syndromes, domain functions of the person and frailty (ref)	
Frailty and functions	**Lifestyle**
– Activities of daily living (ADL) [63]	– Habit of smoking, alcohol, physical activity, social relationships, inadequate nutrition
– Instrumental activities of daily living (IADL) [64]	– AUDIT C [67]
– Electronic Frailty Index [65]	– Fagerstrom [68]
– Fried's frailty phenotype [30]	
– Rockwood Frailty Scale [33]	
– Modified Barthel Index [66]	
– Recent hospital stays	
– Multidimensional Prognostic Index	
Falls and risk for falling	**Gait and balance**
– FRA-HS [69]	– Berg Balance Scale [73]
– FRAX [70]	– 180-degree standing turn strategy (CAT-STS) [74]
– "Get up and go" test [71]	– Timed Up & Go Test [75]
– Evaluation of orthostatic hypotension	– Balance and Gait Evaluation (Tinetti Scale)
– 9-item risk factor checklist [72]	
– Evaluation of home hazards (carpets, low lights, dangerous cables, etc.)	
Sensoric	**Mood**
– Snellen chart	– Yesavage Geriatric Depression Scale [77]
– Audioscope	– Hamilton's Assessment of Anxiety States [78]
– Whisper test [76]	– Montgomery and Asberg Depression Rating Scale (MADRS) [79]
	– The Patient Health Questionnaire-2 (PHQ2/9) [80]
Delirium	**Decubitus**
– 4AT [81]	– Norton Scale [83]
– Single Question in Delirium (SQiD) [82]	– Exton Smith Scale (ESS) [84]
Dysphagia	**Nutrition**
– Daniels Test [85]	– Body Mass Index (BMI)
– Gugging swallowing screen test [86]	– MUST score [87]
	– Mini Nutritional Assessment (MNA) [88]
Pain	**Cognitive impairment**
– Penn Facial Pain Scale [89]	– Mini Mental State Examination (MMSE) [92]
– Pain Assessment in Advanced Dementia Scale (PAINAD-G) [90]	– The Mini-Cog [93]
– Visual Analog scale for pain (VAS pain) [91]	– The GPCOG [94]
– Numeric Rating Scale for Pain (NRS Pain [91]	– Montreal Cognitive Assessment
	– Hodkinson Abbreviated Mental Test Score (AMTS) [95]
	– Short Portable Mental Status Questionnaire [96]

(continued)

Table 9.1 (continued)

How to test geriatric syndromes, domain functions of the person and frailty (ref)	
Frailty and functions	**Lifestyle**
Social assessments	**Polypharmacy**
– Nottingham Extended Activities of Daily Living Scale [97]	– Number of drugs (prescribed + OTC + phytotherapy + alternative therapies) [99]
– BGA Social Questionnaire [29]	– STOPP/START criteria [100]
– BGA Environment Questionnaire [29]	– NO TEARS tool [101]
– Minimum Data Set for Home Care [98]	– Beers Criteria [102]
	– Medication Appropriateness Index [103]
	– Therapeutic reconciliation
	– Anticholinergic Burden Score [104]
	– PRISCUS [105]/ FORTA [106]
Vaccination	**Sarcopenia**
– Registration of vaccinations (influenza, pneumococcal, Zoster) [107]	– The Six-Minute Walk Test (6MWT) [108]
	– Short Physical Performance Battery (SPPB) [109]
	– Chair stand test (CST) [110]
	– Sarc-F-Score [111]
Sleep impairment	**Incontinence**
– Ask for sleep disorders	– Rome III Criteria for the Diagnosis of Irritable Bowel Syndrome [112]
	– The international consultation on incontinence questionnaire (ICIQ) [113]
Advance treatment directives	**Performance status/degree of disability**
– Care plan subscription	– Modified Rankin scale [114]
	– Palliative Performance Scale/ECOG Scale [115]
	– Karnofsky Performance Status [116]

event of abnormalities in a functional area, further specific tests should then follow in order to present and address the specific problems.

The "best" CGA for primary care is widely discussed—it should be easy, time-saving and comprehensive at the same time.

The *Tilburg Frailty Indicator* [117], which contains physical, psychological and social aspects of the older adult, can be assessed by the use of a 15-item checklist.

Another one to mention is the *SHARE-FI* [118], which has been widely used but still requires validation in larger studies in primary healthcare settings. It assesses typical red flag symptoms of the older adult like exhaustion, loss of appetite, weakness, walking difficulties and low physical activity and can be calculated separately for male and female.

One recommended CGA for GP is the *Manageable Geriatric Assessment* (MAGIC), which focuses on common problems of community-dwelling older adults involving nine domains: efficiency in everyday life, sensorial information (seeing, hearing), falls, urinary incontinence, depression, social environment, vaccination and orientation tests for cognitive performance with the clock-test [119]. It was developed out of the STEP assessment, which was shown to be too long for a usual general practice visit [120].

A CGA should be performed when there is a high risk of multidimensional frailty for the individual patient. The CGA is highly desirable in the following situations: when an older person presents to their GP with one or more obvious frailty syndromes; when an older person has an accident (e.g. a fall), which suggests an underlying geriatric morbidity; and when an older person has been discharged from hospital and generally in care homes [29].

In general, CGAs are as heterogenous as the ageing process, but the most common ones can properly identify patients at risk. The choice of the most useful CGA is not an issue – this is up to the general practitioners' experience and knowledge—provided that there is awareness about the multiplicity of instruments available. Testing frailty in a structured way can save time later during the short- and midterm course of life and allows the general practitioner to have an equally good judgement no matter how long he knows the patient [9]. Previous studies, however, showed that the accuracy and sensitivity of the CGA increase when the GP knows the patient for a longer time [59, 121]. But apart of the long-term relationship, performing a CGA delivers new information to the GP and discloses age-associated problems he could have not been aware of before [121], confirming how important the performance of a structured assessment is.

The acceptance of a CGA in general practice has shown to be very good among older adults [122, 123]. The treating GP should be conscious that the medical aspects he focuses on might be different from the issues that the patient worries about. So it seems to be necessary, for increasing the outcome of the CGA, that the GP discusses the relevance of the outcome with the patient [121]. Further research is needed to identify the best practical screening and assessment in general practice, as well as the most effective strategy for implementing CGA or associated prognostic tools [9] in primary care. Even accomplishing the issue of an adequate screening and assessment, there is still a trouble: maintaining a multiprofessional treatment for the selected patients is still extremely hard in usual care.

Providing a good care plan to a patient who was identified with geriatric problems through a CGA needs the development of an effective and comprehensive strategy. This should be achieved throughout the caring process, by adopting shared decision-making strategies in order to set and reset step by step targets and objectives. Goals should be measurable, achievable, relevant and timely and involve carers and family [29].

9.4 Conclusions

In conclusion, there is a high potential in the care of older adults that needs to be activated by policy-makers, carers and doctors. There is a high need to develop and use a structured diagnostic tool for older patients at risk for adverse outcomes to consequently implementing preventive strategies. Since prevention belongs to the field of primary care, and general practitioners are the doctors who are most in touch with older adults, there is the need to perform geriatric diagnostic in general practice. A geriatric screening is useful to screen all adults above the age of 65 years to detect those who need a more detailed geriatric assessment. After a patient is screened positively, there is the need to perform a CGA to assess the whole function and functional limitations of the older person. If some risks or limits are detected, a specific testing of geriatric syndromes can be performed to assess specific targets of intervention. All testing of older patients should be followed by a structured care plan with specific goals. This active care plan should be discussed with the patient to define which problems are indeed relevant to the patient and to arrange a shared action program. After specific goals are addressed, there is the need or a geriatric team to try to intervene to achieve these target points.

Now there is, especially in primary care, a huge gap between what is known to be necessary and its accomplishment, in other words, between evidence and practice. Currently, and unfortunately, barriers against a good and widespread implementation are multiple and strong [124]. Among those barriers, the main are educational gaps in geriatric care, too narrow time windows for testing, insufficient remuneration for geriatric diagnosis or therapy as well as problems with the creation of a geriatric team for an active care plan in the outpatient setting. To overcome those issues, there is the need of more cooperation between specialists and GPs for integrated care and a higher number of studies addressing the problem.

References

1. Bundesvereinigung K. Versichertenbefragung der Kassenärztlichen Bundesvereinigung 2011.
2. Tille F, Gibis B, Balke K, Kuhlmey A, Schnitzer S. Sociodemographic and health-related determinants of health care utilisation and access to primary and specialist care: results of a nationwide population survey in Germany (2006-2016). Z Evid Fortbild Qual Gesundhwes. 2017;126:52–65.
3. Aprile PBE, Brignoli O, Cricelli C, Cricelli I, Lapi F, Medea G, Pasqua A; Pecchioli S, Simonetti M; Lombardo, FP. XII Report Health Search. 2019.
4. Marengoni A, Vetrano DL, Onder G. Target population for clinical trials on multimorbidity: is disease count enough? J Am Med Dir Assoc. 2019;20(2):113–4.
5. Roller-Wirnsberger R, Singler K, Polidori MC. Learning geriatric medicine: a study guide for medical students. Springer International Publishing; 2018.
6. Bergert FWBMFJ, Hüttner U, Kluthe B, Popert U, Seffrin J, Vetter G, Beyer M, Junius-Walker U, Muth C, Schubert I. Hausärztliche Leitline Geriatrisches Assessment in der Hausarztpraxis sowie Praxistipps zu geriatrischen Patienten.
7. Böhm K T-RC, Ziese T. Beiträge zur Gesundheitsberichterstattung des Bundes—Gesundheit und Krankheit im Alter 2009.
8. Ferrucci L, Levine ME, Kuo P-L, Simonsick EM. Time and the metrics of aging. Circ Res. 2018;123(7):740–4.
9. Meyer ASG, Becker I, Betz T, Bödecker AW, Robertz JW, Krause O, Benzing PT, Pilotto A, Polidori MC. The multidimensional prognostic index in general practice: one-year follow-up study. Int J Clin Pract. (accepted pending minor revisions). 2019;
10. Wallace E, Salisbury C, Guthrie B, Lewis C, Fahey T, Smith SM. Managing patients with multimorbidity in primary care. BMJ. 2015;350(jan20 2):h176.
11. Gupta A, Rehman A. Measurement scales used in elderly care. CRC Press; 2017.
12. Heppner HJ. Soft skills : somewhat different doping. Zeitschrift fur Gerontologie und Geriatrie. 2018;51(2):160–4.

13. Osterweil D, Brummel-Smith K, Beck JC. Comprehensive geriatric assessment. McGraw-Hill, Medical Publishing Division; 2000.

14. Stuck AE, Siu AL, Wieland GD, Adams J, Rubenstein LZ. Comprehensive geriatric assessment: a meta-analysis of controlled trials. Lancet. 1993;342(8878):1032–6.

15. Pilotto A, Cella A, Pilotto A, Daragjati J, Veronese N, Musacchio C, et al. Three decades of comprehensive geriatric assessment: evidence coming from different healthcare settings and specific clinical conditions. J Am Med Dir Assoc. 2017;18(2):192. e1- e11

16. Ellis G, Langhorne P. Comprehensive geriatric assessment for older hospital patients. Br Med Bull. 2004;71(1):45–59.

17. Polidori MC. Target and patient-oriented care using the comprehensive geriatric assessment : prognosis estimation for clinical decisions with elderly patients. Zeitschrift fur Gerontologie und Geriatrie. 2017;50(8):706–9.

18. Weinrebe W, Schiefer Y, Weckmuller K, Schulz RJ, Rupp S, Bischoff S, et al. Does the identification of seniors at risk (ISAR) score effectively select geriatric patients on emergency admission? Aging Clin Exp Res. 2019;31:1839.

19. Senin UP, Cherubini A, Mecocci P. Paziente anziano paziente geriatrico Medicina della complessitá. Fondamenti di Gerontologia e Geriatria. Napoli: Edises; 2020.

20. Ferrucci LFE, Walston JD. Frailty. In: JOJG H, Studenski S, High KP, Asthana S, Supiano MA, Ritchie C, editors. Hazzard's geriatric medicine and gerontology, 7e. McGraw-Hill; 2017.

21. Pilotto A, Custodero C, Maggi S, Polidori MC, Veronese N, Ferrucci L. A multidimensional approach to frailty in older people. Ageing Res Rev. 2020;60:101047.

22. Dent E, Martin FC, Bergman H, Woo J, Romero-Ortuno R, Walston JD. Management of frailty: opportunities, challenges, and future directions. Lancet. 2019;394(10206): 1376–86.

23. Polidori MC, Ferrucci L, Benzing T. COVID-19 mortality as a fingerprint of biological age. Ageing Res Rev. 2021;67:101308.

24. Ellis G, Whitehead MA, Robinson D, O'Neill D, Langhorne P. Comprehensive geriatric assessment for older adults admitted to hospital: meta-analysis of randomised controlled trials. BMJ. 2011;343(oct27 1):d6553.

25. Clegg A, Young J, Iliffe S, Rikkert MO, Rockwood K. Frailty in elderly people. Lancet. 2013;381(9868):752–62.

26. Dent E, Kowal P, Hoogendijk EO. Frailty measurement in research and clinical practice: a review. Eur J Intern Med. 2016;31:3–10.

27. Fairhall N, Langron C, Sherrington C, Lord SR, Kurrle SE, Lockwood K, et al. Treating frailty—a practical guide. BMC Med. 2011;9(1):83.

28. Pilotto A, Rengo F, Marchionni N, Sancarlo D, Fontana A, Panza F, et al. Comparing the prognostic accuracy for all-cause mortality of frailty instruments: a multicentre 1-year follow-up in hospitalized older patients. PLoS One. 2012;7(1):e29090.

29. Turner G, Clegg A. Best practice guidelines for the management of frailty: a British Geriatrics Society, Age UK and Royal College of General Practitioners report. Age Ageing. 2014;43(6):744–7.

30. Fried LP, Tangen CM, Walston J, Newman AB, Hirsch C, Gottdiener J, et al. Frailty in older adults: evidence for a phenotype. J Gerontol A Biol Sci Med Sci. 2001;56(3):M146–56.

31. Rolfson DB, Majumdar SR, Tsuyuki RT, Tahir A, Rockwood K. Validity and reliability of the Edmonton Frail Scale. Age Ageing. 2006;35(5):526–9.

32. Morley JE, Malmstrom TK, Miller DK. A simple frailty questionnaire (FRAIL) predicts outcomes in middle aged African Americans. J Nutr Health Aging. 2012;16(7):601–8.

33. Rockwood K, Song X, MacKnight C, Bergman H, Hogan DB, McDowell I, et al. A global clinical measure of fitness and frailty in elderly people. CMAJ. 2005;173(5):489–95.

34. Mende A, Riegel AK, Plumer L, Olotu C, Goetz AE, Kiefmann R. Determinants of perioperative outcome in frail older patients. Dtsch Arztebl Int. 2019;116(5):73.

35. Hoogendijk EO, Afilalo J, Ensrud KE, Kowal P, Onder G, Fried LP. Frailty: implications for clinical practice and public health. Lancet. 2019;394(10206):1365–75.
36. Ellis G, Gardner M, Tsiachristas A, Langhorne P, Burke O, Harwood RH, et al. Comprehensive geriatric assessment for older adults admitted to hospital. Cochrane Database Syst Rev. 2017;9:CD006211.
37. Rakel RE. Textbook of family medicine E-book. Elsevier Health Sciences; 2007.
38. Chen P, Steinman MA. Perception of primary care physicians on the impact of comprehensive geriatric assessment: what is the next step? Isr J Health Policy Res. 2016;5(1):46.
39. Herzog A, Gaertner B, Scheidt-Nave C, Holzhausen M. We can do only what we have the means for' general practitioners' views of primary care for older people with complex health problems. BMC Fam Pract. 2015;16(1):35.
40. Press Y, Punchik B, Kagan E, Barzak A, Freud T. Which factors affect the implementation of geriatric recommendations by primary care physicians? Isr J Health Policy Res. 2017;6(1):7.
41. Stott DJ, Langhorne P, Knight PV. Multidisciplinary care for elderly people in the community. Lancet. 2008;371(9614):699–700.
42. Fischer GC. Geriatrie für die hausärztliche Praxis. Berlin Heidelberg: Springer; 2013.
43. WONCA. 2020.
44. Dagneaux I, Gilard I, De Lepeleire J. Care of elderly people by the general practitioner and the geriatrician in Belgium: a qualitative study of their relationship. J Multidiscip Healthc. 2012;5:17–25.
45. Huss A, Stuck AE, Rubenstein LZ, Egger M, Clough-Gorr KM. Multidimensional preventive home visit programs for community-dwelling older adults: a systematic review and meta-analysis of randomized controlled trials. J Gerontol A Biol Sci Med Sci. 2008;63(3):298–307.
46. Osterweil DB-SK, Beck JC. Comprehensive geriatric assessment. New York: McGraw-Hill; 2000.
47. Mazya AL, Garvin P, Ekdahl AW. Outpatient comprehensive geriatric assessment: effects on frailty and mortality in old people with multimorbidity and high health care utilization. Aging Clin Exp Res. 2019;31(4):519–25.
48. Whitaker PGP. authorGPs are much more than gatekeepers. BMJ. 2016;353:i2751.
49. Hohne A, Jedlitschka K, Hobler D, Landenberger M. General practitioner-centred health-care in Germany. The general practitioner as gatekeeper. Gesundheitswesen. 2009;71(7):414–22.
50. Forssen AS. Humour, beauty, and culture as personal health resources: experiences of elderly Swedish women. Scand J Public Health. 2007;35(3):228–34.
51. Besdine RW, Wetle TF. Opportunities to improve healthcare outcomes for elderly people and reduce re-hospitalization. Aging Clin Exp Res. 2011;23(5–6):427–30.
52. Matthiessen PF. Der Patient als aktiver Partner (2015). Publikationen des Dialogforums. 2015.
53. Clausen G, Borchelt M, Janssen C, Loos S, Mull L, Pfaff H. Patient satisfaction and geriatric care—an empirical study. Zeitschrift fur Gerontologie und Geriatrie. 2006;39(1):48–56.
54. Lauth G. Der Patient als aktiver Partner 1997.
55. Pantel J, Schröder J, Bollheimer C, Sieber C, Kruse A. Praxishandbuch Altersmedizin: Geriatrie—Gerontopsychiatrie—Gerontologie. Kohlhammer Verlag; 2014.
56. Meyer AM, Becker I, Siri G, Brinkkotter PT, Benzing T, Pilotto A, et al. The prognostic significance of geriatric syndromes and resources. Aging Clin Exp Res. 2019;32:115.
57. Meyer AP. Including prognosis evaluation in the management of older patients across different healthcare settings: the Cologne experience. Geriatr Care. 2019;5:3.
58. Mann E, Koller M, Mann C, van der Cammen T, Steurer J. Comprehensive Geriatric Assessment (CGA) in general practice: results from a pilot study in Vorarlberg. Austria BMC Geriatr. 2004;4:4.
59. Meyer AM, Siri G, Becker I, Betz T, Bödecker AW, Robertz JW, et al. The multidimensional prognostic index in general practice: one-year follow-up study. Int J Clin Pract. 2019;
60. Polidori MC. Physiology of aging as basis of complexity in aging medicine and geriatrics. In: Gu DDME, editor. Encyclopedia of gerontology and population aging. Springer International Publishing; 2021.

61. De Lepeleire J, Iliffe S, Mann E, Degryse JM. Frailty: an emerging concept for general practice. Br J Gen Pract. 2009;59(562):e177–e82.
62. Van Kan GA, Rolland Y, Bergman H, Morley JE, Kritchevsky SB, Vellas B. The I.a.N.a. task force on frailty assessment of older people in clinical practice. J Nutr Health Aging. 2008;12(1):29–37.
63. Katz S, Downs TD, Cash HR, Grotz RC. Progress in development of the index of ADL. The Gerontologist. 1970;10(1):20–30.
64. Lawton MP, Brody EM. Assessment of older people: self-maintaining and instrumental activities of daily living. The Gerontologist. 1969;9(3):179–86.
65. Clegg A, Bates C, Young J, Ryan R, Nichols L, Teale EA, et al. Development and validation of an electronic frailty index using routine primary care electronic health record data. Age Ageing. 2017;45:353.
66. Shah S, Vanclay F, Cooper B. Improving the sensitivity of the Barthel Index for stroke rehabilitation. J Clin Epidemiol. 1989;42(8):703–9.
67. Bush K. The AUDIT alcohol consumption questions (AUDIT-C): an effective brief screening test for problem drinking. Arch Intern Med. 1998;158(16):1789.
68. Heatherton TF, Kozlowski LT, Frecker RC, Fagerstrom K-O. The Fagerstrom test for nicotine dependence: a revision of the Fagerstrom tolerance questionnaire. Addiction. 1991;86(9):1119–27.
69. Lapi F, Bianchini E, Michieli R, Pasqua A, Cricelli I, Mazzaglia G, Frediani B, Prieto-Alhambra D, Brandi ML, Cricelli C. Calcif Tissue Int. 2017;100(6):550.
70. Kanis JA, Johnell O, Oden A, Johansson H, McCloskey E. FRAX™ and the assessment of fracture probability in men and women from the UK. Osteoporos Int. 2008;19(4):385–97.
71. Mathias S, Nayak US, Isaacs B. Balance in elderly patients: the "get-up and go" test. Arch Phys Med Rehabil. 1986;67(6):387–9.
72. Nih Consensus Development Panel On Osteoporosis Prevention D, Therapy. Osteoporosis prevention, diagnosis, and therapy. JAMA. 2001;285(6):785–95.
73. Berg KO, Wood-Dauphinee SL, Williams JI, Maki B. Measuring balance in the elderly: validation of an instrument. Can J Public Health. 1992;83(Suppl 2):S7–11.
74. Kobayashi M, Usuda S. Development of a clinical assessment test of 180-degree standing turn strategy (CAT-STS) and investigation of its reliability and validity. J Phys Ther Sci. 2016;28(2):646–53.
75. Shumway-Cook A, Brauer S, Woollacott M. Predicting the probability for falls in community-dwelling older adults using the Timed Up & Go Test. Phys Ther. 2000;80(9):896–903.
76. Macphee GJA, Crowther JA, McAlpine CH. A simple screening test for hearing impairment in elderly patients. Age Ageing. 1988;17(5):347–51.
77. Yesavage JA, Sheikh JI. 9/Geriatric Depression Scale (GDS). Clin Gerontol. 2008;5(1–2):165–73.
78. Hamilton M. The assessment of anxiety states by rating. Br J Med Psychol. 1959;32(1):50–5.
79. Montgomery SA, Asberg M. A new depression scale designed to be sensitive to change. Br J Psychiatry. 1979;134:382–9.
80. Kroenke K, Spitzer RL, Williams JBW. The patient health questionnaire-2. Med Care. 2003;41(11):1284–92.
81. Saller T, Maclullich AMJ, Perneczky R. The 4 AT—an instrument for delirium detection for older patients in the post-anaesthesia care unit. Anaesthesia. 2020;75(3):409–10.
82. Sands M, Dantoc B, Hartshorn A, Ryan C, Lujic S. Single question in delirium (SQiD): testing its efficacy against psychiatrist interview, the confusion assessment method and the memorial delirium assessment scale. Palliat Med. 2010;24(6):561–5.
83. Ek AC, Unosson M, Bjurulf P. The modified Norton scale and the nutritional state. Scand J Caring Sci. 1989;3(4):183–7.
84. Bliss MR, McLaren R, Exton-Smith AN. Mattresses for preventing pressure sores in geriatric patients. Mon Bull Minist Health Public Health Lab Serv. 1966;25:238–68.

85. Daniels R, van Rossum E, Beurskens A, van den Heuvel W, de Witte L. The predictive validity of three self-report screening instruments for identifying frail older people in the community. BMC Public Health. 2012;12(1):69.
86. Warnecke T, Im S, Kaiser C, Hamacher C, Oelenberg S, Dziewas R. Aspiration and dysphagia screening in acute stroke—the Gugging swallowing screen revisited. Eur J Neurol. 2017;24(4):594–601.
87. Murphy J, Mayor A, Forde E. Identifying and treating older patients with malnutrition in primary care: the MUST screening tool. Br J Gen Pract. 2018;68(672):344–5.
88. Sancarlo D, D'Onofrio G, Franceschi M, Scarcelli C, Niro V, Addante F, et al. Validation of a modified-multidimensional prognostic index (m-MPI) including the mini nutritional assessment short-form (MNA-SF) for the prediction of one-year mortality in hospitalized elderly patients. J Nutr Health Aging. 2011;15(3):169–73.
89. Sandhu SK, Lee JY. Measurement of trigeminal neuralgia pain: Penn facial pain scale. Neurosurg Clin N Am. 2016;27(3):327–36.
90. Schuler MS, Becker S, Kaspar R, Nikolaus T, Kruse A, Basler HD. Psychometric properties of the German "pain assessment in advanced dementia scale" (PAINAD-G) in nursing home residents. J Am Med Dir Assoc. 2007;8(6):388–95.
91. Hawker GA, Mian S, Kendzerska T, French M. Measures of adult pain: Visual Analog Scale for Pain (VAS pain), Numeric Rating Scale for Pain (NRS pain), McGill Pain Questionnaire (MPQ), Short-Form McGill Pain Questionnaire (SF-MPQ), Chronic Pain Grade Scale (CPGS), Short Form-36 Bodily Pain Scale (SF). Arthritis Care Res. 2011;63(S11): S240–S52.
92. Trivedi D. Cochrane review summary: Mini-Mental State Examination (MMSE) for the detection of dementia in clinically unevaluated people aged 65 and over in community and primary care populations. Prim Health Care Res Dev. 2017;18(06):527–8.
93. Borson S, Scanlan J, Brush M, Vitaliano P, Dokmak A. The mini-cog: a cognitive ?Vital signs? Measure for dementia screening in multi-lingual elderly. Int J Geriatr Psychiatry. 2000;15(11):1021–7.
94. Brodaty H, Pond D, Kemp NM, Luscombe G, Harding L, Berman K, et al. The GPCOG: a new screening test for dementia designed for general practice. J Am Geriatr Soc. 2002;50(3):530–4.
95. Hodkinson HM. Evaluation of a mental test score for assessment of mental impairment in the elderly. Age Ageing. 1972;1(4):233–8.
96. Pfeiffer E. A short portable mental status questionnaire for the assessment of organic brain deficit in elderly patients. J Am Geriatr Soc. 1975;23(10):433–41.
97. Lincoln NB, Gladman JRF. The extended activities of daily living scale: a further validation. Disabil Rehabil. 1992;14(1):41–3.
98. Landi F, Tua E, Onder G, Carrara B, Sgadari A, Rinaldi C, et al. Minimum data set for home care: a valid instrument to assess frail older people living in the community. Med Care. 2000;38(12):1184–90.
99. Haider SI, Johnell K, Thorslund M, Fastbom J. Analysis of the association between polypharmacy and socioeconomic position among elderly aged ≥77 years in Sweden. Clin Ther. 2008;30(2):419–27.
100. O'Mahony D, O'Sullivan D, Byrne S, O'Connor MN, Ryan C, Gallagher P. STOPP/START criteria for potentially inappropriate prescribing in older people: version 2. Age Ageing. 2015;44(2):213–8.
101. Lewis T. Using the NO TEARS tool for medication review. BMJ. 2004;329(7463):434.
102. American Geriatrics Society 2019 Updated AGS Beers Criteria® for potentially inappropriate medication use in older adults. J Am Geriatr Soc. 2019;67(4):674–94.
103. Samsa GP, Hanlon JT, Schmader KE, Weinberger M, Clipp EC, Uttech KM, et al. A summated score for the medication appropriateness index: development and assessment of clinimetric properties including content validity. J Clin Epidemiol. 1994;47(8):891–6.

104. Kiesel EK, Hopf YM, Drey M. An anticholinergic burden score for German prescribers: score development. BMC Geriatr. 2018;18:1.

105. Pohl-Dernick K, Meier F, Maas R, Schoffski O, Emmert M. Potentially inappropriate medication in the elderly in Germany: an economic appraisal of the PRISCUS list. BMC Health Serv Res. 2016;16(1):109.

106. Wehling M. How to use the FORTA ("fit fOR the aged") list to improve pharmacotherapy in the elderly. Drug Res (Stuttg). 2016;66(2):57–62.

107. Bridges CB, Fukuda K, Uyeki TM, Cox NJ, Singleton JA. Prevention and control of influenza. Recommendations of the advisory committee on immunization practices (ACIP). MMWR Recomm Rep. 2002;51(Rr-3):1–31.

108. Eden MM, Tompkins J, Verheijde JL. Reliability and a correlational analysis of the 6MWT, ten-meter walk test, thirty second sit to stand, and the linear analog scale of function in patients with head and neck cancer. Physiother Theory Pract. 2018;34(3):202–11.

109. Guralnik JM, Simonsick EM, Ferrucci L, Glynn RJ, Berkman LF, Blazer DG, et al. A short physical performance battery assessing lower extremity function: association with self-reported disability and prediction of mortality and nursing home admission. J Gerontol. 1994;49(2):M85–94.

110. Bennell K, Dobson F, Hinman R. Measures of physical performance assessments: Self-Paced Walk Test (SPWT), Stair Climb Test (SCT), Six-Minute Walk Test (6MWT), Chair Stand Test (CST), Timed Up & Go (TUG), Sock Test, Lift and Carry Test (LCT), and Car Task. Arthritis Care Res (Hoboken). 2011;63(Suppl 11):S350–70.

111. Malmstrom TK, Miller DK, Simonsick EM, Ferrucci L, Morley JE. SARC-F: a symptom score to predict persons with sarcopenia at risk for poor functional outcomes. J Cachexia Sarcopenia Muscle. 2016;7(1):28–36.

112. Ford AC, Bercik P, Morgan DG, Bolino C, Pintos-Sanchez MI, Moayyedi P. Validation of the Rome III criteria for the diagnosis of irritable bowel syndrome in secondary care. Gastroenterology. 2013;145(6):1262–70.e1

113. Karmakar D, Mostafa A, Abdel-Fattah M. A new validated score for detecting patient-reported success on postoperative ICIQ-SF: a novel two-stage analysis from two large RCT cohorts. Int Urogynecol J. 2017;28(1):95–100.

114. Wilson JTL, Hareendran A, Grant M, Baird T, Schulz UGR, Muir KW, et al. Improving the assessment of outcomes in stroke: use of a structured interview to assign grades on the modified Rankin scale. Stroke. 2002;33(9):2243–6.

115. Oken MM, Creech RH, Tormey DC, Horton J, Davis TE, McFadden ET, et al. Toxicity and response criteria of the eastern cooperative oncology group. Am J Clin Oncol. 1982;5(6):649–55.

116. Crooks V, Waller S, Smith T, Hahn TJ. The use of the Karnofsky performance scale in determining outcomes and risk in geriatric outpatients. J Gerontol. 1991;46(4):M139–M44.

117. Gobbens RJJ, Van Assen MALM, Luijkx KG, Wijnen-Sponselee MT, Schols JMGA. The Tilburg frailty indicator: psychometric properties. J Am Med Dir Assoc. 2010;11(5):344–55.

118. Romero-Ortuno R, Walsh CD, Lawlor BA, Kenny RA. A frailty instrument for primary care: findings from the Survey of Health, Ageing and Retirement in Europe (SHARE). BMC Geriatr. 2010;10(1):57.

119. Barkhausen T, Junius-Walker U, Hummers-Pradier E, Mueller CA, Theile G. "It's MAGIC" - development of a manageable geriatric assessment for general practice use. BMC Fam Pract. 2015;16(1):4.

120. Junius-Walker U, Krause O. Geriatrisches Assessment—Welche Tests eignen sich für die Hausarztpraxis? DMW—Deutsche Medizinische Wochenschrift. 2016;141(03):165–9.

121. Piccoliori G, Gerolimon E, Abholz HH. Geriatric assessment in general practice using a screening instrument: is it worth the effort? Results of a South Tyrol Study. 2008;37(6):647–52.

122. Garrard JW, Cox NJ, Dodds RM, Roberts HC, Sayer AA. Comprehensive geriatric assessment in primary care: a systematic review. Aging Clin Exp Res. 2019;32:197.

123. Lucchetti G, Granero AL. Use of comprehensive geriatric assessment in general practice: results from the 'Senta Pua' project in Brazil. Eur J Gen Pract. 2011;17(1):20–7.
124. Gladman JRF, Conroy SP, Ranhoff AH, Gordon AL. New horizons in the implementation and research of comprehensive geriatric assessment: knowing, doing and the 'know-do' gap. Age Ageing. 2016;45(2):194–200.

Part III

Older Patients with Geriatric Syndromes: The Role of Family Doctors

Frailty and Sarcopenia in Primary Care: Current Issues

10

Luigi Maria Bracchitta, Daniele Angioni, Stefano Celotto, and Matteo Cesari

Abstract

Frailty consists of an age-related multi-system reduction in reserve capacity that begins early and continues progressively throughout life. The term sarcopenia is used to describe the pathologic age-related loss of muscular mass and strength. These conditions, which are often overlapping, have a multifactorial origin, involving lifestyle habits, disease triggers, and age-dependent biological changes. In this chapter we will describe frailty and sarcopenia and how they are assessed and treated in primary care setting. Family physicians are often the first to experience frailty and sarcopenia because of their long-term relationship with patients. In addition, family physicians are ideally positioned to evaluate and manage frailty among their patients and family caregivers, who may be frail too. Because increased frailty and sarcopenia are associated with increased vulnerability to poor outcomes, early detection may provide an opportunity to prevent or minimize the disabling cascade and to maintain the level of dependence. The new conceptual model physical frailty and sarcopenia (PF&S) that was identified to

L. M. Bracchitta (✉)
Primary Care Department, Local Health Authority ATS Città Metropolitana di Milano, Milan, Italy
e-mail: luigimaria.bracchitta@gmail.com

D. Angioni
Eastern Piedmont, Primary Care Clinic in Novara South-District, Novara, Italy

Diagnostic Medical Sonographer in Vercelli, Vercelli, Italy

S. Celotto
Primary Care Department, Azienda Sanitaria Universitaria Friuli Centrale, Udine, Italy

M. Cesari
Geriatric Unit, Fondazione IRCCS Ca' Granda Ospedale Maggiore Policlinico, Milan, Italy

Department of Clinical Sciences and Community Health, University of Milan, Milan, Italy

© Springer Nature Switzerland AG 2022
J. Demurtas, N. Veronese (eds.), *The Role of Family Physicians in Older People Care*, Practical Issues in Geriatrics, https://doi.org/10.1007/978-3-030-78923-7_10

141

describe a pre-disability age-related condition in which functional impairment is the common core will be presented at the end of the chapter. The dissection of the inflammatory profile of people with PF&S will provide new insights into the role inflammation plays in the disabling cascade and will improve the design of treatment strategies tailored to the patient.

Keywords

Frailty · Sarcopenia · Age-dependent biological changes · Preventive interventions · Disability

Since the last decade, the need for effective solutions to the detrimental effects of age-related conditions (in particular disabilities) on our healthcare systems is growing. In a paper published in 2001, Fried et al. showed that 19.6% of US aged people had functional dependence (i.e., the loss of autonomy of the person); at the same time, this fifth of the population over the age of 70 absorbed almost half (46.3%) of health expenditure [1]. Geriatrics and gerontology researchers have thus made increasing efforts to design, develop, and implement preventive interventions against conditions that determine/drive the disabling cascade. To do so, traditional medicine, based on the idea of diseases, which are identified, diagnosed, and treated as single, independent entities, is important in rejecting. Indeed, population aging has led to a growing clinical complexity among the patients who deal with our health services on a daily basis. The integrated, individually tailored model described by Tinetti and Fried in a milestone work in geriatric medicine (the end of the disease era) needs to be acquired in routine clinical practice [2]. In particular, older persons who are frail or sarcopenic have very high rates of functional deterioration, hospitalization, and death, and recognizing these conditions early would result in interventions aimed at decreasing the disabled cascade and maintaining the level of dependence. The aim of this chapter is to provide the general practitioner with the latest updates on frailty and sarcopenia to manage these medical conditions correctly. Novel perspectives on an integrated view of frailty and sarcopenia will be presented at the end of the chapter.

10.1 Frailty

Frailty can be defined as a state of vulnerability to adverse health outcomes (including falls, hospitalizations, disability, and death), because of a decreased ability to withstand minimal endogenous or exogenous stressors compared with other persons of the same age [3]. This is due to an age-related multi-system reduction in reserve capacity that begins early and continues progressively throughout life. Thus, frailty has grown in importance during the last years, because of a need to better understand how to prevent the disabling cascade and to maintain the level of dependence [4].

Table 10.1 Frailty phenotype. Modified from Fried et al.

Weight loss	Unintentional loss of ≥4.5 kg in the past year
Weakness	Hand-grip strength in the lowest 20% quintile adjusted for sec and body mass index
Exhaustion	Poor endurance and energy, self-reported from the Center for Epidemiologic Studies Depression Scale
Slowness	Walking speed under the lowest quintile adjusted for sex and height
Low physical activity level	Lowest quintile of kilocalories of physical activity during the past week, measured by the Minnesota leisure activity scale

Despite the age-related loss of homeostatic reserve, it has to be distinguished between *chronological* and *biological age*, in order to better identify frail patients among people of the same age. To do so, many instruments and scales have been proposed, and among those, two models remain the cornerstones to better objectify frailty in the clinical and research fields, namely, the so-called frailty phenotype and the Frailty Index [5, 6].

The first, proposed by Fried in 2001 [7], looks at frailty as a syndrome characterized by the presence of signs/symptoms related to the physical dimension of the individual. In order to characterize the concept of frailty, a group of experts, using the data contained in the Cardiovascular Health Study, identified five criteria (*fatigue*, a concept that expresses a person's psychomotor exhaustion; muscle weakness, which, unlike *fatigue*, captures the pure reduction of muscle strength; sedentary behavior, slow gait speed, involuntary weight loss; Table 10.1).

Subsequently, an indication was given to define as "frail" the person who presented three or more criteria, pre-frail the one who had one or two, and robust the one who did not present any. However, on the clinical-operative setting, frailty is not an "all or nothing" condition, but a continuum between different grades of vulnerability to adverse events, expression of a dynamic, continuous process, with a natural tendency to progression/deterioration if not identified early and effectively counteracted. As a matter of fact, many clinical decisions require greater precision than a nonfrail-frail status, and transitions across grades of frailty are common [8].

The second model, the Frailty Index proposed by Mitnitski and Rockwood (again in 2001) [9], makes use of a completely different model. The researchers, in this case, started from the assumption that the aging of the individual is linked to the accumulation of age-related deficits, which can be signs, symptoms, diseases, disabilities, and alterations of biological parameters. According to this model, counting how many deficits have accumulated in an organism provides an objective estimate of its state of frailty. In the operationalization of the Frailty Index (which, in the first validation work, benefited from the Canadian Study of Health and Aging database), the ratio between the number of deficits presented by the person and the number of deficits considered is taken into account. The result (a variable that can range from 0, absence of deficit, to 1, presence of all deficits) represents an estimate of the biological state of the person and a highly predictive parameter of adverse events. Many simplified versions of the Frailty Index exist, evaluating the presence of fewer variables. It is, in fact, possible to obtain a robust instrument as soon as 30 deficits are considered [10], although 20-item Frailty Index has also been used in the

Table 10.2 For each deficit a point is given if present and zero if absent. The result of the Frailty Index is given by the total of the present deficits divided by the number of deficits considered (40 in this case). Modified from Searle et al.

List of 40 variables included in the frailty index	
Help bathing	
Help dressing	Feel everything is an effort
Help getting in/out of chair	Feel depressed
Help walking around house	Feel happy
Help eating	Feel lonely
Help grooming	Have trouble getting going
Help using toilet	High blood pressure
Help up/down stairs	Heart attack
Help lifting 5 kg	Chronic heart failure
Help shopping	Stroke
Help with housework	Cancer
Help with meal preparation	Diabetes
Help taking medication	Arthritis
Help with finances	Chronic lung disease
Lost more than 5 kg in last year	MMSE
Self-rating of health	Peak flow
How health has changed in last year	Shoulder strength
Stayed at bed at least half the day due to health (in last month)	BMI
	Grip strength
Cut down on usual activity (in last month)	
Walk outside	Usual pace
	Rapid pace

literature. For instance, in the case of using 40 variables (Table 10.2), each variable would count for 0.025 (i.e., 1/40). A person with half of the deficits considered (i.e., 20 out of 40) will have a Frailty Index of 0.5 (i.e., 20/40), while another person which has four deficits will have a Frailty Index of 0.1 (i.e., 4/40).

It is extremely rare to have a Frailty Index value above 0.7, and beyond this threshold, the accumulation of deficits would become incompatible with life. This also means that the Frailty Index model gives the same specific weight to the different deficits that have been evaluated, without adequately considering the different clinical relevance of each variable. Nevertheless, the Frailty Index model is based on an arithmetic-quantitative and not a qualitative approach, and therefore, it is extremely unlikely that a "heavy" clinical variable (e.g., feeding dependence) exists in isolation, but it is more likely that it is associated with a cloud of secondary deficits, thus contributing to the increase of the Frailty Index. Furthermore, the Frailty Index often presents an exponential associative pattern with age, meaning that the accumulation of deficits arises exponentially with age increase [10].

There are many other tools to measure frailty, and most of these are based on or are inspired by the two models described above [5]. The *Clinical Frailty Scale* is a visual analogue scale in which some stylized figures of the patient help to estimate the level of frailty. Another tool is based on the acronym *FRAIL*, which is composed by the initials of the words *fatigue*, resistance impairment, aerobic impairment, illnesses, and low physical activity; it generates a score (from 0 to 5) predictive of adverse events. *PRISMA-7* is a questionnaire originally developed for the identification of frail people living at home. The *Edmonton Frail Scale* has been suggested to assess frailty in elective surgical settings. Furthermore, *physical performance measurements* (such as walking speed, Timed Up and Go test, Short Physical Performance Battery) can provide a measure of the individual's state of frailty through the objective quantification of his movement capacity [11, 12]. The *Short Physical Performance Battery (SPPB)* evaluates balance, gait, strength, and endurance by examining an individual's ability to stand with the feet together in side-by-side, semi-tandem, and tandem positions, time to walk 8 ft., and time to rise from a chair and return to the seated position five times. *Usual gait speed* (over a 6-m course) is part of the SPPB, but it can also be used as a single parameter for clinical practice and research, and it is a predictor of adverse health events (severe mobility limitation, mortality). The *timed get-up-and-go (TGUG)* test measures the time needed to complete a series of functionally important tasks, and it serves as an assessment of dynamic balance. The *400-m walk test* predicts mortality and assesses walking ability and endurance. For this test, participants are asked to complete 20 laps of 20 m, each lap as fast as possible, and are allowed up to two rest stops during the test.

Nevertheless, several studies have shown that the agreement between the instruments is rather modest, meaning that, when the instrument changes, different types of people at risk (and, therefore, to be treated) will be obtained. This, of course, is a reason for discussion and greatly impacts with the standardization of clinical practice and research. In the absence of a gold standard instrument for the operationalization of frailty, it becomes fundamental to pay particular attention to the choice of the instrument. In this sense, the Fit for Frailty document produced by the British Geriatric Society in 2014 is interesting to guide the management of frailty in aged subjects living in the community [13]. The document does not offer a single screening tool, and what is important according to the document is the introduction of the frail subject into an intervention system adapted to his needs. This alternative model of intervention is based on comprehensive geriatric assessment and on a multidisciplinary approach, promoting an integrated care model. The model proposed here encourages interactions between the different professional figures that will interface to understand the critical issues of the aged subject and develop a shared, integrated, and multidimensional intervention plan. The reduced homeostasis (or frailty) of the individual becomes a reason to personalize the subsequent intervention on the basis of its resources, needs, and values. Thus, the general concept of frailty goes beyond physical factors to encompass psychological and social dimensions as well, including cognitive status, social support, and other environmental factors.

10.2   Sarcopenia

The term "sarcopenia" (Greek "sarx" or flesh + "penia" or loss) has been introduced by Irwin Rosenberg in the 1990s to describe the pathologic age-related loss of muscular mass and strength [14]. This condition has a multifactorial origin, involving lifestyle habits, disease triggers, and age-dependent biological changes (e.g., chronic inflammation, mitochondrial abnormalities, loss of neuromuscular junctions, reduced satellite cell numbers, hormonal alterations). In a recent review, association between sarcopenia and increased risk of death, disability, and falls presented a highly suggestive evidence, indicating the need of assessing this condition in daily practice [15]. The condition has high personal, social, and economic burdens when untreated. However, the complexity of determining what variables to measure, how to measure them, what cut-off points best guide diagnosis and treatment, and how to best evaluate effects of therapeutic interventions have made sarcopenia for a long time a neglected and undertreated condition [16].

Sarcopenia has long been associated with aging and older people, but the development of sarcopenia is now recognized to begin earlier in life [17]. Sarcopenia can be considered as "primary" (or age-related) or "secondary" depending on whether causal factors other than (or in addition to) aging are evident or not (Fig. 10.1) [18].

While genetic and lifestyle factors can accelerate muscle weakening and progression to functional impairment and disability, these processes appear to be slowed or reversed by interventions including nutrition and exercise training [19]. The relationship between age-related muscle mass reduction and strength is often independent of body mass. It is now clear that changes in muscle composition are also important, and muscle fat infiltration reduces muscle quality and work performance in sarcopenic obese individuals as well as age-related weight loss in sarcopenic cachectic individuals [20]. The prevalence of sarcopenia reaches approximately 10% in older adults, but variations in estimates exist due to different criteria used to diagnose sarcopenia. In this regard, among the numerous proposals, the work that more than others has become more widespread in the literature is probably the one from the European Working Group on Sarcopenia in Older People (EWSGOP), published in 2010 and recently updated (2019), which identifies sarcopenia as a geriatric syndrome [18]. This is due to the prevalence of sarcopenia in older populations, and it has multiple contributing factors such as a less than optimal diet, sedentary lifestyle, chronic diseases, and some drug treatments. In addition, the EWSGOP places greater emphasis on strength rather than quantity of muscle.

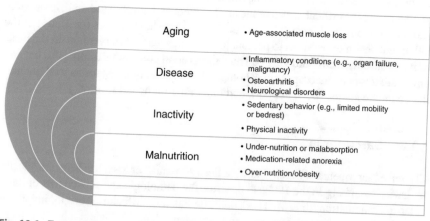

Fig. 10.1 Factors that cause and worsen sarcopenia are categorized as primary (aging) and secondary (disease, inactivity, and poor nutrition). With permission, from A. J. Cruz-Jentoft et al.

Muscle strength is currently the most reliable measure of muscle function, and if low muscle strength is detected, sarcopenia is likely. The choice is likely to be an attempt to facilitate the implementation and coding of sarcopenia in the clinical setting (which also officially has its own code [M62.68] in the ICD-10-CM since 2017). It has recently been shown that muscle strength is also a stronger prognostic factor for adverse events in addition to impacting the quality of life of the person. The measurement of muscle strength is relatively simple and requires only a modern, commercial isokinetic dynamometer compared to the more complicated muscle quantification. Indeed, nuclear magnetic resonance imaging (MRI) and computed tomography (CT) scan (with a cut between the large trochanter's medial margin and the leg's intercondylar fossa) are the most accurate tools for assessing muscle mass. These very specific imaging devices can distinguish fat from other body soft tissues, but at some locations, high cost, limited access to facilities, and radiation exposure concerns restrict the use of these whole-body imaging methods in daily clinical practice. Instruments such as DXA (dual-energy X-ray absorptiometry) and BIA (bioimpedance analysis) are likely to be easier to adopt in the clinical setting and provide an approximate measurement of body muscle mass. Recently, the use of ultrasound in clinical practice has been extended to support sarcopenia diagnosis in older adults as it has been shown to have sufficient accuracy to measure muscle mass compared to DXA, MRI, and CT [21]. In fact, ultrasound has the advantage of being able to measure both the quantity and quality of the muscles. In addition to using a dynamometer, the *chair stand test*, which requires both strength and endurance, can evaluate muscle strength. The chair stand test measures the amount of time it takes for a patient to rise five times from a seated position without using his or her arms and can therefore be used as a proxy for the strength of the muscles of the legs (quadriceps). EWGSOP proposes a conceptual staging as "presarcopenia," "sarcopenia," and "severe sarcopenia." The stage of "presarcopenia" is characterized by low muscle mass without affecting muscle strength or performance. Only techniques that accurately measure muscle mass can define this level. Low muscle mass, plus low muscle strength or low physical performance, characterizes the "sarcopenia" phase. "Severe sarcopenia" is the stage where all three definition criteria (low muscle mass, low muscle strength, and low physical performance) are met. As an outcome variable, physical performance can be used to categorize the severity of sarcopenia, and it can be evaluated by *physical performance measurements*. In particular, gait speed (i.e., the *4-m usual walking speed test*) has been shown to predict adverse outcomes related to sarcopenia, and it is widely used in practice as it is considered a fast and highly reliable sarcopenia test. EWGSOP recommends a single cut-off speed of ≤ 0.8 m/s as an indicator of severe sarcopenia. Case-finding can begin in clinical practice when a patient reports sarcopenia symptoms or signs (i.e., falling, feeling weak, slow walking speed, difficulty rising from a chair, or weight loss). Further sarcopenia testing is recommended in such cases. EWGSOP suggests using the SARC-F, a 5-item questionnaire, as a means of obtaining patients' self-reports on symptoms indicative of sarcopenia (Table 10.3) [22, 23]. Responses are based on the perception of the patient's strength limitations, walking ability, rising from a chair, climbing stairs, and fall experiences. To predict low muscle strength,

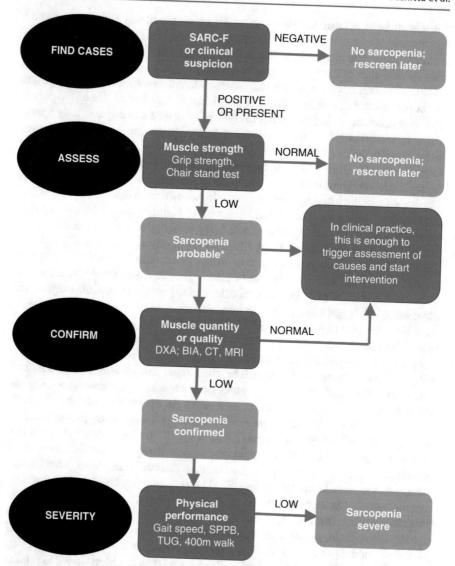

Fig. 10.2 EWGSOP2 algorithm for case-finding, making a diagnosis and quantifying severity in practice. The steps of the pathway are represented as find-assess-confirm-severity or F-A-C-S. *Consider other reasons for low muscle strength (e.g., depression, stroke, balance disorders, peripheral vascular disorders). With permission, from A. J. Cruz-Jentoft et al.

SARC-F has a low to moderate sensitivity and a very high specificity. SARC-F is an inexpensive and convenient way to introduce sarcopenia screening, evaluation, and treatment into clinical practice and can be used effectively in community healthcare and other medical settings. The Ishii screening test is another method that uses an equation-derived score based on three variables – age, grip strength, and calf

Table 10.3 SARC-F screen for sarcopenia. Modified from Malmstrom TK et al.

Component	Question	Scoring
Strength	How much difficulty do you have in lifting and carrying 5 kg	None = 0 Some = 1 A lot or unable = 2
Assistance in walking	How much difficulty do you have walking across a room?	None = 0 Some = 1 A lot, use aids, or unable = 2
Rise from a chair	How much difficulty do you have transferring from a chair or bed?	None = 0 Some = 1 A lot or unable without help = 2
Climb stairs	How much difficulty do you have climbing a flight of 10 stairs?	None = 0 Some = 1 A lot or unable = 2
Falls	How many times have you fallen in the past year?	None = 0 1–3 falls = 1 4 or more falls = 2

circumference – to estimate the likelihood of sarcopenia [24]. Finally, EWGSOP updated its algorithm for sarcopenia case-finding, diagnosis, and severity determination (Fig. 10.2).

Another important proposal comes from the Foundation for the National Institutes of Health Biomarkers Consortium—Sarcopenia Project (FNIH) [25]. By analyzing data from nine international cohort studies (more than 26,000 participants), the researchers provided the mass and muscle strength measurements that were best able to predict the onset of functional limitations. Among the many measurements tested, the *handgrip strength* and the *appendicular lean mass* were the best parameters to qualify and quantify the muscle; for these variables, precise sex-specific cut-points were calculated (Table 10.4).

10.3 Physical Frailty and Sarcopenia (PF&S): A New Conceptual Model

Despite sarcopenia and frailty have been studied in parallel and separately since the beginning, the common aspects between the two conditions have been recently highlighted in order to identify the biological (muscle-specific) substrate of a phenotypic manifestation of clinical relevance. In fact, frailty and sarcopenia are often overlapping conditions; most frail older people have sarcopenia, and some older people with sarcopenia are frail as well (Fig. 10.3) [26]. Although physical frailty (PF) is only part of the frailty spectrum, it is the most widely used and presents a pathophysiological background that is well characterized. In addition, it has been shown that the PF condition depicted by the frailty phenotype predicts major negative health-related outcomes. On this basis, the physical frailty and sarcopenia (PF&S) construct was identified to describe a pre-disability age-related condition in

Table 10.4 Definition of low muscle mass and poor muscle function, according to FNIH recommendations. ALM, appendicular lean mass; BMI, body mass index

Parameter		
Muscle weakness	**Men**	**Women**
Hand grip strength	<26 kg	<16 kg
BMI-adjusted hand grip strength (alternate)	<1.0 kg	<0.56 kg
Low muscle mass	**Men**	**Women**
BMI-adjusted ALM (recommended)	<0.789	<0.56
ALM (alternate)	<19.75 kg	<15.02 kg

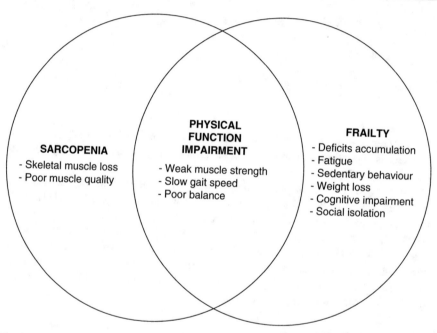

Fig. 10.3 Relationship among sarcopenia, frailty, and physical function impairment. From Cesari et al. (2014)

which functional impairment is the common core [27]. According to Cesari et al. [26], both conditions are (1) highly prevalent in the old age, (2) related to adverse health events, (3) potentially reversible, and (4) relatively easy to implement in clinical practice. Disability secondary prevention can therefore be accomplished by acting in this preclinical phase of the disease.

A frequently encountered element in PF&S is the presence of a chronic, low-grade inflammation, which is a hallmark of aging and is associated with changes in body composition and declining physical function. Dysregulation of the cytokine network is acknowledged as a major driver of aging and related conditions. Thus, the circulating inflammatory profile that characterizes older people with PF&S has been recently described for the first time [28]. In particular, the "core" inflammatory signature of PF&S was defined by higher levels of P-selectin, C-reactive protein (CRP), and interferon γ-induced protein 10 and a decrease in levels of myeloperoxidase (MPO), interleukin (IL) 8, monocyte chemoattractant protein 1 (MCP-1), macrophage inflammatory protein 1-α, and platelet-derived growth factor (PDGF) BB. In addition, PF&S has been characterized by gender-specific inflammatory fingerprints, identifying peculiar patterns of relationships for men and women. The dissection of the inflammatory profile of people with PF&S will provide new insights into the role inflammation plays in the disabled cascade and will improve the design of treatment strategies tailored to the patient. Other possible biomarkers might include neuromuscular junction markers, muscle protein turnover, behavior-mediated pathways, redox-related factors, hormones, or other anabolic factors [29]. Developing a panel of biomarkers could provide a means of stratifying sarcopenia and frailty risk, facilitating the identification of a worsening condition, and monitoring the effectiveness of treatment.

10.4 The Role of the General Practitioner in Managing Frailty and Sarcopenia

Frailty is recognized as a multidimensional phenomenon with complex interrelated factors that affect a person's physiological equilibrium in the physical, psychological, social, and environmental domains [3–4]. Recognition of frailty is important because of its increasing prevalence and its most noticeable clinical variation in primary care. Family physicians are often the first to experience frailty because of their long-term relationship with patients. In addition, family physicians are ideally positioned to evaluate and manage frailty among their patients and family caregivers, who may be frail too [30]. Because increased frailty is associated with increased vulnerability to poor outcomes, early detection may provide an opportunity to prevent or minimize subsequent destabilization of the health. Interventions could then be aimed at those identified as frail, in order to improve adverse outcomes [31]. For example, this has been shown with high-intensity exercise training, which has been shown to increase frailty rates and subsequent survival [32]. Frailty recognition can also assist healthcare providers in providing adequate advice to patients and family members on the risks associated with some medical interventions. Clinicians may also have the opportunity to better handle coexisting conditions underlying frailty and minimize stressors that may precipitate adverse outcomes, with the goal of preventing potentially avoidable emergency department visits and hospitalizations, caregiver distress, premature institutionalization, and early mortality.

Sarcopenia is increasingly recognized as a correlate of aging and is associated with increased probability of adverse outcomes including falls, fractures, frailty, and mortality [15]. In clinical trials several tools were recommended to evaluate muscle mass, muscle strength, and physical performance. While in investigational settings these tools have proven to be accurate and reliable, many are not easily applied to everyday practice [16]. Healthcare providers, particularly in primary care, should consider an assessment of sarcopenia in individuals at increased risk using simple, rapid, and inexpensive tools [33]. Sarcopenia treatment should be predominantly patient-centered and include integrating resistance- and endurance-based exercise programs with or without dietary interventions [34]. The ability to prevent further decline and reduce adverse outcomes with proactive interventions highlights the importance of early detection and intervention for frailty and sarcopenia.

10.5 To Sum up

- *Frailty* consists of an age-related multi-system reduction in reserve capacity that begins early and continues progressively throughout life.
- Despite many instruments and scales have been proposed, two models remain the cornerstones to better objectify frailty in the clinical and research fields, namely, the *frailty phenotype* and the Frailty Index. The first looks at frailty as a syndrome characterized by the presence of signs/symptoms related to the physical dimension of the individual, while the second provides an objective estimate of an individual's state of frailty by counting how many deficits have accumulated.
- The term *sarcopenia* is used to describe the pathologic age-related loss of muscular mass and strength. This condition has a multifactorial origin, involving lifestyle habits, disease triggers, and age-dependent biological changes.
- Several tools were recommended to evaluate muscle mass, muscle strength, and physical performance. While many tools can only be applied in investigational settings, others can easily be used in everyday practice.
- Both frailty and sarcopenia, which are often overlapping conditions, have been associated with an increased risk of disability, death, and hospitalizations, indicating the need of assessing these conditions in daily practice.

References

1. Fried TR, Bradley EH, Williams CS, Tinetti ME. Functional disability and health care expenditures for older persons. Arch Intern Med. 2001.
2. Tinetti ME, Fried T. The end of the disease era. Am J Med. 2004.
3. Clegg A, Young J, Iliffe S, Rikkert MO, Rockwood K. Frailty in elderly people. Lancet. 2013;381:752–62.
4. Cesari M, Calvani R, Marzetti E. Frailty in older persons. Clin Geriatr Med. 2017;33:293–303.
5. Buta BJ, Walston JD, Godino JG, Park M, Kalyani RR, Xue QL, et al. Frailty assessment instruments: systematic characterization of the uses and contexts of highly-cited instruments. Ageing Res Rev. 2016.
6. Cesari M, Gambassi G, Abellan van Kan G, Vellas B. The frailty phenotype and the frailty index: different instruments for different purposes. Age Ageing. 2014;43:10–2.
7. Fried LP, Tangen CM, Walston J, Newman AB, Hirsch C, Gottdiener J, et al. Frailty in older adults: evidence for a phenotype. J Gerontol Ser A Biol Sci Med Sci. 2001;56:M146–57.
8. Cesari M, Pérez-Zepeda MU, Marzetti E. Frailty and multimorbidity: different ways of thinking about geriatrics. J Am Med Dir Assoc. 2017;18:361–4.

9. Mitnitski AB, Mogilner AJ, Rockwood K. Accumulation of deficits as a proxy measure of aging. Sci World J. 2001;1:323–36.
10. Searle SD, Mitnitski A, Gahbauer EA, Gill TM, Rockwood K. A standard procedure for creating a frailty index. BMC Geriatr. 2008.
11. Evans WJ, Bhasin S, Cress E, Espeland MA, Ferrucci L, Fried LP, et al. Functional outcomes for clinical trials in frail older persons: time to be moving. J Gerontol—Ser A Biol Sci Med Sci. 2008.
12. Beaudart C, Rolland Y, Cruz-Jentoft AJ, Bauer JM, Sieber C, Cooper C, et al. Assessment of muscle function and physical performance in daily clinical practice. Calcif Tissue Int. 2019;105:1–14.
13. British Geriatric society. Fit for frailty- consensus best practice guidance for the care of older people living in community and outpatient settings. Br Geriatr Soc. 2014.
14. Rosenberg IH. Summary comments: epidemiological and methodological problems in determining nutritional status of older persons. Am J Clin Nutr. 1989.
15. Veronese N, Demurtas J, Soysal P, Smith L, Torbahn G, Schoene D, et al. Sarcopenia and health-related outcomes: an umbrella review of observational studies. Eur Geriatr Med. 2019.
16. Han A, Bokshan S, Marcaccio S, DePasse J, Daniels A. Diagnostic criteria and clinical outcomes in sarcopenia research: a literature review. J Clin Med. 2018.
17. Sayer AA, Syddall H, Martin H, Patel H, Baylis D, Cooper C. The developmental origins of sarcopenia. J Nutr Heal Aging. 2008.
18. Cruz-Jentoft AJ, Bahat G, Bauer J, Boirie Y, Bruyère O, Cederholm T, et al. Sarcopenia: revised European consensus on definition and diagnosis. Age Ageing. 2019;48:16–31.
19. Bloom I, Shand C, Cooper C, Robinson S, Baird J. Diet quality and sarcopenia in older adults: a systematic review. Nutrients. 2018.
20. Hubbard RE, Lang IA, Llewellyn DJ, Rockwood K. Frailty, body mass index, and abdominal obesity in older people. J Gerontol—Ser A Biol Sci Med Sci. 2010.
21. Perkisas S, Baudry S, Bauer J, Beckwée D, De Cock AM, Hobbelen H, et al. Application of ultrasound for muscle assessment in sarcopenia: towards standardized measurements. Eur Geriatr Med. 2018.
22. Malmstrom TK, Miller DK, Simonsick EM, Ferrucci L, Morley JE. SARC-F: a symptom score to predict persons with sarcopenia at risk for poor functional outcomes. J Cachexia Sarcopenia Muscle. 2016.
23. Malmstrom TK, Morley JE. SARC-F: A simple questionnaire to rapidly diagnose sarcopenia. J Am Med Dir Assoc. 2013.
24. Ishii S, Tanaka T, Shibasaki K, Ouchi Y, Kikutani T, Higashiguchi T, et al. Development of a simple screening test for sarcopenia in older adults. Geriatr Gerontol Int. 2014.
25. Studenski SA, Peters KW, Alley DE, Cawthon PM, McLean RR, Harris TB, et al. The FNIH sarcopenia project: rationale, study description, conference recommendations, and final estimates. J Gerontol Ser A. 2014;69:547–58.
26. Cesari M, Landi F, Vellas B, Bernabei R, Marzetti E. Sarcopenia and physical frailty: two sides of the same coin. Front Aging Neurosci. 2014.
27. Bernabei R, Martone AM, Vetrano DL, Calvani R, Landi F, Marzetti E. Frailty, physical frailty, sarcopenia: a new conceptual model. Stud Health Technol Inform. 2014.
28. Marzetti E, Picca A, Marini F, Biancolillo A, Coelho-Junior HJ, Gervasoni J, et al. Inflammatory signatures in older persons with physical frailty and sarcopenia: the frailty "cytokinome" at its core. Exp Gerontol. 2019;122:129–38.
29. Curcio F, Ferro G, Basile C, Liguori I, Parrella P, Pirozzi F, et al. Biomarkers in sarcopenia: a multifactorial approach. Exp Gerontol. 2016.
30. Lee L, Patel T, Hillier LM, Maulkhan N, Slonim K, Costa A. Identifying frailty in primary care: a systematic review. Geriatr Gerontol Int. 2017.
31. Lee L, Heckman G, Molnar FJ. Frailty: identifying elderly patients at high risk of poor outcomes. Can Fam Physician. 2015;61:227.

32. Theou O, Stathokostas L, Roland KP, Jakobi JM, Patterson C, Vandervoort AA, et al. The effectiveness of exercise interventions for the management of frailty: a systematic review. J Aging Res. 2011.

33. Beaudart C, McCloskey E, Bruyère O, Cesari M, Rolland Y, Rizzoli R, et al. Sarcopenia in daily practice: assessment and management. BMC Geriatr. 2016.

34. Peterson MD, Sen A, Gordon PM. Influence of resistance exercise on lean body mass in aging adults: a meta-analysis. Med Sci Sports Exerc. 2011.

Approach the Older Patients with Cognitive Impairment in Primary Care

11

Neziha Ulusoylar, Fatma Sena Dost, Pinar Soysal, and Ahmet Turan Isik

Abstract

Forgetfulness has many reasons and even more causes. Advancing age has relative increased risks. Although loss of memory is often a prime reason of dementia, forgetfulness, and cognitive impairment, these are not synonymous terms. Cognitive impairment that includes memory, orientation, paying attention, using language, visio-spatialability, and psychomotor speed is used to describe any impairment of intellectual abilities. They include inadequacy in social or occupational activities. Mild cognitive impairment (MCI) that estimates from 3% to 42% in adults aged 65 years or older is different from dementia. In MCI cases the cognitive impairment is not severe enough to interfere with instrumental activities of daily life. MCI is important because it constitutes a high-risk group for dementia. Dementia is decline of cognition that is significant enough to interfere with independent daily functioning. But it should be noted that some diseases can lead to dementia-like conditions. Therefore, since the prime purpose of the case evaluation is to conclude the treatable causes, detailed anamnesis, family interview, comprehensive physical examination, and appropriate blood tests as well as additional cognitive screening tests should be performed. There are several cognitive screening tools to be used in the primary care setting, and the appropriate one should be selected according to the patient's literacy and educational level. Finally, it is crucial that a patient with cognitive complaints should

N. Ulusoylar · F. S. Dost · A. T. Isik (✉)
Department of Geriatric Medicine, Faculty of Medicine, Dokuz Eylul University, Izmir, Turkey
e-mail: atisik@yahoo.com

P. Soysal
Department of Geriatric Medicine, Faculty of Medicine, Bezmialem Vakif University, Istanbul, Turkey

© Springer Nature Switzerland AG 2022
J. Demurtas, N. Veronese (eds.), *The Role of Family Physicians in Older People Care*, Practical Issues in Geriatrics, https://doi.org/10.1007/978-3-030-78923-7_11

be referred to the reference memory center for differential diagnosis, after initial appropriate clinical and biochemical evaluations and screening for cognitive impairment in the elderly.

Keywords

Forgetfulness · Cognitive impairment · Primary care setting · Older adults

Aging, although defined as age-related structural changes in the brain, in behaviors, and in cognitive functions, is generally seen as a period of time in human life without specific dysfunction [1, 2]. It is accepted as one of the advanced stages of the natural process that starts with birth and continues with childhood and is seen as a natural process that is reached sooner or later as long as the organism is alive. The process applies to all organs and functions as well as to the brain and cognitive functions. The brain is the earliest organ to begin aging compared to other organs [3].

The synapse rate of ten million neurons present in developmental birth rises in time, and myelinization also increases. Therefore, the size of the brain is 4–5 times higher than in adults. However, time does not only affect the development of the brain in a positive way. There is a 5% loss in brain weight every 10 years after the age of 40 [4, 5]. There is a decrease in the size and volume of the aging brain, an expansion of the ventricles, and an increase in the amount of intracranial space. There is also an increase in cerebrospinal fluid (CSF). Meanwhile, the sulcus expands, and the gyrus loses its bombing. These are accompanied by microscopic, biochemical, and electrophysiological changes [6]. It has been reported that the brain of an older person (80–90 years) has less neurons than younger adult brains (20–30 years) and that cortex volumes, synapse, and receptor numbers as well as cortical metabolic rate and blood flow are lower [3]. These changes are also reflected in cognitive functions. The general approach is that some cognitive functions diminish with age, while others are protected. Older people often complain about the decrease in cognitive skills, especially in the memory area. A decrease in memory functions is expected with advancing age, in which period there is also a decrease in other cognitive habits, including slowdown in response, prolonged complex reaction time, reduced channel capacity, and reduced creativity [7]. Cognitive processes, which are also considered as crystalline intelligence or wisdom, including word production, historical knowledge, and previously acquired skills, are preserved until very old ages. With advancing age, the number of cognitively normal older adults gradually decreases. Cognitive impairment develops in approximately half of the cases, and dementia is detected in 20% of patients over 85 years of age. Although 1/3 of the patients over 90–100 years of age are under normal expectations, 1/3 of them are mildly moderate, and 1/3 of them have severe dementia [8, 9].

Memory changes are features of normal aging. However, some components of the memory are resistant to change, while others vary significantly with age. Ordinary simple forgetfulness is taken more seriously by older adults than young people, because it is perceived as harbingers (predictors) of dementia [9, 10]. The deterioration of intellectual abilities that is quite common in older people was thought to be inevitable for a long time, although it is one of the changes observed in the normal aging process [11]. While some older adults have enough memory performance to make young people jealous, the advancing age generally affects memory functions in various aspects. It has been shown in recent studies that it is difficult even for older patients, who usually do not have any significant disease, to learn new information. When older adults are given the chance to repeat enough to learn new information, they remember a significant portion of the data, but both the slowdown in learning curves and the low amount of knowledge learned are important. It has been reported that individuals with subjective memory complaints cannot find the things in the place where they search, take frequent notes not to forget, cannot find the right word, and have general forgetfulness [12].

Although the amount of post-learning delayed recall is decreased in older people, the more remarkable is the decrease in those cases' learning speed. In the delayed memory tests performed within 15–60 min of the onset, it should be kept in mind that although the amount of recall is reduced due to aging, a significant portion of the data learned at the beginning is usually remembered by older adults. In a study using the story recall scale in cases over 85 years of age, it was found that 90% of them remember at least 50% of it [12–14] Even though this may be test-specific, the aging process has a small but significant negative effect on delayed learning, especially in visual memory tests, which may be due to a discrepancy in learning style caused by differences between generations. Indeed, the use of memory strategies reduces the negative effects of aging on free recall. In addition, long-term (remote) memory, such as sensory memory, is not affected by age. Moreover, it should be noted that although aging is accompanied by many diseases that cause physical limitations, procedural memory is preserved by healthy aging. In addition, semantic memory, including general vocabulary and general information about the world, is preserved up to advanced ages [13, 14].

Semantic skills include the ability to reorganize and name long-term preserved knowledge. There is a regular increase in vocabulary during the middle adulthood, which typically remains constant in later years. However, the most common complaint in older adults is the phenomenon "I know it very well, but I cannot remember now," in which they make extreme efforts to find words spontaneously. However, unlike dysnomia, which is often associated with dementia, such changes appear as a result of the difficulties in evaluating rather than storing the data, and therefore, when clues are given, a significant improvement occurs. Verbal fluency, which means the rate at which a person can produce a word spontaneously in relation to a single phonetic and semantic category, varies slightly with age. While phonetic fluency (can you tell me all the words starting with "F" you know/remember in a minute?) remains generally stable, many research findings support a reduction in semantic fluency (can you tell me all the animal names you remember in a minute?). Therefore, older individuals rely on structural vocabulary more than the meaning of the word [15].

Table 11.1 Etiology of correctable and neurodegenerative dementia

Correctable	Neurodegenerative
Depression	Alzheimer's disease
Delirium	Frontotemporal dementia
Endocrine disorders	Dementia with Lewy body
Vitamin deficiency (vitB12, VitD)	Parkinson disease
Organ dysfunction	Multisystem atrophy
İnfections (HIV, JC virus, tuberculosis, etc.)	Corticobasal degeneration
Normal pressure hydrocephalus	Progressive supranuclear palsy
Head trauma and diffuse brain damage	Huntington's disease

In the absence of any disease, cognitive changes can be compensated for by using clues (notes, appointment registrations) and other strategies, so that overall memory performance can be normalized [16]. Researchers have reported that cognitive changes associated with a truly healthy aging do not cause any decrease in functionality, nor do they lead to any significant change in daily functionality. None of the cognitive functional changes considered normal in healthy aging is excessive and does not prevent the people from continuing their normal daily life in a cognitive way. Regardless of memory complaints, a relative's assertion that the patient can easily do the usual work helps to identify the older person without dementia. Although a moderate decline in memory functions is normally observed with advancing age, this can be compensated for, as executive functions remain intact, and the person can take the necessary steps to plan his/her tasks and to put them into action [17]. In 1958 the term "well-intentioned forgetfulness" was first used to describe the decline in memory functions that occur due to advancing age [18]. It seems to have arisen as a result of evaluation problems rather than the storage of the data, and therefore there is a significant improvement when clues are given. Mild cognitive impairment (MCI), which has been developed to represent cognitive dysfunction between normal aging and dementia in the last 20 years, is a clinical condition in which measurable cognitive impairment exists but basic daily life activities are preserved. The MCI table, by which daily living activities are also affected, progresses to dementia between 8% and 15% per year. Therefore, the diagnosis and treatment management is of great importance [19]. As for the dementia clinic, the fact that progressive decrease in cognitive functions gradually deteriorates daily life activities and increases caregiver dependence is one of the main features of the disease. The most common cause of dementia occurring in 5–10% over the age of 65 years is the dementia of Alzheimer's disease accompanied by degenerative process [4, 5]. There are also other types of dementia that are neurodegenerative and nondegenerative (Table 11.1) [20].

11.1 Anamnesis

As usual, a detailed anamnesis is the most important step in patients who present with "forgetfulness." When deepening the anamnesis, the factors that may cause cognitive effects should be questioned. These include mainly the chemical or herbal agents used by the patient, the presence of trauma leading to consciousness turbidity, frequency of falls, urinary incontinence, constipation, pain, sleep disturbances, depression, visual or auditory deficiencies, the presence of infection, and vitamin deficiencies. Although dementia is a disease evaluated according to diagnostic criteria, physical, cognitive health, and daily living activities of the older people are affected by many variables. It is not possible to reach a healthy diagnosis without excluding the role of these factors in patients with a large number of concomitant diseases and using a large number of drugs. Therefore, evaluation of the patient should be carried out meticulously in all aspects. As is the case here, the most important part in the diagnosis is getting the right anamnesis. During the anamnesis to evaluate forgetfulness, the patient should be asked about changes in cognitive processes, sleep problems, behavior patterns, and daily life activity influences. This assessment should be supported by a relative who spends time with the patient and observes him/her well. If the patient has movement problems, the medication used and the timing of the complaints should be questioned in detail. Another important part is to provide a comprehensive history of memory complaints, which will help us to diagnose acute or chronic causes of cognitive timing symptoms. For example, delirium is an acute potentially life-threatening condition characterized by inattention, generalized cognitive impairments, and disturbances in consciousness mainly affecting elderly inpatients Cognitive deficits such as memory, language, perception, and impairment of consciousness may accompany the syndrome, and delirium is common in the elderly, but unfortunately underdiagnosed [21]. In contrast, dementia, the most common form being Alzheimer's disease (AD), is characterized by insidious onset, normal level of consciousness, and a chronic or slowly progressive irreversible decline in cognitive function [22, 23].

It is known that depression, which is one of the chronic processes, with increasing frequency and accepted as pseudo-dementia, leads to cognitive impairment. Although there are many hypotheses to identify the relationship between dementia and depression, the presence of depression alone is an independent risk factor for dementia. On the other hand, the cognitive impairment brought about by the presence of dementia can lead to depression [24–26]. Changes in the sleep-wakefulness cycle and various behavioral disorders can be seen in different clinical pictures of delirium or depression just as in dementia. Therefore, it is important to evaluate the sleep-wakefulness cycles to be asked both in the family interview and in the CV. Sleep disorders are among the most disruptive factors of total quality of life, since they degrade cognitive and behavioral functions secondary to dementia syndromes and may affect daily life rather negatively. When evaluating sleep, the distribution of the total sleep duration during the day should be determined. In addition, total sleep time, fitness to biological rhythm, presence of apnea, restless leg syndrome, and rapid eye movement (REM) sleep behavior disorder are the topics to be asked. Patients with REM sleep behavior disorder, a parasomnia manifested by vivid, often frightening dreams associated with simple or complex motor behavior during REM sleep, appear to "act out their dreams," in which the exhibited behaviors mirror the content of the dreams, and the dream content often involves a chasing or attacking theme [18, 27–29].

Another important factor in the history is the monitoring of existing systemic diseases and controlling the symptoms. Also, the presence of an underlying cancer or the management of the negative effects of the existing cancer is another important step in the cognitive assessment. For example, it would not be appropriate to evaluate the cognitive function of a patient with impaired sleep-wakefulness cycle due to restless legs or a patient suffering from fracture due to osteoporosis [30]. A detailed sensorimotor neurological examination should be performed after the systemic examination following a comprehensive anamnesis. Visual impairment and hearing difficulties should be recorded both in terms of inducing stimulus deficiency and related systemic diseases. Basic examination of the respiratory system and cardiovascular system must be performed. For example, it should be remembered that confusion may occur due to lethargy or chronic constipation, which may cause agitation or pneumonia burden due to hypoxia [31–33]. The second part of the evaluation is the neurological examination. In the basic neurological examination, mental status, cranial nerve examination, motor examination, sensory-neural examination, reflexes, and balance and gait evaluation are important. First, the orientation for the person, place, time, and alertness should be questioned. Cranial nerve, mental status examination, and motor deficits are guiding factors in the identification of acute intracranial events. Balance and gait assessment is important for the diagnosis of normal pressure hydrocephalus (NPH), the cause of reversible dementia. NPH includes urinary incontinence, gait apraxia, broad-based gait, and trunk imbalance [34]. While a "Timed Up and Go" test (TUG) is valid for measuring functional mobility, it also does not require special equipment or training [35]. The patient is lifted from the seat while in the sitting position and made to walk in a total of 3 m. All mobility is observed and timed, including returning and sitting time. This assessment will ensure the patient to be managed properly. In addition to these severe conditions, it should be kept in mind that due to a simple vitamin B12 deficiency, there may be abnormal findings in the gait and balance system and other neurological systems [36, 37] (algorithm 1) (Fig. 11.1).

11.2 Laboratory and Imaging

The processes leading to dementia are examined in a wide spectrum of common and local pathologies. Exclusion of dementia-like clinical manifestations should be one of the main objectives. Some of these processes (normal pressure hydrocephalus, subdural hematoma, hypothyroidism, vitamin B12 deficiency, lead exposure, etc.) can lead to a progressive but treatable impairment in cognition. Therefore, the laboratory and other examinations to be planned after the examination should be determined according to the patient's clinical status, history, and physical examination. Metabolic dysfunction, such as a simple decrease in kidney and liver function, can lead to cognitive impairment with aging. Firstly, the laboratory tests to be evaluated are complete blood count (CBC), renal function tests, serum electrolytes, hepatic function tests, thyroid function tests, and vitamin B12 level. In addition, all patients with memory complaints should be screened for syphilis and human

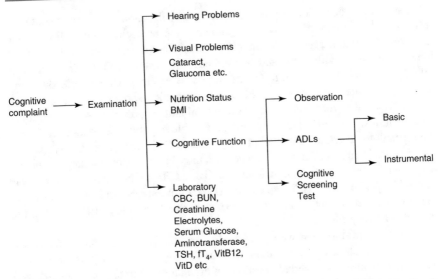

Fig. 11.1 Algorithm of cognitive assessment (modified by [38] th reference). *BUN* blood urea nitrogen, *CBC* complete blood counts, *fT₄* free T₄ (thyroxine), *TSH* thyroid-stimulating hormone, *VitB12* vitamin B12, *VitD* vitamin D, *ADLs* activities of daily living

immunodeficiency virus, as well as vitamin D and serum glucose levels [39–42]. Acute hypoglycemia affects complex cognitive activities in both diabetic and non-diabetic people [43]. Diabetic patients who are not aware of hypoglycemia are more likely to have cognitive impairment than those who are aware of it [16]. In addition, HbA1c levels may be misleading in patients with frequent or profound hypoglycemia attacks [44–47]. Additionally, patients with cognitive impairment have a higher risk of acute mental changes [48].

Infections can cause urinary tract infections and delirium, and the most common is pneumonia in older patients [49]. A complete urine test and urine culture, chest X-ray, and C-reactive protein (CRP) are helpful in diagnosing the underlying cause. Dementia is a clinical diagnosis in which distinctive features are unacceptable cognitive decline and impaired ADLs. However, the role of structural and neuro-imaging in dementia patients primarily supports the diagnosis. Therefore, many guidelines recommend imaging to exclude other anatomical disorders such as tumors, hydrocephalus, or intracranial hemorrhage [50].

11.3 Screening Tests

The part that requires the most time and experience in assessing patients with cognitive impairment is mental status examination. There are several tests for differential diagnosis as well as some other tests used to evaluate the patient's memory adequacy. Attention, memory, language, visual spatial skills, and administrative-executive functions should be evaluated in accordance with the age and education of the patient, in order to identify which areas are problematic. There are several tests used to screen cognitive activities. Following the physician's evaluation of the memory complaints reported by the patient and/or her relatives and of their effects on daily living activities, it would be appropriate to evaluate suitable cases in terms of cognitive impairment, and this issue should be evaluated with an effective diagnostic procedure. Ideally, a detailed clinical evaluation should be performed with the patient and his/her family for 2–4 h in total and supported by some laboratory examinations. However, this is not always possible in polyclinic conditions. It may be difficult to determine the level of forgetfulness of the patient with only existing symptoms. Therefore, detailed anamnesis, family interview, comprehensive physical examination, and appropriate tests as well as additional cognitive screening tests should be performed [51]. There are several cognitive screening tools to be used in the primary care setting, and the appropriate one should be selected according to the patient's literacy and educational level.

Among them, the most widely used Mini Mental State Examination (MMSE), which was developed by Folstein et al. in 1975, consists of two parts. In the first part, the patient is asked verbal questions of orientation, memory, and attention and asked for answers. In the second part, the patient is requested to perform verbal and written commands, to write a spontaneous sentence, and to copy two nested pentagons. The maximum score is 30. The test, which lasts for an average of 10–15 min, is considered normal between 24 and 30 points [52]. The validity and reliability study of the version (MMSE-E) for the illiterate was also conducted [52].

Additionally, the Cognitive Assessment Test (COST) was developed in 2012 for the illiterate [53]. Although there are several versions of MMSE for the uneducated, there is no clear consensus. The most important advantage of COST is that the same version can be used for both educated and uneducated populations. Unlike MMSE, COST also provides a detailed assessment of more cognitive domains and language functions such as retrograde memory, general current knowledge, apraxia, agnosia, and executive functions. The highest score from eleven sub-units is 30. It takes approximately 10–15 min. The higher the score, the better the cognitive function [53].

The Montreal Cognitive Assessment (MOCA) test can also be used to detect particularly early stages of cognitive dysfunction [54]. Application time is approximately 10 min. It includes items that measure attention, concentration, executive function, memory, language, visual-spatial skills, abstract thinking, and calculation. The highest score is 30. The scores 21 and above are considered normal.

The Saint Louis University Mental Status Exam (SLUMS) is used for cognitive assessment in individuals over the age of 60 [55]. Reliability and validity are available in many cultures and languages such as Chinese and Arabic. It mainly aims to differentiate HKB and dementia from the cognitively normal geriatric population. It consists of 11 items and the highest score is 30. According to the educational level of the patient, the evaluation of the scores varies [56].

Another practical cognitive screening test for primary health care is Rapid Cognitive Screening (RCS). This test, which can be applied in about 5 min, contains three titles, which are clock drawing, remembering, and insight. The highest score is 10. The validation study was also made in Turkey [57]. Mini-cog, the General Practitioner Assessment of Cognition (GPCOG), and Memory Impairment Screen (MIS) are some of the choices. Mini-cog is a 3-min screening test that can increase the detection of cognitive impairment in older adults [58]. It consists of a three-point recall test and a simple rated clock drawing. These tests are easily performed by non-physician healthcare professionals. It is considered to be relatively independent from education, language, and culture [10]. In Table 11.2, other tests that can be applied in primary healthcare institutions are briefly mentioned.

Additionally, because the development of easily applicable, time-saving, and cost-effective screening methods has allowed identifying the individuals that require further evaluation among the patients who apply to especially primary care settings for memory loss, some methods, such as applause sign (AS), head turning sign (HTS), and attended alone sign (AAS), were reported by which the physicians decide to screen for cognitive impairment in older adults [59–63]. The evaluation of AS is as follows: the patient was asked to clap three times as fast as possible after the examiner. If the patient clapped three times, they were considered negative for AS; if the patient clapped more than three times, they were considered positive for AS. Patients who clapped less than three times were considered as pathologic and having positive for AS, as reported previously [64–66]. HTS was assessed while the patient's caregiver sat silently at a 450 angle, approximately 1 m behind the patient. The patient was encouraged in a conversation about their cognitive function history. If the patient turned her/his head away from the collocutor and toward the caregiver

Table 11.2 Cognitive function screening tests used in primary healthcare

Tests	Features
RCS [57]	It is applied in about 5 min, contains 3 titles that are clock drawing, remembering, and insight
Triple [63]	It consists of the attended alone sign, head turning sign, and applause sign
RCS-Triple [67]	RCS plus triple test
Mini-cog [58]	It is a 3-min screening test. It consists of a three-point recall test and a simple rated clock drawing. It has high sensitivity
SPMSQ [68]	It consists of 10 questions. High specificity. Applicable to all levels of education
6CIT [69]	It consists of 6 questions. High specificity. Applicable to all levels of education
AMT [70]	It consists of 10 questions. High specificity. Applicable to all levels of education
CDT [71]	It has high specificity and sensitivity. It is sufficient to be literate; it can be applied to all education levels
GPCOG [72]	It consists of two parts, both for the patient and the caregiver. High sensitivity and specificity. A certain level of education is required
MIS [73]	It consists of 6 questions. It has high sensitivity and specificity. Applicable to all levels of education

AS applause sign, *AAS* attended alone sign, *AMT* Abbreviated Mental Test, *CDT* clock drawing test, *GPCOG* General Practitioner Assessment of Cognition, *HTS* head turning sign, *MIS* Memory Impairment Screen, *Mini-cog* mini cognitive test, *RCS* Rapid Cognitive Screen Test, *SPMSQ* Short Portable Mental Status Questionnaire, *6CIT* 6-item Cognitive Impairment Test person(s) for help, the patient was considered positive for HTS; if the patient did not seek help, they were considered negative for HTS [60, 61, 63]. AAS was evaluated based on whether the patient attended the clinic with a family member, caregiver, or friend. If the patient was accompanied, they were considered negative for attended alone sign [61, 63, 65, 66]. Our study group demonstrated that the combination of these three signs, named Triple test, has been shown to be a simple, rapid, and effective screening tool for detecting cognitive impairment and deterioration of daily living activities in elderly adults [63]. Furthermore the combination of RCS and Triple test has the ability to identify the cognitively healthy older adults with subjective memory complaints, while those with poor performance for any of them may require further neurocognitive evaluation for cognitive impairment [67]. In other words, the combination of both tests could serve as an indicator in need of further neurocognitive analysis, especially in daily busy clinical practice.

Loss of memory disrupting daily life, difficulties in planning or solving problems, difficulty in completing known tasks, confusion in time or place, difficulty in understanding visual images and spatial relationships, new problems with words when speaking or writing, placing things in the wrong place and losing the ability to follow the steps, difficulty in decision-making, withdrawal from work or social activities, and changes in mood and personality are particularly stimulating findings for Alzheimer's type dementia [22, 74]. For the differential diagnosis of MCI and dementia, it should be evaluated whether there is a deterioration in daily and instrumental life activities. It may be possible to understand this by asking the following questions [15, 22, 74, 75]:

- Have you ever experienced any confusion or loss of consciousness in the last 12 months?
- Did you need help in the past 7 days for any activity such as eating, bathing, using the toilet, or dressing?
- Did you need any help from someone else in the past 7 days, except for cleaning the house, using a telephone, preparing food, traveling, shopping, or taking your medication?

11.4 Management

That the primary healthcare physicians make a differential diagnosis in a patient coming to say "I'm forgetful" and manage treatment for correctable causes is one of the desired goals. In addition, it is crucial that primary physicians should play a more active role in combating polypharmacy and potentially inappropriate medications due to potentially negative effects on cognitive functions [76]. Additionally, since delirium is an acute alteration of cognition, it is important to develop primary and secondary prevention and therefore close contact with the patient, ensuring adequate vision, hearing, nutrition, hydration, and sleep; informing the caregivers about delirium for recognizing early symptoms of delirium, mobilizing the patient as early as possible, and managing the pain are strongly recommended in the primary care setting [21].

Finally, it is crucial that a patient with cognitive complaints should be referred to the reference memory center for differential diagnosis, after initial appropriate clinical and biochemical evaluations and screening for cognitive impairment in the elderly.

References

1. Petersen RC, Smith GE, Waring SC, Ivnik RJ, Tangalos EG, Kokmen E. Mild cognitive impairment: clinical characterization and outcome. Arch Neurol. 1999;56(3):303–8.
2. Drachman DA. Aging and the brain: a new frontier. Ann Neurol. 1997;42(6):819–28.
3. Mesulam M. Aging, Alzheimer's disease and dementia. In: Mesulam M, editor. Clinical and neurobiological perspectives. Principles of behavioral and cognitive neurology. 2nd ed. New York: Oxford University Press; 2000. p. 439–522.
4. Craik FI, Bialystok E. Cognition through the lifespan: mechanisms of change. Trends Cogn Sci. 2006;10:131–8.
5. Yankner BA, Lu T, Loerch P. The aging brain. Annu Rev Pathol. 2008;3:41–66.
6. Lezak MD, Howieson DB, Loring DW, Fischer JS. Neuropsychological assessment. USA: Oxford University Press; 2004.
7. Sternberg RJ, Lubart TI. Wisdom and creativity. In: Birren JE, Schaie KW, editors. Handbook of the psychology of aging. 5th ed. San Diego: Academic Press; 2001.
8. Salthouse TA. Theories of cognition. In: Bengtson VL, Schaie KW, editors. Handbook of theories of aging; 1999. p. 196–208.
9. Drachman DA. Aging of the brain, entropy, and Alzheimer disease. Neurology. 2006;67(8):1340–52.
10. Cordell CB, Borson S, Boustani M, Chodosh J, Reuben D, Verghese J, et al. Alzheimer's Association recommendations for operationalizing the detection of cognitive impairment during the Medicare Annual Wellness Visit in a primary care setting. Alzheimers Dement. 2013;9(2):141–50.
11. Ritchie K, Leibovici D, Ledésert B, Touchon J. A typology of sub-clinical senescent cognitive disorder. Br J Psychiatry. 1996;168(4):470–6.
12. Schmand B, Jonker C, Hooijer C, Lindeboom J. Subjective memory complaints may announce dementia. Neurology. 1996;46(1):121–5.
13. Malec JF, Ivnik RJ, & Smith GE. Neuropsychology and normal aging: the clinician's perspective. In: Parks RW, Zec RF, & Wilson RS, editors. Neuropsychology of alzheimer's disease and other dementias, Oxford University Press; 1993:81–111.
14. Craft S, Cholerton B, Reger M. Cognitive changes associated with normal and pathologic aging [chapter 62]. Hazzard's geriatric medicine and gerontology, 7e. 7th ed. New York: McGraw-Hill Education; 2017.
15. Troyer AK, Moscovitch M, Winocur G. Clustering and switching as two components of verbal fluency: evidence from younger and older healthy adults. Neuropsychology. 1997;11(1):138.
16. Artegiani B, Calegari F. Age-related cognitive decline: can neural stem cells help us? Aging (Albany NY). 2012;4(3):176.
17. Costa PT. Recognition and initial assessment of Alzheimer's disease and related dementias (No. 97). US Department of Health and Human Services, Public Health Service, Agency for Health Care Policy and Research. 1996.
18. Isik AT. Her Yönüyle Alzheimer Hastalığı. Turkey: SomKitap; 2012.
19. DeCarli C, Massaro J, Harvey D, Hald J, Tullberg M, Au R, et al. Measures of brain morphology and infarction in the Framingham heart study: establishing what is normal. Neurobiol Aging. 2005;26(4):491–510.

20. Kandiah N. Overview of dementia and diagnosis of dementia. The Singapore Family Physician. 2013;39(2 (Supplement)):8–14.
21. Soysal P, Kaya D, Isik AT. Current concepts in the diagnosis, pathophysiology, and treatment of delirium: a European perspective. Curr Geriatr Rep. 2015;4(4):284–9.
22. Isik AT. Late onset Alzheimer's disease in older people. Clin Interv Aging. 2010;5:307–11.
23. Isik AT. Delirium superimposed dementia. In: Isik AT, Grossberg GT, editors. Delirium in elderly patients. Springer Nature; 2018. p. 39–48.
24. Martínez MF, Flores JC, de las Heras SP, Lekumberri AM, Menocal MG, Imirizaldu JJZ. Risk factors for dementia in the epidemiological study of Munguialde County (Basque Country-Spain). BMC Neurol. 2008;8(1):39.
25. Sheline YI, Barch DM, Garcia K, Gersing K, Pieper C, Welsh-Bohmer K, et al. Cognitive function in late life depression: relationships to depression severity, cerebrovascular risk factors and processing speed. Biol Psychiatry. 2006;60(1):58–65.
26. Panza F, Frisardi V, Capurso C, D'Introno A, Colacicco AM, Imbimbo BP, et al. Late-life depression, mild cognitive impairment, and dementia: possible continuum? Am J Geriatr Psychiatry. 2010;18(2):98–116.
27. Boeve BF. REM sleep behavior disorder: updated review of the core features, the RBD-neurodegenerative disease association, evolving concepts, controversies, and future directions. Ann N Y Acad Sci. 2010;1184:15.
28. Pagel JF, Parnes BL. Medications for the treatment of sleep disorders: an overview. Prim Care Companion J Clin Psychiatry. 2001;3(3):118.
29. Sateia MJ, Buysse DJ, Krystal AD, Neubauer DN, Heald JL. Clinical practice guideline for the pharmacologic treatment of chronic insomnia in adults: an American Academy of sleep medicine clinical practice guideline. J Clin Sleep Med. 2017;13(02):307–49.
30. Pendergrass JC, Targum SD, Harrison JE. Cognitive impairment associated with cancer: a brief review. Innov Clin Neurosci. 2018;15(1–2):36.
31. Liao W, Hamel RE, Rikkert MGO, Oosterveld SM, Aalten P, Verhey FR, et al. A profile of the clinical course of cognition and comorbidity in mild cognitive impairment and dementia study (the 4C study): two complementary longitudinal, clinical cohorts in the Netherlands. BMC Neurol. 2016;16(1):242.
32. Lyketsos CG, Toone L, Tschanz J, Rabins PV, Steinberg M, Onyike CU, et al. Population-based study of medical comorbidity in early dementia and "cognitive impairment, no dementia (CIND)": association with functional and cognitive impairment: the Cache County Study. Am J Geriatr Psychiatry. 2005;13(8):656–64.
33. Eshkoor SA, Hamid TA, Mun CY. Correlation of cognitive impairment with constipation and renal failure. Sains Malaysiana. 2016;45(9):1357–61.
34. Adams RD, Fisher CM, Hakim S, Ojemann RG, Sweet WH. Symptomatic occult hydrocephalus with normal cerebrospinal-fluid pressure: a treatable syndrome. N Engl J Med. 1965;273(3):117–26.
35. Barry E, Galvin R, Keogh C, Horgan F, Fahey T. Is the timed up and go test a useful predictor of risk of falls in community dwelling older adults: a systematic review and meta-analysis. BMC Geriatr. 2014;14(1):14.
36. Dharmarajan TS, Adiga GU, Norkus EP. Vitamin B12 deficiency. Recognizing subtle symptoms in older adults. Geriatrics (Basel, Switzerland). 2003;58(3):30–4.
37. Hin H, Clarke R, Sherliker P, Atoyebi W, Emmens K, Birks J, et al. Clinical relevance of low serum vitamin B12 concentrations in older people: the Banbury B12 study. Age Ageing. 2006;35(4):416–22.
38. Geldmacher DS, Whitehouse PJ. Evaluation of dementia. N Engl J Med. 1996;335(5):330–6.
39. Knopman DS, DeKosky ST, Cummings JL, Chui H, Corey-Bloom J, Relkin N, Small GW, Miller B, Stevens JC. Practice parameter: diagnosis of dementia. American Academy of Neurology; 2000.
40. Gold AE, MacLeod KM, Deary IJ, Frier BM. Hypoglycemia-induced cognitive dysfunction in diabetes mellitus: effect of hypoglycemia unawareness. Physiol Behav. 1995;58(3):501–11.

41. Small SA, Stern Y, Tang M, Mayeux R. Selective decline in memory function among healthy elderly. Neurology. 1999;52:1392.
42. Carrière I, Fourrier-Reglat A, Dartigues JF, et al. Drugs with anticholinergic properties, cognitive decline, and dementia in an elderly general population: the 3-city study. Arch Intern Med. 2009;169:1317.
43. Chinta SJ, Woods G, Rane A, Demaria M, Campisi J, Andersen JK. Cellular senescence and the aging brain. Exp Gerontol. 2015;68:3–7.
44. Knopman DS, DeKosky ST, Cummings JL, Chui H, Corey-Bloom J, Relkin N, et al. Practice parameter: diagnosis of dementia (an evidence-based review): report of the Quality Standards Subcommittee of the American Academy of Neurology. Neurology. 2001;56(9):1143–53.
45. Tsoi KK, Chan JY, Hirai HW, Wong SY, Kwok TC. Cognitive tests to detect dementia: a systematic review and meta-analysis. JAMA Intern Med. 2015;175(9):1450–8.
46. Knopman DS. The initial recognition and diagnosis of dementia. Am J Med. 1998;104(4):2S–12S.
47. Weytingh MD, Bossuyt PMM, Van Crevel H. Reversible dementia: more than 10% or less than 1%? J Neurol. 1995;242(7):466–71.
48. Fick DM, Agostini JV, Inouye SK. Delirium superimposed on dementia: a systematic review. J Am Geriatr Soc. 2002;50(10):1723–32.
49. Setters B, Solberg LM. Delirium. Prim Care. 2017;44(3):541–59.
50. Narayanan L, Murray AD. What can imaging tell us about cognitive impairment and dementia? World J Radiol. 2016;8(3):240.
51. Janssen J, Koekkoek PS, van Charante EPM, Kappelle LJ, Biessels GJ, Rutten GE. How to choose the most appropriate cognitive test to evaluate cognitive complaints in primary care. BMC Fam Pract. 2017;18(1):101.
52. Babacan-Yıldız G, Ur-Özçelik E, Kolukısa M, Işık AT, Gürsoy E, Kocaman G, & Çelebi A Eğitimsizler İçin Modifiye Edilen Mini Mental Testin (Mmse-E) Türk Toplumunda Alzheimer Hastalığı Tanısında Geçerlik Ve Güvenilirlik Çalışması. 2015.
53. Babacan-Yildiz G, Isik AT, Ur E, Aydemir E, Ertas C, Cebi M, et al. COST: cognitive state test, a brief screening battery for Alzheimer disease in illiterate and literate patients. Int Psychogeriatr. 2013;25(3):403–12.
54. Nasreddine ZS, Phillips NA, Bédirian V, Charbonneau S, Whitehead V, Collin I, et al. The Montreal cognitive assessment, MoCA: a brief screening tool for mild cognitive impairment. J Am Geriatr Soc. 2005;53(4):695–9.
55. Tariq SH, Tumosa N, Chibnall JT, Perry MH III, Morley JE. Comparison of the Saint Louis University mental status examination and the mini-mental state examination for detecting dementia and mild neurocognitive disorder—a pilot study. Am J Geriatr Psychiatry. 2006;14(11):900–10.
56. Kaya D, Isik AT, Usarel C, Soysal P, Ellidokuz H, Grossberg GT. The Saint Louis University Mental Status Examination is better than the Mini-Mental State Examination to determine the cognitive impairment in Turkish elderly people. J Am Med Dir Assoc. 2016;17(4):370–e11.
57. Okudur SK, Dokuzlar O, Usarel C, Soysal P, Isik AT. Validity and reliability of rapid cognitive screening test for Turkish older adults. J Nutr Health Aging. 2019;23(1):68–72.
58. Borson S, Scanlan J, Brush M, Vitaliano P, Dokmak A. The mini-cog: a cognitive 'vital signs' measure for dementia screening in multi-lingual elderly. Int J Geriatr Psychiatry. 2000;15(11):1021–7.
59. Larner AJ. "Who came with you?" a diagnostic observation in patients with memory problems? J Neurol Neurosurg Psychiatry. 2005;76(12):1739.
60. Larner AJ. Head turning sign: pragmatic utility in clinical diagnosis of cognitive impairment. J Neurol Neurosurg Psychiatry. 2012;83(8):852–3.
61. Larner AJ. Screening utility of the "attended alone" sign for subjective memory impairment. Alzheimer Dis Assoc Disord. 2014;28(4):364–5.
62. Soysal P, Usarel C, Ispirli G, Isik AT. Attended with and head-turning sign can be clinical markers of cognitive impairment in older adults. Int Psychogeriatr. 2017;29(11):1763–9.

168

N. Ulusoylar et al.

63. Isik AT, Soysal P, Kaya D, Usarel C. Triple test, a diagnostic observation, can detect cognitive impairment in older adults. Psychogeriatrics. 2018;18(2):98–105.
64. Wu LJ, Sitburana O, Davidson A, Jankovic J. Applause sign in parkinsonian disorders and Huntington's disease. Mov Disord. 2008;23(16):2307–11.
65. Isella V, Rucci F, Traficante D, Mapelli C, Ferri F, Appollonio IM. The applause sign in cortical and cortical-subcortical dementia. J Neurol. 2013;260(4):1099–103.
66. Larner AJ. Dementia in clinical practice: a neurological perspective: pragmatic studies in the cognitive function clinic. Springer Science & Business; 2014.
67. Koc Okudur S, Dokuzlar O, Kaya D, Soysal P, Isik AT. Triple test plus rapid cognitive screening test: a combination of clinical signs and a tool for cognitive assessment in older adults. Diagnostics. 2019;9(3):97.
68. Erkinjuntti T, Sulkava R, Wikström J, Autio L. Short portable mental status questionnaire as a screening test for dementia and delirium among the elderly. J Am Geriatr Soc. 1987;35(5):412–6.
69. Brooke P, Bullock R. Validation of a 6 item cognitive impairment test with a view to primary care usage. Int J Geriatr Psychiatry. 1999;14(11):936–40.
70. Hodkinson HM. Evaluation of a mental test score for assessment of mental impairment in the elderly. Age Ageing. 1972;1(4):233–8.
71. Shulman KI. Clock-drawing: is it the ideal cognitive screening test? Int J Geriatr Psychiatry. 2000;15(6):548–61.
72. Brodaty H, Pond D, Kemp NM, Luscombe G, Harding L, Berman K, Huppert FA. The GPCOG: a new screening test for dementia designed for general practice. J Am Geriatr Soc. 2002;50(3):530–4.
73. Buschke H, Kuslansky G, Katz M, Stewart WF, Sliwinski MJ, Eckholdt HM, Lipton RB. Screening for dementia with the memory impairment screen. Neurology. 1999;52(2):231.
74. Alzheimer's Association. 2010 Alzheimer's disease facts and figures. Alzheimers Dement. 2010;6(2):158–94.
75. Prince M, Guerchet M, & Prina M. Alzheimer's Disease International. Policy brief for heads of government: the global impact of dementia 2013–2050. Alzheimer's Disease International. 2013.
76. Derksen E, Vernooij-Dassen M, Gillissen F, Olde Rikkert M, Scheltens P. Impact of diagnostic disclosure in dementia on patients and carers: qualitative case series analysis. Aging Ment Health. 2006;10(5):525–31.

The Older Patient with Psychiatric Illness   12

Alessandro Miola, Alessandro Brunini, Jacopo Demurtas, and Marco Solmi

Abstract

Demographic composition of societies is aging and the prevalence of mental illness is high in older patients and associated with a poor outcome. Compared with younger age groups, manifestations of mental disorders may be different in the elderly. Moreover, there are several difficulties in separating symptoms of mental disorders from those occurring in normal aging. Many factors linked to psychiatric disorders increases with age, including loss of close relatives, social network, previous status in society, sensory functions, functional ability. In addition, psychosocial risk factors as well as organic factors increase the risk and can complicate the development of psychiatric disorders in such population.

Thus, it is crucial to investigate and recognize psychiatric disorders among the elderly patients because of their consequences that include social deprivation, poor quality of life, cognitive decline, disability, increased risk for somatic disorders, suicide, and increased non-suicidal mortality

A. Miola
Neurosciences Department, University of Padova, Padua, Italy

A. Brunini
Primary Care Department—Geriatric Unit, Azienda USL Toscana Sud Est, Grosseto, Italy

J. Demurtas
Primary Care Department, USL Toscana Sud Est, Grosseto, Italy

M. Solmi (✉)
Department of Psychiatry, University of Ottawa, Ottawa,ON, Canada
e-mail: marco.solmi83@gmail.com

© Springer Nature Switzerland AG 2022
J. Demurtas, N. Veronese (eds.), *The Role of Family Physicians in Older People Care*, Practical Issues in Geriatrics, https://doi.org/10.1007/978-3-030-78923-7_12

Keywords

Depressive disorder · Anxiety disorder · Hypochondriasis · Alcohol use disorder
Bipolar disorder · Psychosis · Older people · Primary care · Psychiatry
Mental health

12.1 Epidemiology of Major Psychiatric Disorders in the Older People

Human longevity is increasing, and the demographic composition of societies is aging. Between 2015 and 2050, global life expectancy at birth is expected to increase from 70 to 77 years [1].

By 2050, the proportion of the world's population aged older than 60 years is projected to double, and the proportion aged older than 80 years is projected to triple [2, 3]. So, many studies estimate that the global prevalence of major depressive disorder (MDD) is in the range of 1% to 5% among adults aged 65 years or older 4–10 [4–9].

Global estimate of the prevalence of clinically significant depressive symptoms (CSDSs), which do not meet the full criteria for MDD, among adults aged 65 years or older is around 15% [4, 9–12].

The prevalence of major depressive disorder and clinically significant depressive symptoms in older adults is similar to that of middle-aged adults, and in the older people, this problem is a public health priority [12, 13] given that the consequences of depression are more severe among older adults. Depression in older people increases the risk for many adverse outcomes such as physical health problems, suicide, mortality, and reduced physical, cognitive, and social functioning [4, 6, 12, 14–18].

A frequent psychiatric illness in older people is anxiety [19–22]. Prevalence rates of anxiety disorders among older adults are 1.2–15% in community samples and 1–28% in clinical samples of older adults [23–25].

With age, anxiety and depression comorbidity seems to increase, with about half of depressed older adults meeting criteria for a coexisting anxiety disorder [26–29].

The coexistence of anxiety and dementia is common too [30]. The development of anxiety in these patients is often associated with memory impairment or confusion [30]; may be a mark of agitation, a typical feature in the behavioral manifestation of dementia [31]; and is not always detected, because of their inability to report their own subjective experiences accurately [32, 33].

Alcohol use disorder is also a common but underrecognized problem among older adults. Alcohol use disorders (AUDs) afflict 1–3% of older subjects [34]. One third of older alcoholic persons develop a problem with alcohol in later life, while the other two thirds grow older with the medical and psychosocial sequelae of early-onset alcoholism [35].

A systematic review of the prevalence of BD in population-based studies revealed heterogeneous findings concerning the prevalence of BD, ranging from 0.1% to 7.5% [36], related to the consideration of subthreshold criteria upon diagnosis, differences in study design, and psychiatric assessment.

Psychosis is one of the most common conditions in later life with a lifetime risk of 23%. Despite its high prevalence, late-onset psychosis remains a diagnostic and treatment dilemma. In fact there are no reliable pathognomonic signs to distinguish primary or secondary psychosis that affects approximately 60% of older patients with newly incident psychosis [37].

12.2   Major Psychiatric Disorders in Older People

12.2.1 Depressive Disorder in the Older People

Mood disorders are frequent in the older people, and depression is the most common psychiatric disorder. When depression occurs in subjects older than 65 years old, it's called late-life depression (LLD) [38].

In older people, depression can worsen comorbid medical conditions and can cause a relevant burden impacting on caregivers and the family in general [39]. Depression is associated with increased morbidity and mortality [40].

According to DSM-5, depressive disorders include major depressive disorder (major depression – DM), persistent depressive disorder (dysthymia), a substance–/drug-induced depressive disorder, depressive disorder due to another medical condition, otherwise specified depressive disorder, and the depressive disorder without specification [41].

The common characteristic of the aforementioned disorder is the presence of sad mood or loss of interest and pleasure, accompanied by somatic modifications and cognitive impairments that significantly affect the individual functioning [42]. To receive a diagnosis of major depressive disorder, patients should have depressed mood and/or loss of interest plus four or more associated symptoms, including (1) changes in appetite, (2) sleep disturbance, (3) psychomotor agitation or retardation, (4) fatigue, (5) inappropriate guilt or feelings of worthlessness, (6) poor concentration or indecisiveness, and (7) recurrent thoughts of death or suicidal ideation.

These symptoms must be present nearly every day for at least 2 weeks and cause clinically significant distress or functional impairment [41].

The clinical picture of DM varies considerably along the life span, particularly among those who have an early onset depression (EOD) or late-onset depression (LOD), after 50 years. LOD is characterized by apathy and neuropsychological deficits, including executive dysfunction, as well as psychomotor modifications [43, 44].

In addition to depressed mood and/or loss of interest, depressive symptoms in LLD can be distinguished in vegetative, cognitive, and psycho-somatic. Vegetative symptoms include sleep disorders (early awakenings, intermediate insomnia), loss of appetite, constipation, loss of libido, and asthenia. Cognitive symptoms include decreased attention and motivation, insecurity, slowdown of thought, reduced concentration, and continuous brooding. Most common psychosomatic symptoms are asthenia, osteoarticular migrant pain, palpitations, tachycardia, headaches, abdominal pain, empty head and confused, dyspnea, sense of suffocation, low back pain, gastrointestinal disorders, and, importantly, anhedonia, as well as Beck's triad (negative view of the world, of themselves, and of the future), meaning of guilt, self-denigration, and feelings of despair and of impotence [39, 45].

Depression in the older people is heterogeneous and manifests in more complex pictures than adulthood; however no specific section is dedicated in DSM-5. LLD is frequently underrecognized, underestimated, and undertreated. Anxiety, irritability, and physical symptoms, including pain, frequently manifest LLD [46]. Many psychological, relational, and socio-environmental factors are obstacle for LLD diagnosis. Social isolation, mourning, loneliness, and sensory deficits (in particular sight and hearing) can limit older people individuals' access to mental health care. Also, chronic medical conditions can cause physical symptoms which can frequently also be a manifestation of LLD (i.e., gastrointestinal symptoms, pain, among others) [47].

Finally, cognitive deficits can also be prominent and catalyze clinical attention, with depressive symptoms being masked and ending up being neglected [38]. Cognitive symptoms can also be the only manifestation of LLD, which can mimic dementia (pseudodementia), yet just being a manifestation of depression and responding well to antidepressants.

About the pathogenesis of LOD, it is shown that vascular and neurodegenerative factors contribute to the variety of phenotypic manifestations [48].

Recognition of risk factors for depression can aid in making the diagnosis. Risk factors can be categorized as biological or psychosocial. The most significant risk factors for depression in the older people include female gender, past history of depression, sleep disturbance, disability, and bereavement. Protective factors include physical health, self-efficacy, good social networks, and religious involvement [4, 49].

Biological risk factors are female gender, history of depression, chronic medical illness, chronic pain, sleep disturbance, and medications (i.e., opioids, BDZ, beta blockers). Psychosocial risk factors are social isolation, being divorced or widowhood, bereavement, caregiver role, low socioeconomic status, and poor perceived health.

Most commonly reported psychiatric comorbidities, which influence the course and the outcome of depression, are anxiety disorders, alcoholism, and cluster B and C personality disorders [50, 51].

As any other psychiatric condition, symptoms of depression can be measured. Depression rating scales do not replace clinical diagnosis but can be useful as screening tools and as a measure of efficacy. The most commonly used in the geriatric age are the Geriatric Depression Scale (GDS), the Hamilton Depression Rating Scale (HRSD), the Cornel Scale for Depression in Dementia (CDS), the "Center for Epidemiologic Studies Depression Scale" (CES-D), the Self Rating Depression Scale (SDS), the Beck Depression Inventory (BDI), and Patient Health Questionnaire-9 (PHQ-9) [52].

Two common depression rating scales utilized by general practitioner are the Geriatric Depression Scale (GDS) and the Patient Health Questionnaire-9 (PHQ-9). GDS is a 30-item instrument developed specifically for older adults. The scale utilizes a Yes/No format and can be self-administered or clinician administered [53]. One advantage of the GDS lies in its focus on psychological and cognitive aspects of depression rather than neurovegetative symptoms that may overlap with medical illnesses common in older adults.

The PHQ-9 is a nine-item self- or clinician-administered screening tool designed for use in primary care. The nine items on this scale correspond to the DSM-5 criteria for major depression. Both versions have approximately 80% sensitivity and specificity in detecting depression. An added advantage of PHQ-9 over GDS is that it can be useful in monitoring treatment response over time [54].

Moreover, a functional assessment is especially important in the evaluation of the impact and severity of LLD. Basic activities of daily living (ADLs) include bathing, dressing, grooming, toileting, and self-transferring. Instrumental activities of daily living (IADLs) include more complex daily activities such as preparing meals, administering medications, driving, managing finances, and using simple electronics such as the telephone or remote control [55]. (I)ADL should also be measured in subjects with LLD and in particular in subjects with medical comorbidities.

Suicidality can range from passive thoughts of death and wishing that one were not alive to active thoughts of self-harm with plan and intent. A suicide assessment begins with inquiring about the presence of suicidal thoughts, plans, and intent. A complete suicide assessment requires attention to suicide risk factors, protective factors, and warning signs of impending suicide. Risk factors for suicide in the older adult include mood disorders, chronic medical illnesses and associated functional impairment, chronic pain, and psychosocial factors such as social isolation [56]. Warning signs of impending suicide may indicate preparations for suicide and include feelings of hopelessness or lack of purpose, feeling trapped, talking about death, threatening suicide, agitation, social withdrawal, increased substance use, and reckless behavior [57].

The diagnostic process should investigate eventual underlying illness, so a physical examination should be performed first. In fact the condition that most frequently leads to depression is the presence of a physical illness with consequent disability, loss of autonomy, and dependence. Secondly a complete blood exam should search eventual cause of LLD. Recommended blood tests are RBC, Na, K, Mg, BUN, creatinine, Vit B12, iron deficiency, folate, and a complete thyroid hormone exam.

First-level neuroimaging is CT scan of the brain. In fact neuroimaging may reveal signs of cerebrovascular disease which can predispose, precipitate, or perpetuate depression in older adults.

Pharmacological and psychosocial interventions for depressions are both crucial to treat LLD and sustain patients' caregivers.

The pharmacological management of depression in late life is complicated by age-related changes, higher sensitivity to develop side effects, concomitant medical disorders with drug interaction phenomena, and compliance problems [46]. However, even an untreated depressive disorder can be detrimental, given the detrimental impact it can have on an individual's daily activities with loss of independence and on the adherence to eventually comorbidities' treatment.

The choice of antidepressant must be based on the best side effect profile and on the lowest risk of drug interactions [58].

Use of selective serotonin reuptake inhibitors (SSRIs) and serotonin noradrenaline reuptake inhibitors (SNRIs) represents a frequent choice among a wide range of antidepressants. Among SSRIs, escitalopram and citalopram have less side effects in terms of sedation and cognitive impairment and should be considered first, while fluoxetine and paroxetine should be third choice given their long half-life and anticholinergic effects, respectively. Among SNRIs, both duloxetine and venlafaxine are valid options.

Although most of the clinical studies have been conducted on SSRIs and SNRIs, there are other classes of antidepressants that are equally effective: noradrenergic and specific serotonergic antidepressant (NaSSA) like mirtazapine [59] and reuptake inhibitors of noradrenaline (NaRI) including reboxetine [60], mianserin [61], and trazodone [62, 63]. Yet, these latter medication can have sedative side effects.

Vortioxetine is also a novel antidepressant with multimodal activity (5-HT3, 5-HT7, and 5-HT1D receptor antagonist, 5-HT1B receptor partial agonist, 5-HT1A receptor agonist and serotonin (5-HT) transporter (SERT) inhibitor) and procognitive effects [64, 65].

The use of TCAs, nortriptyline, and desipramine, for instance, is currently indicated as a third-line therapy and can be considered in cases of resistance to treatment with new-generation drugs in the absence of comorbidity [66–68].

Exercise should supplement pharmacological treatment, given the body of evidence supporting its efficacy on depressive symptoms and specifically in the older people [69].

Moreover, psychosocial support including family members and pro-socializing support should also be performed, given the detrimental effects loneliness can have on physical and mental health [70].

Participant ID#:   Date:
Geriatric depression scale
Instructions: Choose the best answer for how you felt over the past week.
Note: When asking the participant to complete the form, provide the self-rated form.

	A	B
1. Are you basically satisfied with your life?	No	Yes
2. Have you dropped many of your activities and interests?	Yes	No
3. Do you feel that your life is empty?	Yes	No
4. Do you often get bored?	Yes	No
5. Are you hopeful about the future?	No	Yes
6. Are you bothered by thoughts that you just can't get out of your head?	Yes	No
7. Are you in good spirits most of the time?	No	Yes
8. Are you afraid that something bad is going to happen to you?	Yes	No
9. Do you feel happy most of the time?	No	Yes
10. Do you often feel helpless?	Yes	No
11. Do you often get restless and fidgety?	Yes	No
12. Do you prefer to stay home at night, rather than go out and do new things?	Yes	No
13. Do you frequently worry about the future?	Yes	No
14. Do you feel that you have more problems with memory than most?	Yes	No
15. Do you think that it is wonderful to be alive now?	No	Yes
16. Do you often feel downhearted and blue?	Yes	No
17. Do you feel pretty worthless the way you are now?	Yes	No
18. Do you worry a lot about the past?	Yes	No
19. Do you find life very exciting?	No	Yes
20. Is it hard for you to get started on new projects?	Yes	No
21. Do you feel full of energy?	No	Yes
22. Do you feel that your situation is hopeless?	Yes	No
23. Do you think most persons are better off than you are?	Yes	No
24. Do you frequently get upset over little things?	Yes	No
25. Do you frequently feel like crying?	Yes	No
26. Do you have trouble concentrating?	Yes	No
27. Do you enjoy getting up in the morning?	No	Yes
28. Do you prefer to avoid social gatherings?	Yes	No
29. Is it easy for you to make decisions?	No	Yes
30. Is your mind as clear as it used to be?	No	Yes

Score: Count responses circled in column A. A total greater than 12 may indicate depression. Short form consists of 15 questions including items 1–4, 7–9, 12, 14, 15, 17, and 21–23. A total greater than 4 column A responses may indicate depression.

Yesavage JA, Brink TL, Rose TL, et al. Development and validation of a geriatric depression screening scale: a preliminary report. J Psychiatr Res. 1983;17:37–49.

**Over the last 2 weeks, how often have you
been bothered by any of the following problems?**

(Use " ✔" to indicate your answer"

	Not at all	Several days	More than half the days	Nearly every day
1. Little interest or pleasure in doing things...............	0	1	2	3
2. Feeling down, depressed, or hopeless.................	0	1	2	3
3. Trouble falling or staying asleep, or sleeping too much..	0	1	2	3
4. Feeling tired or having little energy.......................	0	1	2	3
5. Poor appetite or overeating...................................	0	1	2	3
6. Feeling bad about yourself—or that you are a failure or have let yourself or your family down......................	0	1	2	3
7. Trouble concentrating on things, such as reading the newspaper or watching television.............................	0	1	2	3
8. Moving or speaking so slowly that other people could have noticed? Or the opposite —being so fidgety or restless that you have been moving. around a lot more than usual..	0	1	2	3
9. Thoughts that you would be better off dead or of hurting yourself in some way......	0	1	2	3

Column totals   ___ + ___ + ___ + ___

= Total Score _____

Kroenke K, Spitzer RL, Williams JB. The PHQ-9: validity of a brief depression severity measure. J Gen Intern Med 2001;16:606–613.

12.3 Anxiety Disorder

Anxiety is a frequent negative emotional state involving more than temporary worry or fear and characterized by excessive and persistent sense of apprehension, accompanied by specific somatic, cognitive, neurobiological, and behavioral manifestations [71].

It can cause clinically significant distress or impairment in social, occupational, and other important areas of functioning and is characterized by intense fear, anxious arousal, irrational thought, and avoidance. Until the fifth edition of the *Diagnostic and Statistical Manual of Mental Disorders* (DSM-5), anxiety disorder included GAD (general anxiety disorder), phobia (social phobia, agoraphobia, and specific phobia), panic disorder, obsessive-compulsive disorder (OCD), and post-traumatic stress disorder (PTSD), but the two latter are no longer considered as anxiety disorders [72, 73].

Anxiety disorders not only have a high prevalence, but there's also a frequent comorbidity with somatic manifestations as well as other mental disorders [74]. Older people with anxiety disorders frequently have physical illness such as cardiovascular disease, hypertension, diabetes, asthma, and chronic pain [75, 76]. Conversely, in clinical settings (e.g., patients with diabetes, cancer, cardiovascular, respiratory, or neurological disease), the prevalence of anxiety is reported to be high, reaching over 50% [77–79], and can contribute to the onset or increased severity of somatic diseases. Depressive and anxiety disorders frequently coexist across the lifespan [80].

Anxiety is also associated with cognitive impairment (understanding and communicating), difficulty in social interaction, life activities, and participation in social networks. The disability levels are particularly high for social anxiety disorder and mixed anxiety disorder [81]. Anxiety disorders, especially in the older people, are not only chronic and with high recurrence rates but also frequently accompanied with low compliance with medical treatment which also contributes to high disability level and thus an increased risk of mortality [74].

Generalized anxiety disorder (GAD) is characterized by chronic, uncontrollable worry that interferes with function and is accompanied by restlessness, irritability, muscle tension, easily fatigue, impaired concentration, and disturbed sleep [82]. GAD is a distressing chronic illness and is often accompanied by somatic anxiety symptoms, so most patients are not recognized in primary care [83].

Patients with anxiety disorder had received adequate treatment whatever in 50% of case, and less than 25% of patients with anxiety or depression reported adequate treatment in primary care [84].

This happens because patients with anxiety disorder and with GAD search treatment in general practitioners specially for somatic symptoms (e.g., restlessness, being easily fatigued, irritability, difficulty concentrating, dyssomnia, and muscle tension) rather than worrying. That's true in particular for older people who also suffer from chronic diseases. Hence these patients tend to be under-detected, under-treated, or treated inappropriately, and the rates of full remission tend to be low [85]. The prevalence of GAD in persons over 65 years of age is lower than in younger adults, with a range in older people of 1–2% [86].

PD is characterized by episodic, unexpected panic attacks that occur without a clear trigger [82]. Panic attacks are defined by the rapid onset of intense fear (typically peaking within about 10 min) that evidence physical and cognitive dysfunction. Another requirement for the diagnosis of PD is that the patient worries about further attacks or modifies his or her behavior in maladaptive ways to avoid them. The most common physical symptom accompanying panic attacks is palpitations [87].

Social phobia is characterized by marked anxiety about one or more social situations in which the individual is exposed to possible scrutiny by others such as social interactions or being observed while eating or performing in public [88]. Core symptoms of abovementioned disorder are anxiety associated with thinking about social situations, being in the social situation, remaining in the social situation too long, and avoiding such occasions. Additional concerns involve self-evaluations of being more nervous than others and having greater fear or avoidance than is reasonable [89]. People 65 years and older experience less social phobia than those who are younger.

Specific phobia is an anxiety disorder that represents exaggerated or irrational fear related to a specific object or situation [90], and the prevalence and course of specific phobia decrease in the older people. One common example of specific phobia is fear of falling that is especially frequent among older individuals and occurs in up to 50% of those in long-term facilities [91].

When evaluating a patient for a suspected anxiety disorder, it is important to exclude medical conditions with similar presentations (e.g., endocrine conditions such as hyperthyroidism, pheochromocytoma, or hyperparathyroidism; cardiopulmonary conditions such as arrhythmia or obstructive pulmonary diseases; neurologic diseases such as temporal lobe epilepsy or transient ischemic attacks). Other psychiatric disorders (e.g., other anxiety disorders, major depressive disorder, bipolar disorder); use of substances such as caffeine, albuterol, levothyroxine, or decongestants; or substance withdrawal may also present with similar symptoms and should be ruled out.

Psychotherapy is optioned for treatment of GAD with the advantage of being side effect free.

CBT (cognitive behavioral therapy) is considered the gold standard psychotherapeutic treatment focusing on challenging cognitive biases through cognitive restructuring and behaviors through graded exposure, teaching the patients specific skills to rerun in their daily routine as well as relaxation training. The cognitive interventions aim to modify maladaptive cognitions, self-statements, or beliefs, but their efficacy is also contingent on the ability of the therapist, the severity of the disorder, and the length of therapy [92].

Exposure therapy is recommended for patients with specific phobias [93].

Drug treatment often has better efficacy than psychotherapy alone in people with late-life anxiety [94].

Antidepressants are generally the first-line medical treatment option for anxiety disorders and include SSRI or serotonin-norepinephrine reuptake inhibitor (SNRI) drugs [95]. SSRIs have been shown to be the best-tolerated medications, and response rates are significantly higher than for placebos [92]. This class of medications includes escitalopram, paroxetine, and sertraline.

Among SSRI class paroxetine has important anticholinergic effects, so it is not indicated in patients that have cognitive impairment or that can develop it. Moreover SSRI class may show adverse effects such as agitation, sleep disturbances, and nervousness at the beginning of treatment. These effects may be controlled with benzodiazepines drugs.

All these medications should be initially administrated at low doses and gradually augmented to the therapeutic levels so we can prevent anxiety exacerbation, especially in older people patients.

Another drug indicated in general anxiety disorder is pregabalin that is a synthetic gamma-aminobutyric acid (GABA) analog with anticonvulsant, anxiolytic, and analgesic activities. Compared to SSRIs pregabalin improves not only psychic symptoms but also somatic symptoms of GAD, and it does not appear to have the withdrawal symptoms associated with benzodiazepines, but dizziness and somnolence are frequently reported especially at the beginning of treatment [96, 97].

Benzodiazepines are used for relieving acute anxiety on a short-term basis (up to 4 weeks), but benzodiazepine side effects in the older people must be considered, cognitive impairment, psychomotor impairment, excessive sedation, instability of gait, falls, and fractures, so these drugs have limited use [98–100]. Long-term use of benzodiazepines can lead to substance dependence, tolerance effects, as well as severe withdrawal symptoms when stopping this treatment.

Box 12.1 Overview of Anxiety Syndromes and Treatments

Disorders	Treatments
Specific phobia	Exposure therapy, as in cognitive behavioral therapy (CBT), is recommended as treatment for specific phobia; when CBT is unavailable, benzodiazepines may be utilized if there is no history of or current substance abuse; benzodiazepines should not be prescribed concurrently with opioids
Social phobia	CBT is effective; patients preferring medication may be treated with second-generation antidepressant drugs; propranolol may be prescribed for those with infrequent performance anxiety, such as for public speaking
Generalized anxiety disorder	CBT is effective; patients preferring medication may be treated with second-generation antidepressant drugs
Panic disorder	Second-generation antidepressant drugs are efficacious for patients with panic disorder but should be started at low doses; benzodiazepines have more rapid onset of effects but are not prescribed for those with substance use concerns due to dependency risks

---

12.3.1 Hypochondriasis in the Older People

Old patients previously diagnosed with hypochondriasis may be diagnosed as having illness anxiety disorder, in which the somatic symptoms are not present or they are only mild, or most frequently with somatic symptom disorder (SSD).

SSD is a recently defined diagnosis in the *Diagnostic and Statistical Manual of Mental Disorders*, fifth edition (DSM-V), and it is the manifestation of one or more physical symptoms accompanied by excessive thoughts, emotion, and/or behavior related to the symptom, which causes significant distress and/or dysfunction [101, 102].

According to the DSM-5, three criteria have been identified for the diagnosis of somatic syndrome disorders (SSDs):

- Somatic symptom(s) that cause significant distress or disruption in daily living.
- One or more thoughts, feelings, and/or behaviors that are related to the somatic symptoms which are persistent, excessive, associated with a high level of anxiety, and result in the devotion of excessive time and energy.
- Symptoms lasting for more than 6 months.

The prevalence of somatic symptom disorder (SSD) is estimated to be 5–7% of the general population, with higher female representation (female-to-male ratio 10:1), and can occur in childhood, adolescence, or adulthood [103]. The prevalence increases to approximately 17% of the primary care patient population [104].

The diagnosis of SSD and a concomitant organic disease are not mutually exclusive and often occur together.

It is important to make a differential diagnosis with other psychiatric diseases: in particular anxiety disorders (DAP, GAD), depressive disorders, delusional disorders, body dysmorphic disorder, and obsessive-compulsive disorder. In addiction the diffuse, non-specific symptoms in somatic syndrome disorder (SSD) may confound and mimic presentations of other medical illnesses, making diagnosis and treatment difficult.

The primary care provider should schedule regular visits to reinforce that symptoms are not suggestive of a life-threatening or disabling medical condition [105].

Diagnostic procedures and invasive surgical treatment are not recommended, and sedative medications, or narcotic analgesics, should be avoided. Conversely early psychiatric treatment is recommended. Studies have shown that cognitive-behavioral therapy is associated with significant improvement in patient-reported functioning and somatic symptoms [106]. Pharmacologic approaches should be limited: antidepressants can be initiated to treat psychiatric comorbidities (anxiety, depressive symptoms, obsessive-compulsive disorder). Selective serotonin reuptake inhibitors (SSRIs) and serotonin-norepinephrine reuptake inhibitors (SNRIs) have shown efficacy with an improvement of SSD compared to placebo [107]. However, medications should be initiated at the lowest dose and increased slowly to achieve a therapeutic effect as patients with SSD may have a low threshold for perceiving adverse effects, introducing another source of concern.

12.3.2 Alcohol Use Disorder in the Older People

Alcohol use disorder is a condition characterized by compulsive heavy alcohol use, loss of control over alcohol intake, and a negative emotional state when not drinking, which can follow a chronic, relapsing course. Alcohol use disorders are some of the most prevalent mental disorders globally, affecting 8.6% of men and 1.7% of women in 2016, predominantly affecting men still five times that in women. It is associated with high mortality and burden of disease, mainly due to medical consequences [108].

Despite their high prevalence, alcohol use disorders are undertreated partly because of the high stigma associated with them but also because of insufficient systematic screening in primary healthcare [108].

Managing alcohol use disorders among older patients is complicated by the increased effect of alcohol associated with pharmacologic changes in the older people; by the interactions between alcohol and drugs, prescription and over-the-counter; and by the physiologic changes related to aging that can alter the presentation of medical complications of alcoholism [35].

Alcohol use disorders are defined by the *Diagnostic and Statistical Manual of Mental Disorders* (DSM) and the International Classification of Disease (ICD) by operational criteria: continued alcohol use despite negative psychological, biological, behavioral, and social consequences, of which a minimum number must be met during the same 12-month period to qualify for the diagnosis. Depending on the number of criteria met, it is classified in mild, moderate, or severe disorder.

It is possible to distinguish three different phases that characterize the alcohol addiction cycle: (1) binge or intoxication; (2) withdrawal or negative affect; and (3) preoccupation or craving [109].

Patients, their families, and society in general should be informed that alcohol use disorders are not a result of any individual weakness or moral failing, but it is caused by a complex interaction of individual, social, cultural, and biological factors.

Screening instruments can be used by family physicians to identify older patients who have problems related to alcohol: CAGE, SMAST-G, and AUDIT (or AUDIT-C, the short form of the AUDIT comprising only the three consumption items) are the most common and validated questionnaires used to identify AUDs in the older people. The ten-item WHO AUDIT is useful in detection of problem drinking in a range of clinically and culturally diverse population (sensitivity and specificity typically 80–90%).

Clinical assessment should obtain a detailed history of alcohol use, the symptoms of alcohol use disorder, and the details of last drinking session. The use of other substances, social situation, and their insight and motivation to change their drinking habits should be assessed. Physical examination should begin by assessment of intoxication (slurred speech, ataxia, and inappropriate affect) and withdrawal symptoms (restlessness, tachycardia, and fine action tremor). A neurological assessment should look for signs of Wernicke's encephalopathy characterized by the classic triad of confusion, ataxia, and nystagmus. Orientation, short-term memory, and mental state should be evaluated [110].

Some laboratory markers of alcohol abuse (AST, ALT, GGT, MCV, and CDT) may also be helpful. In particular, the sensitivity of MCV or GGT in detecting alcohol misuse is higher in older than in younger populations [34]. Tell-tale indicators have been described, such as the smell of alcohol on a patient's breath, the presence of red eyes, and findings of raised liver enzymes or other comorbidities, rather than on official criteria [111].

Chronic alcohol abuse is associated with tissue damage to several organs. An increased level of blood pressure is more frequent in the older people than in younger adults, and a greater vulnerability to the onset of alcoholic liver disease and an increasing risk of breast cancer in menopausal women have been described. The incidence of medical and neurological complications during alcohol withdrawal syndrome in older alcoholic people is higher than in younger alcoholics, including seizures and delirium.

In addition, the prevalence of dementia in older alcoholic people is almost five times higher than in non-alcoholic older people individuals, about 25% of older people patients with dementia are also alcoholics, and almost 20% of individuals aged 65 and over with a diagnosis of depression have a co-occurring AUD [34].

Psychosocial treatments such as brief counselling, motivational enhancement therapy, the community reinforcement approach, guided self-change, behavior contracting, and social skills training were among the top ten most effective interventions for alcohol use disorders, together with some pharmacological interventions [112]. Alcoholics Anonymous is also a widely used intervention for alcohol use disorders.

Acute management involves airway protection; hydration; monitoring of seizures, blood glucose, and ketoacidosis; and intramuscular sedation in the emergency department if patients manifest an aggressive behavior. The most widely used drugs for management of alcohol withdrawal are benzodiazepines [113].

Different pharmacotherapies for relapse prevention have been approved to treat alcohol use disorders by maintenance of abstinence: naltrexone, acamprosate, and disulfiram. Nalmefene has been approved to reduce alcohol use rather than achieve abstinence. It is taken when the patients are at risk of drinking [114]. Previous meta-analyses showed that acamprosate and disulfiram might be better choice for abstinence-oriented treatment; conversely naltrexone and nalmefene should be used when reduced or controlled drinking is the goal [110]. In alcohol-dependent populations, little evidence is also associated to telephone-based interventions or Internet-based interventions [115, 116].

12.3.3 Bipolar Disorders in the Older People

Bipolar disorder (BD) is a major affective disorder marked by recurrent episodes of mania/hypomania or depression as described in DSM-5 [73]. The subtypes of BD include bipolar disorder I (BD-I) and bipolar disorder II (BD-II). Patients with BD-I experience manic episodes and nearly always experience major depressive and hypomanic episodes, whereas BD-II is marked by at least one hypomanic episode, at least one major depressive episode, and the absence of manic episodes. To satisfy a clinical diagnosis of BD, the abnormal mood episodes should have a detrimental effect on individual's social and occupational functioning.

A systematic review of the prevalence of BD in population-based studies showed prevalence of BD ranged from 0.1% to 7.5% [36]. Identifying BD in the older people is of prominent clinical importance, given the long-term outcomes of patients with BD including cognitive deficits [117, 118], impaired functioning, and increased risk of dementia and ultimately premature death [119, 120].

Older age bipolar disorder (OABD) refers to patients older than 60 years with bipolar disorder (BD) [121].

Globally among all patients with BD, 25% are older than 60 years [122], with expected increasing rates up to 50% in 2030 [123], due to aging of the general population among other factors [124]. Patients with OABD can be categorized into three groups. First, subjects may have been diagnosed with BD in early life and survived to old age (early onset). Second, they may have become manic in later life after previous depressive episodes (converter). Third, approximately 10% of patients with OABD develop new-onset mania later in life, often associated with vascular changes or other brain disorders (late onset) [125].

> **Box 12.2 Primary and Secondary Mania**
> Disorders in which manic symptoms may present
> *Mental disorders*
> 1. BD
> 1a. Converter (subjects with previous depressive episodes and first manic episode in older age)
> 1b. Late-life BD (subjects with previous manic episodes)
> 1c. Late-onset mania: New-onset BD in late life
> 2. Schizoaffective disorder
> *Other disorders—Secondary mania*
> Caused by underlying somatic illness or medication
> Caused by underlying neurologic illness
> Cause by substance abuse
> Caused by medications

Box 12.3 Diagnostic Assessment for OABD

History	Somatic and psychiatric history
	Medications, including over-the-counter medications
	Collect history with an informant (spouse)
	Exclude alcohol and illicit drug use
	Family history for mood illness or other psychiatric disorders
	Dramatic changes in functioning lifetime
Physical examination	With a specific focus on neurological examination
Cognition	MMSE, full neuropsychological examination if indicated
Laboratory studies	Vitamin B, folic acid, full blood count, electrolytes, creatinine,
	GFR, thyroid and liver function tests
	Serum blood levels of current medications such as lithium and
	Anticonvulsant medications
	HIV and lues serology if indicated
	Substances (alcohol, cocaine, others)
Imaging	MRI scan of the brain
	EEG

Box 12.4 Red Flags of Secondary Mania

Red flags—signs and symptoms associated with secondary mania

Dementia—Associated with neuropsychological deficits, or visual hallucinations, or neurological deficits

Substance abuse—Evidence of substance use in biological samples, or medical history, or as referred by relevant others

Medications—Check whether the subject is taking corticosteroids, or other CNS active medications recently introduces before manic symptoms

Thyroid dysfunction—Evidence of other signs of thyroid dysfunction, including gastrointestinal, heart rate, weight changes

Brain tumors—Evidence of associated neurological deficits, or abrupt major behavioral changes with associated confusion, headache, fever, sensory alterations

Delirium—Prominent confusing symptoms, including eventual signs of alcohol abstinence (delirium tremens)

While retrospective studies of OABD found that about half of all patients experience depression as their first mood episode [126–128], manic episodes also virtually always require major clinical attention. In the older people, manic symptoms can occur in the context of the three aforementioned clinical pictures (early onset, converter, and late-onset BD), as well as in the context of a schizoaffective disorder, but can also be caused by a specific medical condition.

The presentation, severity, and prevalence of manic and depressive symptoms in OABD do not differ that much from those in adults younger than 60 years of age [124, 129]. Also, no significant differences were found between early-onset and late-onset OABD [121]. However, given that BD associates with a number of medical conditions, including cardiovascular disease, diabetes, hypertension, hyperlipidemia, and obesity [130], and given that incidence of these comorbidities clearly increases with age, the role of medical comorbidities is particularly relevant in OABD. This is particularly important given the association between the cumulative number of illnesses and the estimated relative risk of suicide [131].

An assessment of older adults presenting with symptoms of mania, depression, or mood episodes with mixed characteristics requires a thorough examination and differential diagnostic evaluation, including identifying any potentially treatable medical conditions that may contribute to the manic/depressive symptoms. Assessment should include family history and careful characterization of prior mood episodes. A complete physical and neurologic examination should be conducted. Laboratory workup should include a comprehensive metabolic panel, complete blood cell count, thyroid function, toxicology screen, and more specialized assessments eventually indicated by the medical history, physical, or neurologic examination [132]. Differential diagnosis can be challenging and should include a number of medical conditions or substances. Neuroimaging to rule out acute CNS pathology should be complemented by more specific procedures (i.e., electroencephalogram, lumbar puncture), depending on the clinical presentation. In particular, neuroimaging is indicated in the case of abrupt behavioral changes or in the presence of headache, fever, and neurological signs. Also, blood panel should be requested in particular when symptoms are confusing, including deficit in orientation or fluctuating level of consciousness, as well as changes in memory, or language, all of which are more characteristic of delirium than mania. Also, while BD and OABD are associated with specific cognitive deficits (attention, cognitive flexibility, processing speed, memory [133], and fluency [117] in 40% to 50% of patients with OABD in the euthymic phase) [133, 134], a frank cognitive decline with dementia can in some cases mimic manic symptoms. Of course, clinical history can help in differential diagnosis with dementia. In addition to medical conditions, corticosteroids and dopamine-related drugs, as well as some antiepileptics (levetiracetam) among others, can induce manic symptoms (secondary mania) [132].

Alterations in pharmacokinetics and dynamics, increasing comorbidity, drug interactions, and the subsequent polypharmacy combined with functional and cognitive limitations related to aging condition could modify the response to mood stabilizers [135].

Research on pharmacotherapy in OABD is limited because older adults are often excluded from randomized controlled registration trials because of the increasing risk of medical complications with advancing age. Most guidelines recommend that first-line treatment of OABD should be similar to that of BD, with specific attention to vulnerability to side effects and somatic comorbidity [136].

Integrated treatment focusing simultaneously on psychiatric and medical outcomes may offer substantial advantages over usual care, which is often fragmented.

Lithium still remains a pharmacological cornerstone for the prevention of manic and depressive recurrences in BD [137]. It has been previously suggested that lithium may also have neuroprotective abilities and may reduce the risk of developing dementia [138].

Lithium is indicated in both manic and depressive episodes in BD, as well as in maintenance phase. Also, lithium has proven to be effective in suicide prevention [139, 140].

Considering the narrow therapeutic window of lithium and the well-known harmful adverse effects of chronic lithium intoxication, lithium concentration monitoring should be warranted [135]. Comorbidities and polypharmacy related to the aged could also result in instability of serum lithium concentrations. For instance, a variety of antihypertensives (thiazide diuretics, angiotensin-converting enzyme inhibitors) and nonsteroidal anti-inflammatory agents, which are common medications in older people patients, can increase lithium concentrations [141].

Additional pharmacological agents have shown to be effective in BD. In a network meta-analysis, carbamazepine, valproate, haloperidol, lithium, olanzapine, quetiapine, and risperidone were more effective than placebo in adult BD, manic episode [142]. In a further network meta-analysis, lurasidone, valproate, quetiapine, and the combinations of fluoxetine with olanzapine and olanzapine and lamotrigine were significantly more effective than placebo for the treatment of bipolar depression in adult BD [143]. The use of antidepressants in BD remains controversial and should be cautiously prescribed [144]. Also, pharmacological treatment should be supplemented with psychoeducation [125].

12.4 Psychosis in the Older People

Psychosis classically describes a mental state involving a loss of contact with reality and, according to the fifth edition of the *Diagnostic and Statistical Manual of Mental Disorders* (DSM-5), aligns with the ICD-10, is defined by the presence of delusions, hallucinations, disorganized thinking (speech), grossly disorganized or abnormal motor behavior (including catatonia), or negative symptoms [145].

Late-life psychosis is notably prevalent in older adults, presenting in 5–15% of older people geropsychiatric inpatients, 10–62% of nursing home patients, and as high as 27% of community-dwelling psychiatric outpatients [146, 147]. Despite its widespread prevalence in older adults, late-onset psychosis frequently represents a diagnostic and treatment dilemma [37].

Psychoses can be distinguished as primary (idiopathic or caused by a psychiatric disorder) or secondary (due to a known medical illness or substance use).

Primary psychosis in older adults may occur in the context of early-onset schizophrenia that persists into later life, late-onset schizophrenia, delusional disorder, mood disorders with psychotic features, and various dementias (most notably, Alzheimer's, Lewy body, vascular, and Parkinson's dementia). Secondary psychosis can occur conversely as a result of drug use and withdrawal, both prescription and illicit, and in the context of delirium, autoimmune disorders, stroke, brain tumors, metabolic disturbances, central nervous system (CNS) infections, and various chronic neurological disorders [148].

Late-life schizophrenia simply refers to schizophrenia in older adults, regardless of age of onset: it is commonly categorized into early-onset (EOS) and late-onset schizophrenia (LOS); onset after age 40 or 45 years is commonly considered late onset [149]. The lifetime prevalence of schizophrenia is estimated to be 1.0% for those between the ages of 45 and 64 years and 0.3% for those over age 65 years [150]. Patients with late-onset schizophrenia have similar symptoms to those with early-onset schizophrenia, but they are more likely to refer hallucinations (visual, olfactory, and tactile; when auditory hallucinations with an accusatory nature or involve a third-person running commentary), persecutory delusions, and partition delusions. On the other hand, they are less likely to show formal thought disorder, affective flattening, or blunting than their earlier-onset counterparts [151].

According to DSM-5, delusional disorder is characterized by the presence of at least one delusion for at least 1 month. Additionally, the individual cannot ever met the criteria for a diagnosis of schizophrenia, cannot be markedly functionally impaired or exhibit odd/bizarre behavior, and cannot ever have had depressive or manic episodes that are anything but brief in relation to the duration of delusions, and their symptoms cannot be due to substance use, a medical condition, or another psychiatric disorder [145]. As such, in keeping with the early- versus late-onset dichotomy of schizophrenia, delusional disorder can be considered a disorder of older adults with a lifetime prevalence of 0.18% [148].

Schizoaffective disorder, according to DSM-5, is characterized by a depressed episode (with depressed mood) or a manic episode in the presence of an uninterrupted psychotic illness. Additionally, mood episodes must be present for the majority of illness duration, and in contrast to depressive or bipolar disorder with psychotic features, at some point during the course of schizoaffective disorder, hallucinations or delusions must occur for at least a 2-week period in the absence of a depressive or manic episode. That is, there must be a period with persistent psychotic symptoms but no major mood symptoms [145]. The lifetime prevalence of schizoaffective disorder is estimated to be 0.32% [152].

In addition to their prominence in abovementioned psychiatric disorders, psychotic symptoms are also very common in the setting of Alzheimer's disease and certain other dementias, in particular in Lewy body, vascular, and Parkinson's dementias.

A variety of risk factors associated with aging make older adults more prone to psychosis [37, 153]:

- Sensory deficits.
- Social isolation.
- Cognitive decline.
- Medical comorbidities.
- Polypharmacy.
- Age-related changes in pharmacokinetics and pharmacodynamics.
- Comorbid psychiatric illnesses such as dementia and delirium.
- Age-related changes in cerebral structures such as frontotemporal cortices.
- Neurochemical changes associated with aging.

Clinical presentations that should increase suspicion of secondary psychosis include [37, 154] the following:

- Unusual age of onset of the presenting psychiatric symptoms.
- An absence of family history of mental illness.
- An absence of past psychiatric history.
- Limited response to psychiatric treatment.
- Symptoms more severe than might be expected.
- Psychopathology developed following an abrupt personality change.
- Comorbid medical condition(s) with a known association with mental illness (psychosis).
- Abnormalities of cognition, particularly memory, and consciousness.

An accurate diagnosis of psychosis in older populations is essential, particularly given the presence of serious medical disorders that may masquerade as psychotic illness. Because there are no pathognomonic signs to easily distinguish primary from secondary psychotic disorders, the diagnosis and treatment of primary late-life psychotic disorders should proceed only after the evaluation for secondary late-life psychotic disorders is complete. Clinicians should remember the pre-diagnostic probability in the older people – three fifths of psychoses are secondary psychoses—and be willing to revisit their assessments as more information becomes available [37].

Secondary psychosis can result from a wide variety of disorders, including traumatic brain injury, autoimmune disorders, stroke, CNS malignancies, CNS infections, other neurodegenerative disorders (in addition to those already discussed), seizure disorders, endocrine disorders, metabolic disorders, and drug use (both licit and illicit). General features that help to distinguish secondary psychoses from primary disorders include the following: atypical presentation of psychosis (a later age of onset, the presence of visual hallucinations, or multimodality hallucinations, altered states of consciousness), presence of accompanying medical symptoms, temporal relation to detectable medical cause, prescription or over-the-counter medication or substance use, evidence of direct physiological causal relationship to the etiological agent, and absence of evidence to support a diagnosis of a primary psychotic illness [148, 155].

Older people patients with late-life-onset psychosis require careful evaluation. A history and physical examination are essential for workup of a psychotic disorder. It is necessary conduct a complete blood count (CBC) and comprehensive metabolic panel (CMP) but also add thyroid-stimulating hormone (TSH), vitamin B12, folate, rapid plasma regain (RPR), and erythrocyte sedimentation rate (ESR). Autoimmune antibody screens, HIV testing, and toxicology may be done when indicated. Often, a head MRI or CT scan is done; EEG and polysomnography are to be considered if indicated by history (Box 12.5) [37, 155].

Treatment is oriented toward the specific cause of psychosis and shaped based on comorbid conditions. Frequently, environmental and psychosocial interventions are first-line treatments in late-life psychoses. Prudence should be used in all older people patients when initiating pharmacotherapy for psychosis, particularly antipsychotic medications because of their association with drug-drug interaction in the context of polypharmacy, adverse events, and increased morbidity and mortality [37].

Traditionally, antipsychotics have been the most commonly used treatment for psychotic symptoms. Their usefulness in treating chronic and late-onset schizophrenia is well established, and the atypical antipsychotics (such as aripiprazole, risperidone, paliperidone, olanzapine, and quetiapine, among others) should be preferred over first-generation antipsychotics. More recently, there have been increasing concerns about their safety in psychoses due to dementia. The debate about their use is still ongoing, but it has highlighted the need for adopting and developing non-pharmacological interventions [156].

Box 12.5 Secondary Psychoses

Approach to investigating patients to rule out secondary psychoses
First-line assessments (to be routinely considered in all first psychotic episode patients)
Detailed medical and neurological/psychiatric history
Physical/neurological examination
Neuropsychological tests (MMSE)
Laboratory tests: Complete and differential blood count, erythrocyte sedimentation rate, glucose, electrolytes, thyroid function tests, liver function tests, urinary drug screen
Second line assessments (to be considered when above assessments raise specific diagnostic possibilities)
Laboratory tests: Rapid plasma reagin to rule out syphilis; HIV testing; serum heavy metals; copper and ceruloplasmin levels; serum calcium levels; autoantibody titers (e.g., antinuclear antibodies for lupus); B12, folate levels; arylsulfatase-A levels; urine: Culture and toxicology, drug screen
Neuroimaging: Computed tomography, magnetic resonance imaging, positron emission tomography, single proton emission tomography
Electroencephalography, polysomnography, evoked potentials
Cerebrospinal fluid investigations: Glucose, protein, cultures, cryptococcal antigen
Karyotyping

12.5 Delirium

Delirium, defined as an acute disorder of attention and cognition, is a common, life-threatening, and often preventable clinical syndrome in older persons. Often occurring after acute illness, surgery, or hospitalization, the development of delirium starts a series of events culminating in loss of independence, increased morbidity and mortality, institutionalization, and high healthcare costs. Delirium remains underrecognized and rates of identification have not improved significantly over time [157]. Delirium is common in the acute care setting but should never be considered a normal part of aging. It is estimated that greater than 40% of all hospitalized older adult patients experience delirium.

Delirium also frequently occurs in long-term care facilities and in retirement home in the community as well, where the diagnosis is more likely to be missed clinically. Because there's a great heterogeneity among older adults, individuals have variable susceptibility to this condition [158].

Delirium and dementia are associated with higher rates of depression that may be a predictor for cognitive decline. This relationship is important for the primary care provider to recognize and understand because more than 10% of older adults seen in primary care offices suffer from depressive disorders. Of all the office-based visits made for depression, 64% are to primary care physicians [159].

12.5.1 The Role of Family Physician

Due to its peculiarities, family practice exposes the GP to a broad number of consultations, in which the reason for encounter is often represented by a psychological/psychiatric issue.

It has to be highlighted that many of the psychiatric disorder cared in general practice may be underpinned by several organic contingencies (i.e., dysionemia) and sometimes organ failure (i.e., kidney failure) or tumors (i.e., depression in pancreatic cancer).

Therefore, when facing any of these disturbs in general practice, notably in delirium, which is common in older patients, especially in nursing homes or at home, family physicians should try to understand the cause of the condition, instead of merely treating it with medications. Not resolving the organic conditions which led to the psychiatric manifestation may impair all treatment.

The family doctor should try to investigate during the consultation with patient and sometimes relatives the characteristics of the psychiatric disorder, use his knowledge of patient and his skill to understand whether it may be secondary or primary, refer patient to the psychiatrist, or consult the geriatrician if necessary.

12.6 Conclusion

The prevalence of mental disorders is high among older patients and is associated with a poor outcome in the elderly. The presence of many factors linked to mental disorders increases with age, including loss of close relatives, social network, previous status in society, sensory functions, functional ability, and health. Moreover, organic factors involving cerebral neurodegeneration and cerebrovascular disease, as well as psychosocial risk factors, increase the risk and can complicate the development of psychiatric disorders in such population.

Manifestations of mental disorders may be different in the elderly, compared with younger age groups, and there may be difficulties in separating symptoms of mental disorders from those occurring in normal aging. For example, there is an overlap in symptoms of depression and those occurring in physical disorders and in normal aging (loss of appetite, tiredness, and sleep disturbances).

It is therefore crucial to investigate and recognize psychiatric disorders among the elderly patients because of their consequences that include social deprivation, poor quality of life, cognitive decline, disability, increased risk for somatic disorders, suicide, and increased non-suicidal mortality.

References

1. United Nations. World Urbanization Prospects: The 2014 Revision, Highlights (ST/ESA/SER.A/352). 2014.
2. UN. Department of Economic and Social Affairs, Population Division (2015). World Population Prospects: The 2015 Revision, Key Findings and Advance Tables. Working Paper No. ESA/P/WP.241. 2015.
3. UN. World Population Prospects: The 2017 Revision (Department of Economic and Social Affairs). 2017.
4. Fiske A, Wetherell JL, Gatz M. Depression in older adults. Annu Rev Clin Psychol. 2009.
5. Hasin DS, Goodwin RD, Stinson FS, Grant BF. Epidemiology of major depressive disorder: results from the National Epidemiologic Survey on alcoholism and related conditions. Arch Gen Psychiatry. 2005.
6. Alexopoulos GS. Depression in the elderly. Lancet. 2005.
7. Blazer D. Depression in the elderly. N Engl J Med. 1989.
8. Djernes JK. Prevalence and predictors of depression in populations of elderly: a review. Acta Psychiatr Scand. 2006.
9. Sutin AR, Terracciano A, Milaneschi Y, An Y, Ferrucci L, Zonderman AB. The trajectory of depressive symptoms across the adult life span. JAMA Psychiat. 2013.
10. Blazer DG. Depression in late life: review and commentary. J Gerontol Ser A Biol Sci Med Sci. 2003.
11. Beekman ATF, Copeland JRM, Prince MJ. Review of community prevalence of depression in later life. Br J Psychiatry. 1999.
12. Meeks TW, Vahia IV, Lavretsky H, Kulkarni G, Jeste DV. A tune in "a minor" can "b major": a review of epidemiology, illness course, and public health implications of subthreshold depression in older adults. J Affect Disord. 2011.
13. Haigh EAP, Bogucki OE, Sigmon ST, Blazer DG. Depression among older adults: a 20-year update on five common myths and misconceptions. Am J Geriatr Psychiatry. 2018.
14. Kok RM, Reynolds CF. Management of depression in older adults: a review. JAMA—J Am Med Assoc. 2017.
15. Mitchell AJ, Subramaniam H. Prognosis of depression in old age compared to middle age: a systematic review of comparative studies. Am J Psychiatry. 2005.
16. Chui H, Gerstorf D, Hoppmann CA, Luszcz MA. Trajectories of depressive symptoms in old age: integrating age-, pathology-, and mortality-related changes. Psychol Aging. 2015.
17. Cole MG, Bellavance F, Mansour A. Prognosis of depression in elderly community and primary care populations: a systematic review and meta-analysis. Am J Psychiatry. 1999.
18. Chapman DP, Perry GS. Depression as a major component of public health for older adults. Prev Chronic Dis. 2008.

19. El-Gabalawy R, Mackenzie CS, Thibodeau MA, Asmundson GJG, Sareen J. Health anxiety disorders in older adults: conceptualizing complex conditions in late life. Clin Psychol Rev. 2013.

20. Cully JA, Stanley MA. Assessment and treatment of anxiety in later life. Handb Emot Disord Later Life. 2015.

21. Kessler RC, Angermeyer M, Anthony JC, De Graaf R, Demyttenaere K, Gasquet I, et al. Lifetime prevalence and age-of-onset distributions of mental disorders in the World Health Organization's World Mental Health Survey Initiative. World Psychiatry 2007.

22. Baxter AJ, Scott KM, Vos T, Whiteford HA. Global prevalence of anxiety disorders: a systematic review and meta-regression. Psychol Med. 2013.

23. Wolitzky-Taylor KB, Castriotta N, Lenze EJ, Stanley MA, Craske MG. Anxiety disorders in older adults: a comprehensive review. Depress Anxiety. 2010.

24. Bryant C, Jackson H, Ames D. Depression and anxiety in medically unwell older adults: prevalence and short-term course. Int Psychogeriatr. 2009.

25. Norton J, Ancelin ML, Stewart R, Berr C, Ritchie K, Carrière I. Anxiety symptoms and disorder predict activity limitations in the elderly. J Affect Disord. 2012.

26. Beekman ATF, De Beurs E, Van Balkom AJLM, Deeg DJH, Van Dyck R, Van Tilburg W. Anxiety and depression in later life: co-occurrence and communality of risk factors. Am J Psychiatry. 2000.

27. Meeks S, Woodruff-Borden J, Depp CA. Structural differentiation of self-reported depression and anxiety in late life. J Anxiety Disord. 2003.

28. Yochim BP, Mueller AE, June A, Segal DL. Psychometric properties of the geriatric anxiety scale: comparison to the beck anxiety inventory and geriatric anxiety inventory. Clin Gerontol. 2011.

29. Stanley MA, Novy DM, Bourland SL, Beck JG, Averill PM. Assessing older adults with generalized anxiety: a replication and extension. Behav Res Ther. 2001.

30. Carstensen LL, Edelstein BA, Dornbrand L, editors. The practical handbook of clinical gerontology. Pract Handb Clin Gerontol 1996.

31. Seignourel PJ, Kunik ME, Snow L, Wilson N, Stanley M. Anxiety in dementia: a critical review. Clin Psychol Rev. 2008.

32. Kogan JN, Edelstein BA, McKee DR. Assessment of anxiety in older adults: current status. J Anxiety Disord. 2000.

33. Badrakalimuthu VR, Tarbuck AF. Anxiety: a hidden element in dementia. Adv Psychiatr Treat. 2012.

34. Caputo F, Vignoli T, Leggio L, Addolorato G, Zoli G, Bernardi M. Alcohol use disorders in the elderly: a brief overview from epidemiology to treatment options. Exp Gerontol. 2012.

35. Rigler SK. Alcoholism in the elderly. Prim Care Companion J Clin Psychiatry. 2000.

36. Dell'Aglio JC Jr, Basso LA, de Argimon L II, Arteche A. Systematic review of the prevalence of bipolar disorder and bipolar spectrum disorders in population-based studies. Trends Psychiatry Psychother. 2013.

37. Reinhardt MM, Cohen CI. Late-life psychosis: diagnosis and treatment. Curr Psychiatry Rep. 2015.

38. Rozzini R, Vampini C, Ferranini L. La depressione nella persona che invecchia. Psicogeriatria 2015.

39. Dudek D, Rachel W, Cyranka K. Depression in older people. Encycl Biomed Gerontol. 2019.

40. Mitchell PB, Harvey SB. Depression and the older medical patient—when and how to intervene. Maturitas. 2014.

41. American Psychiatric Association. Diagnostic and Statistical Mental Disorders (DSM 5). 2013.

42. Uher R, Payne JL, Pavlova B, Perlis RH. Major depressive disorder in DSM-5: implications for clinical practice and research of changes from DSM-IV. Depress Anxiety. 2014.

43. Naismith SL, Norrie LM, Mowszowski L, Hickie IB. The neurobiology of depression in later-life: clinical, neuropsychological, neuroimaging and pathophysiological features. Prog Neurobiol. 2012.

44. Weisenbach SL, Kumar A. Current understanding of the neurobiology and longitudinal course of geriatric depression. Curr Psychiatry Rep. 2014.

45. Taylor WD. Depression in the elderly. N Engl J Med. 2014.

46. Altamura AC, Cattaneo E, Pozzoli S, Bassetti R. Inquadramento diagnostico e gestione farmacologica della depressione senile. Ital J Psychopathol. 2006.

47. Scaglione F, Vampini C, Parrino L, Zanetti O. Managing insomnia in the older people patient: from pharmacology to subthreshold depression. Riv Psichiatr. 2018;53(1):5–17.

48. Sachdev PS, Mohan A, Taylor L, Jeste DV. DSM-5 and mental disorders in older individuals: An overview. Harv Rev Psychiatry. 2015.

49. Cole MG, Dendukuri N. Risk factors for depression among elderly community subjects: a systematic review and meta-analysis. Am J Psychiatry. 2003.

50. Devanand DP. Comorbid psychiatric disorders in late life depression. Biol Psychiatry. 2002.

51. Alexopoulos GS, Buckwalter K, Olin J, Martinez R, Wainscott C, Krishnan KRR. Comorbidity of late life depression: an opportunity for research on mechanisms and treatment. Biol Psychiatry. 2002.

52. Richardson TM, He H, Podgorski C, Tu X, Conwell Y. Screening depression aging services clients. Am J Geriatr Psychiatry. 2010.

53. Yesavage JA, Brink TL, Rose TL, Lum O, Huang V, Adey M, et al. Development and validation of a geriatric depression screening scale: a preliminary report. J Psychiatr Res. 1982.

54. Spitzer RL, Kroenke K, Williams JBW. Validation and utility of a self-report version of PRIME-MD: the PHQ primary care study. J Am Med Assoc. 1999.

55. Pinals SL. The American Psychiatric Publishing Textbook of Geriatric Psychiatry, 3rd edition. J Nerv Ment Dis. 2005.

56. Van Orden K, Conwell Y. Suicides in late life. Curr Psychiatry Rep. 2011.

57. Rudd MD, Berman AL, Joiner TE, Nock MK, Silverman MM, Mandrusiak M, et al. Warning signs for suicide: theory, research, and clinical applications. Suicide Life-Threatening Behav. 2006.

58. Mottram PG, Wilson K, Strobl JJ. Antidepressants for depressed elderly. Cochrane Database Syst Rev. 2006.

59. Croom KF, Perry CM, Plosker GL. Mirtazapine: a review of its use in major depression and other psychiatric disorders. CNS Drugs. 2009.

60. Eyding D, Lelgemann M, Grouven U, Härter M, Kromp M, Kaiser T, et al. Reboxetine for acute treatment of major depression: systematic review and meta-analysis of published and unpublished placebo and selective serotonin reuptake inhibitor controlled trials. BMJ. 2010.

61. Karlsson I, Godderis J, De Mendonça Lima CA, Nygaard H, Simányi M, Taal M, et al. A randomised, double-blind comparison of the efficacy and safety of citalopram compared to mianserin in elderly, depressed patients with or without mild to moderate dementia. Int J Geriatr Psychiatry. 2000.

62. Mendelson WB. A review of the evidence for the efficacy and safety of trazodone in insomnia. J Clin Psychiatry. 2005.

63. Fagiolini A, Comandini A, Dell'Osso MC, Kasper S. Rediscovering trazodone for the treatment of major depressive disorder. CNS Drugs. 2012.

64. Sanchez C, Asin KE, Artigas F. Vortioxetine, a novel antidepressant with multimodal activity: review of preclinical and clinical data. Pharmacol Ther. 2015.

65. Pan Z, Grovu RC, Cha DS, Carmona NE, Subramaniapillai M, Shekotikhina M, et al. Pharmacological treatment of cognitive symptoms in major depressive disorder. CNS Neurol Disord—Drug Targets. 2018.

66. Alexopoulos GS, Katz IR, Reynolds CF, Carpenter D, Docherty JP. The expert consensus guideline series. Pharmacotherapy of depressive disorders in older patients. Postgrad Med. 2001.

67. Katz PR. Clinical geriatric psychopharmacology. J Am Geriatr Soc. 1993.

68. Roose SP, Schatzberg AF. The efficacy of antidepressants in the treatment of late-life depression. J Clin Psychopharmacol. 2005.

69. Stubbs B, Vancampfort D, Firth J, Schuch FB, Hallgren M, Smith L, et al. Relationship between sedentary behavior and depression: a mediation analysis of influential factors across the lifespan among 42,469 people in low- and middle-income countries. J Affect Disord. 2018.
70. Liu L, Gou Z, Zuo J. Social support mediates loneliness and depression in elderly people. J Health Psychol. 2016.
71. Nuss P. Anxiety disorders and GABA neurotransmission: a disturbance of modulation. Neuropsychiatr Dis Treat. 2015.
72. American Psychiatric Association. American Psychiatric Association: diagnostic and statistical manual of mental disorders, fourth edition, text revision. Am Psychiatr Assoc. 2000.
73. American Psychiatric Association. American Psychiatric Association: diagnostic and statistical manual of mental disorders, 5th edition. 2013.
74. Leray E, Camara A, Drapier D, Riou F, Bougeant N, Pelissolo A, et al. Prevalence, characteristics and comorbidities of anxiety disorders in France: results from the " mental health in general population" survey (MHGP). Eur Psychiatry. 2011.
75. Gili M, Comas A, García-García M, Monzón S, Antoni SB, Roca M. Comorbidity between common mental disorders and chronic somatic diseases in primary care patients. Gen Hosp Psychiatry. 2010.
76. Hasan SS, Clavarino AM, Dingle K, Mamun AA, Kairuz T. Diabetes mellitus and the risk of depressive and anxiety disorders in Australian women: a longitudinal study. J Women's Health. 2015.
77. Lin EHB, Von Korff M. Mental disorders among persons with diabetes-results from the world mental health surveys. J Psychosom Res. 2008.
78. Linden W, Vodermaier A, MacKenzie R, Greig D. Anxiety and depression after cancer diagnosis: prevalence rates by cancer type, gender, and age. J Affect Disord. 2012.
79. Tovilla-Zárate C, Juárez-Rojop I, Jimenez Y, Jiménez MA, Vázquez S, Bermúdez-Ocaña D, et al. Prevalence of anxiety and depression among outpatients with type 2 diabetes in the Mexican population. PLoS One. 2012.
80. King-Kallimanis B, Gum AM, Kohn R. Comorbidity of depressive and anxiety disorders for older Americans in the national comorbidity survey-replication. Am J Geriatr Psychiatry. 2009.
81. Hendriks SM, Spijker J, Licht CMM, Beekman ATF, Hardeveld F, De Graaf R, et al. Disability in anxiety disorders. J Affect Disord. 2014.
82. Association AP. American Psychiatric Association, 2013. Diagnostic and statistical manual of mental disorders (5th ed.). 2013.
83. Kessler RC, Avenevoli S, Costello EJ, Georgiades K, Green JG, Gruber MJ, et al. Prevalence, persistence, and sociodemographic correlates of DSM-IV disorders in the National Comorbidity Survey Replication Adolescent Supplement. Arch Gen Psychiatry. 2012.
84. Fernández A, Haro JM, Martinez-Alonso M, Demyttenaere K, Brugha TS, Autonell J, et al. Treatment adequacy for anxiety and depressive disorders in six European countries. Br J Psychiatry. 2007.
85. Hoge EA, Ivkovic A, Fricchione GL. Generalized anxiety disorder: diagnosis and treatment. BMJ. 2012.
86. Flint AJ. Generalised anxiety disorder in elderly patients: epidemiology, diagnosis and treatment options. Drugs Aging. 2005.
87. Craske MG, Kircanski K, Epstein A, Wittchen HU, Pine DS, Lewis-Fernández R, et al. Panic disorder: a review of DSM-IV panic disorder and proposals for DSM-V. Depress Anxiety. 2010.
88. Black DW, Grant JE. DSM-5® guidebook: the essential companion to the diagnostic and statistical manual of mental disorders. Am Psychiatr Publ. 2014.
89. Miloyan B, Bulley A, Pachana NA, Byrne GJ. Social phobia symptoms across the adult lifespan. J Affect Disord. 2014.
90. LeBeau RT, Glenn D, Liao B, Wittchen HU, Beesdo-Baum K, Ollendick T, et al. Specific phobia: a review of DSM-IV specific phobia and preliminary recommendations for DSM-V. Depress Anxiety. 2010.

91. Lach HW, Parsons JL. Impact of fear of falling in long term care: an integrative review. J Am Med Dir Assoc. 2013.
92. Bandelow B, Reitt M, Röver C, Michaelis S, Görlich Y, Wedekind D. Efficacy of treatments for anxiety disorders: a meta-analysis. Int Clin Psychopharmacol. 2015.
93. Pachana NA, Woodward RM, GJA B. Treatment of specific phobia in older adults. Clin Interv Aging. 2007.
94. Gonçalves DC, Byrne GJ. Interventions for generalized anxiety disorder in older adults: systematic review and meta-analysis. J Anxiety Disord. 2012.
95. Baldwin DS, Anderson IM, Nutt DJ, Bandelow B, Bond A, Davidson JRT, et al. Evidence-based guidelines for the pharmacological treatment of anxiety disorders: recommendations from the British Association for Psychopharmacology. J Psychopharmacol. 2005.
96. Holsboer-Trachsler E, Prieto R. Effects of pregabalin on sleep in generalized anxiety disorder. Int J Neuropsychopharmacol. 2013.
97. Pande AC, Crockatt JG, Feltner DE, Janney CA, Smith WT, Weisler R, et al. Pregabalin in generalized anxiety disorder: a placebo-controlled trial. Am J Psychiatry. 2003.
98. Gray SL, LaCroix AZ, Hanlon JT, Penninx BW, Blough DK, Leveille SG, et al. Benzodiazepine use and physical disability in community-dwelling older adults. J Am Geriatr Soc. 2006.
99. Petrov ME, Sawyer P, Kennedy R, Bradley LA, Allman RM. Benzodiazepine (BZD) use in community-dwelling older adults: longitudinal associations with mobility, functioning, and pain. Arch Gerontol Geriatr. 2014.
100. Wetherell JL, Stoddard JA, White KS, Kornblith S, Nguyen H, Andreescu C, et al. Augmenting antidepressant medication with modular CBT for geriatric generalized anxiety disorder: a pilot study. Int J Geriatr Psychiatry. 2011.
101. Witthöft M, Jasper F. Somatic symptom disorder. Encycl Ment Health Second Ed. 2016.
102. Kurlansik SL, Maffei MS. Somatic symptom disorder. Am Fam Physician. 2016.
103. Harris AM, Orav EJ, Bates DW, Barsky AJ. Somatization increases disability independent of comorbidity. J Gen Intern Med. 2009.
104. Creed F, Barsky A. A systematic review of the epidemiology of somatisation disorder and hypochondriasis. J Psychosom Res. 2004.
105. Den Boeft M, Claassen-Van Dessel N, Van Der Wouden JC. How should we manage adults with persistent unexplained physical symptoms? BMJ. 2017.
106. Allen LA, Woolfolk RL, Escobar JI, Gara MA, Hamer RM. Cognitive-behavioral therapy for somatization disorder: a randomized controlled trial. Arch Intern Med. 2006.
107. Kleinstäuber M, Witthöft M, Steffanowski A, van Marwijk H, Hiller W, Lambert MJ. Pharmacological interventions for somatoform disorders in adults. Cochrane Database Syst Rev. 2014.
108. Carvalho AF, Heilig M, Perez A, Probst C, Rehm J. Alcohol use disorders. Lancet. 2019.
109. Koob GF, Volkow ND. Neurobiology of addiction: a neurocircuitry analysis. Lancet Psychiatry. 2016.
110. Connor JP, Haber PS, Hall WD. Alcohol use disorders. Lancet. 2016.
111. Rehm J, Allamani A, Vedova R, Della EZ, Jakubczyk A, Landsmane I, et al. General practitioners recognizing alcohol dependence: a large cross-sectional study in 6 European Countries. Ann Fam Med. 2015.
112. Miller WR, Wilbourne PL. Mesa Grande: a methodological analysis of clinical trials of treatments for alcohol use disorders. Addiction. 2002.
113. Perry EC. Inpatient management of acute alcohol withdrawal syndrome. CNS Drugs. 2014.
114. Sinclair J, Chick J, Sørensen P, Kiefer F, Batel P, Gual A. Can alcohol dependent patients adhere to an "As-needed" medication regimen? Eur Addict Res. 2014.
115. Danielsson AK, Eriksson AK, Allebeck P. Technology-based support via telephone or web: a systematic review of the effects on smoking, alcohol use and gambling. Addict Behav. 2014.
116. White A, Kavanagh D, Stallman H, Klein B, Kay-Lambkin F, Proudfoot J, et al. Online alcohol interventions: a systematic review. J Med Internet Res. 2010.
117. Samamé C, Martino DJ, Strejilevich SA. A quantitative review of neurocognition in euthymic late-life bipolar disorder. Bipolar Disord. 2013.

118. Schouws SNTM, Stek ML, Comijs HC, Beekman ATF. Risk factors for cognitive impairment in elderly bipolar patients. J Affect Disord. 2010.
119. Kessing LV, Andersen PK. Does the risk of developing dementia increase with the number of episodes in patients with depressive disorder and in patients with bipolar disorder? J Neurol Neurosurg Psychiatry. 2004.
120. Almeida OP, Hankey GJ, Yeap BB, Golledge J, Norman PE, Flicker L. Mortality among people with severe mental disorders who reach old age: a longitudinal study of a community-representative sample of 37892 men. PLoS One. 2014.
121. Depp CA, Jeste DV. Bipolar disorder in older adults: a critical review. Bipolar Disord. 2004.
122. Sajatovic M. Maintenance treatment outcomes in older patients with bipolar I disorder. Am J Geriatr Psychiatry. 2005.
123. Jeste DV, Alexopoulos GS, Bartels SJ, Cummings JL, Gallo JJ, Gottlieb GL, et al. Consensus statement on the upcoming crisis in geriatric mental. Research agenda for the next 2 decades. Arch Gen Psychiatry. 1999.
124. Almeida OP, Fenner S. Bipolar disorder: similarities and differences between patients with illness onset before and after 65 years of age. Int Psychogeriatr. 2002.
125. Dols A, Beekman A. Older age bipolar disorder. Psychiatr Clin North Am. 2018.
126. Snowdon J. A retrospective case-note study of bipolar disorder in old age. Br J Psychiatry. 1991;
127. Shulman KI, Tohen M, Satlin A, Mallya G, Kalunian D. Mania compared with unipolar depression in old age. Am J Psychiatry. 1992.
128. Broadhead J, Jacoby R. Mania in old age: a first prospective study. Int J Geriatr Psychiatry. 1990.
129. Kessing LV. Diagnostic subtypes of bipolar disorder in older versus younger adults. Bipolar Disord. 2006.
130. McIntyre RS, Konarski JZ, Soczynska JK, Wilkins K, Panjwani G, Bouffard B, et al. Medical comorbidity in bipolar disorder: implications for functional outcomes and health service utilization. Psychiatr Serv. 2006.
131. Juurlink DN, Herrmann N, Szalai JP, Kopp A, Redelmeier DA. Medical illness and the risk of suicide in the elderly. Arch Intern Med. 2004.
132. Sajatovic M, Chen P. Geriatric bipolar disorder. Psychiatr Clin North Am. 2011.
133. Schouws SNTM, Comijs HC, Stek ML, Beekman ATF. Self-reported cognitive complaints in elderly bipolar patients. Am J Geriatr Psychiatry. 2012.
134. Gildengers AG, Butters MA, Seligman K, McShea M, Miller MD, Mulsant BH, et al. Cognitive functioning in late-life bipolar disorder. Am J Psychiatry. 2004.
135. Rise IV, Haro JM, Gjervan B. Clinical features, comorbidity, and cognitive impairment in elderly bipolar patients. Neuropsychiatr Dis Treat. 2016.
136. Dols A, Kessing LV, Strejilevich SA, Rej S, Tsai SY, Gildengers AG, et al. Do current national and international guidelines have specific recommendations for older adults with bipolar disorder? A brief report. Int J Geriatr Psychiatry. 2016.
137. Rybakowski JK, Abramowicz M, Chłopocka-Wozniak M, Czekalski S. Novel markers of kidney injury in bipolar patients on long-term lithium treatment. Hum Psychopharmacol. 2013.
138. Kessing LV, Forman JL, Andersen PK. Does lithium protect against dementia? Bipolar Disord. 2010.
139. Cipriani A, Hawton K, Stockton S, Geddes JR. Lithium in the prevention of suicide in mood disorders: updated systematic review and meta-analysis. BMJ. 2013.
140. Geddes JR, Burgess S, Hawton K, Jamison K, Goodwin GM. Long-term lithium therapy for bipolar disorder: systematic review and meta-analysis of randomized controlled trials. Am J Psychiatry. 2004.
141. Dunner DL. Drug interactions of lithium and other antimanic/mood-stabilizing medications. J Clin Psychiatry. 2003.
142. Cipriani A, Barbui C, Salanti G, Rendell J, Brown R, Stockton S, et al. Comparative efficacy and acceptability of antimanic drugs in acute mania: a multiple-treatments meta-analysis. Lancet. 2011.

143. Zimmerman M, Morgan TA, Hayati Rezvan P, Lee KJ, Simpson JA, National Institute for Health and Care Excellence (NICE). Bipolar disorder: assessment and management. Clinical guideline 185. Dialogues Clin Neurosci. 2015.
144. Pacchiarotti I, Bond DJ, Baldessarini RJ, Nolen WA, Grunze H, Licht RW, et al. The International Society for Bipolar Disorders (ISBD) task force report on antidepressant use in bipolar disorders. Am J Psychiatry. 2013.
145. American Psychiatric Association. DSM-5 diagnostic classification. Diagnostic and Statistical Manual of Mental Disorders. 2013.
146. Holroyd S, Laurie S. Correlates of psychotic symptoms among elderly outpatients. Int J Geriatr Psychiatry. 1999.
147. Webster J, Grossberg GT. Late-life onset of psychotic symptoms. Am J Geriatr Psychiatry. 1998.
148. Colijn MA, Nitta BH, Grossberg GT. Psychosis in later life: a review and update. Harv Rev Psychiatry. 2015.
149. Iglewicz A, Meeks TW, Jeste DV. New wine in old bottle: late-life psychosis. Psychiatr Clin North Am. 2011.
150. Psychiatric disorders in America: the epidemiologic catchment area study. Choice Rev Online. 1991.
151. Byeong KY, Hong N. Late-onset psychosis. Psychiatry Investig. 2007.
152. Perälä J, Suvisaari J, Saarni SI, Kuoppasalmi K, Isometsä E, Pirkola S, et al. Lifetime prevalence of psychotic and bipolar I disorders in a general population. Arch Gen Psychiatry. 2007.
153. Brunelle S, Cole MG, Elie M. Risk factors for the late-onset psychoses: a systematic review of cohort studies. Int J Geriatr Psychiatry. 2012.
154. Marsh CM. Psychiatric presentations of medical illness. Psychiatr Clin North Am. 1997.
155. Keshavan MS, Kaneko Y. Secondary psychoses: an update. World Psychiatry. 2013.
156. Karim S, Byrne EJ. Treatment of psychosis in elderly people. Adv Psychiatr Treat. 2005.
157. Inouye SK, Westendorp RGJ, Saczynski JS. Delirium in elderly people. Lancet. 2014.
158. Fong TG, Tulebaev SR, Inouye SK. Delirium in elderly adults: diagnosis, prevention and treatment. Nat Rev Neurol. 2009.
159. Fong TG, Davis D, Growdon ME, Albuquerque A, Inouye SK. The interface between delirium and dementia in elderly adults. Lancet Neurol. 2015.

Managing Urinary Incontinence

13

Pinar Soysal, Lee Smith, Luigi Maria Bracchitta,
Damiano Pizzol, and Carlos Verdejo-Bravo

Abstract

Urinary incontinence (UI) is the involuntary leakage of urine that has a multifactorial etiology and is common in the general population, increasing significantly with aging. The main causes are neurological disorders, delirium, urinary infections, atrophic urethritis and vaginitis, drugs as diuretics and psychoactive medications, psychological disorders, restricted mobility, and stool impaction. Considering the impact that UI may have on quality of life, it is crucial to make the diagnosis correctly, both by anamnesis collection and test performance, to provide effective treatment. The treatment, after exclusion and removal of reversible causes, includes lifestyle changes, behavioral and other non-pharmacological approaches, and pharmacological and surgical interventions.

Keywords

Urinary incontinence · Involuntary leakages · Geriatric urology · Urogynecologist

P. Soysal
Department of Geriatric Medicine, Faculty of Medicine, Bezmialem Vakif University,
Istanbul, Turkey

L. Smith
The Cambridge Centre for Sport & Exercise Sciences, Anglia Ruskin University,
Cambridge, UK

L. M. Bracchitta
Primary Care Department, Local Health Authority ATS Città Metropolitana di Milano,
Milan, Italy

D. Pizzol (✉)
Italian Agency for Development Cooperation, Khartum, Sudan
e-mail: damianopizzol8@gmail.com

C. Verdejo-Bravo
Department of Geriatrics, Hospital Universitario Clínico San Carlos, Madrid, Spain

© Springer Nature Switzerland AG 2022
J. Demurtas, N. Veronese (eds.), *The Role of Family Physicians in Older People Care*, Practical Issues in Geriatrics, https://doi.org/10.1007/978-3-030-78923-7_13

13.1   Introduction

Urinary incontinence (UI) is a geriatric syndrome with a multifactorial etiology, and its prevalence increases with aging. According to the International Continence Society (ICS), UI is defined as "the complaint of any involuntary leakage of urine" [1]. It is rarely expressed by the patient because it is considered a natural consequence of aging as well as a sense of shame. For these reasons, it is important that the physician questions and evaluates the condition adequately and accurately. Preventing, detecting, and treating UI increase quality of life and reduce morbidity and health expenditures.

13.2   Anatomy and Physiology

Cognitive, neurological, muscular, and urological system must be robust to maintain continence. Knowing the anatomy and physiology of these systems will facilitate the perception of pathophysiology [2–6].

The bladder consists of two functional units: the bladder body and the base. The bladder neck, placed in the base, is contracted during the filling of the bladder and allows the excretion of urine by opening simultaneously with the contraction of the detrusor muscle during the voiding. The urethra is about 3 cm long for women and about 20 cm long for men, and the sphincter zones allow the urine to be stored with continuous tonic activity and the voiding to start by relaxing at the appropriate time. The sphincter unit, located in the membranous urethra, has both intrinsic and extrinsic mechanisms. The neural stimuli of the filling, storage, and emptying functions of the bladder are complex. Peripheral nervous system stimuli of the bladder and urethra consist of sympathetic and parasympathetic autonomic stimuli and somatic stimuli. Bladder emptying occurs due to parasympathetic stimulation of cholinergic receptors by the contraction of detrusor muscle. The somatic nervous system controls the extrinsic urethral sphincter and pelvic floor muscles consisting of striated muscles. The central nervous system, especially the rostral pons and pontine voiding center, plays a fundamental role in the integration and coordination of the bladder and sphincter activities.

13.3   Changes in the Lower Urinary System with Age

The role of aging in the development of UI is more pronounced in women; as a result, the incidence of UI has a more rapid increase in older women than in men. In a study of nulliparous women, the incidence increased from 3% between 25 and 34 years to 7% between 55 and 64 years [7]. Changes in the lower urinary system (LUS) in both genders with aging are shown in Table 13.1 [8].

In women, the decrease in post-menopausal estrogen hormone levels is one of the important reasons that facilitate the development of UI. Lack of estrogen can

Table 13.1 Changes in lower urinary system with aging [8]

Ascending	Descending
Urinary flow rate	Residual volume after voiding
Detrusor contraction rate	Urinary frequency
Maximum bladder capacity	Obstruction of the bladder outlet pathway (in men)
Functional bladder capacity	
Bladder filling sensation	
Collagen-detrusor ratio (in women)	

Table 13.2 Results of age-related changes facilitating UI [14]

Alteration	The results
Detrusor muscle overactivity	Frequency, urgency, nocturia, UI
Benign prostatic hyperplasia	Output obstruction with frequency, urgency and nocturia, increased postvoid residual volume, overflow type UI
Excessive urine output at night	Nocturia, nocturnal UI
Atrophic vaginitis, urethritis	Thinning, irritation, urge and stress in the urethral mucosa UI, UTI
Increased postvoidal residue	Frequency, nocturia, UI
Reduction in retention of micturation	Frequency, urgency, nocturia, UI
Decrease in bladder capacity	Frequency, urgency, nocturia, UI
Decreased detrusor contractility	Decreased flow rate, increased postvoid residual volume, hesitancy, UI

lead to atrophy of the urethral mucosa, vaginal atrophy, stress, and urge-type incontinence due to decreased supportive tissue surrounding the urethra [8, 9].

The incidence of benign prostatic hyperplasia (BPH) increasing with age is one of the main factors involved in the development of UI in men. With the growth of the prostate gland, decrease in urinary flow rate, increase in residual volume after voiding, increase in urinary frequency, and obstruction of the bladder outlet pathway may occur [8, 10]. The risk of acute urinary retention in an untreated man with symptomatic BPH was found to be 2.5% per year [11].

Nocturia is a symptom that is seen in 25–50% of older healthy people, with its important consequences due to deterioration of sleep quality and falls. Its prevalence and episodes increase with age. The overall prevalence of nocturia is reported to increase by an average of 2–3% per year after the age of 60 years [12, 13].

Changes in age-related immune functions, hormonal changes, deterioration of hygiene conditions, and increasing incidence of comorbid diseases may facilitate urinary tract infections that are among the correctable causes of UI (Table 13.2) [15].

13.4   Epidemiology of Urinary Incontinence

Lower urinary tract symptoms (LUTS) and UI are common in the general population, and the incidence increases with age. In the EPIC study, 19,000 men and women aged 40 years and over were included, and the number of participants with at least one LUTS was >60% [16]. The most common LUTS was reported as nocturia. The incidence of LUTS (nocturia, urgency, frequency) and UI has been shown to increase with age in both genders. In a study conducted in nulliparous women, the incidence of UI in those aged 25–34 years increased from 3% to 7% in those aged 55–64 years [7]. When the prevalence of moderate-severe UI in community-dwelling women was examined, it was reported that it was 7%, 17%, 23%, and 32% in those aged 20–39, 40–49, 60–79, and ≥80 years, respectively [17]. When the individuals living in nursing homes were examined, it was shown that the prevalence of UI was 54.5% and that it was higher in women (59.8%) than in men (39.2%) [18]. In the studies involving both genders, the prevalence of UI was found to be between 11% and 34% in men older than 65 years and about twice the frequency in women [19], This frequency increases significantly in individuals living in nursing homes and varies between 43% and 77%. In the studies, 45 different risk factors were identified. Specifically, it has been shown that there is a relationship between UI and gender, age, dementia, and mobility ability [20]. When older people with and without UI are compared, it is seen that individuals with incontinence have a higher risk of being placed in an institution [21].

In a study conducted in older individuals in Turkey, in which the prevalence of UI was 44.2%, incontinence rate was 57.1% in women and 21.5% in men [22]. It was reported that mixed-type incontinence affected 70.1% of women (urge and stress type) and urge type incontinence affected 56.4% of men; these are the most common clinical types of UI. Approximately 62% of women and 73% of men included in the study were shown to have psychosocial effects due to UI. Stress incontinence is the most common type of UI in young women, while the incidence of urge and mixed-type UI increases in older women [23, 24]. In males, urge UI is the most common type in almost all age groups [25].

13.5   Quality of Life in UI

The main negative effect of UI is on quality of life and can lead to loss of self-confidence and social isolation. It is estimated that about 20% of community-dwelling older adults have incontinence to limit their daily life activities. Often, affected individuals deny and hide urinary incontinence, which results in physical and psychosocial restrictions to the enjoyment in life. It is also known that UI can be associated with major neurological damage which can be functional or iatrogenic. In older people with incontinence, negative results such as anxiety, depression, deterioration in sexual life, and decrease in physical activity may occur [26]. When the relationship with major depression is examined, it is seen that urge UI carries a greater risk than stress UI [24]. In addition to its medical and social adverse effects, the high economic cost of UI is also an important factor to be considered. It is estimated that approximately $32 billion is spent annually in the United States (US) for the diagnosis and treatment of UI, which costs greater than the sum of money spent on dialysis and coronary by-pass surgery. The cost of adult diapers is estimated to be around $6 billion, which is almost doubled per decade. It is estimated that approximately 1 h a day is spent for UI and the care for every patient with incontinence, especially for patients staying in nursing homes, and its annual cost is approximately $10,000 per patient [26, 27].

13.6 Etiology of Urinary Incontinence

Cognitive, neurological, muscular, and urological system must be robust to maintain continence. Consciousness, motivation, comprehension, and attention processes must be harmonized in order for voiding to take place at the appropriate time. Muscle and joint systems also play an important role in reaching the bathroom. Muscle and joint disorders that affect mobility may also result in incontinence.

Age-related changes in the urinary system may also predispose to incontinence in a continent old patient. Fluid intake, self-mobility, and diuretic treatment may influence diuresis and thus UI. As in almost every problem in older people, more than one cause may be involved in the etiology of UI. As with all medical conditions, the cause(s) should be elucidated for an effective treatment plan. For a clinical approach to UI, it may be useful to distinguish the etiology as acute or transient and chronic or persistent causes.

13.7 Acute and Transient Causes of Urinary Incontinence

If acute causes are eliminated, UI can improve. These factors can be recalled briefly by using a mnemonic device with the initials of their English equivalents ("DIAPPERS") and are shown in Table 13.3 [28].

Delirium: A patient with delirium may not be aware of the fullness of the bladder or the need for voiding. It can also be difficult for the patient to find the bathroom in time. Delirium can often be due to infections, metabolic disorders, or drugs. As a result of the elimination of the underlying cause, the delirium picture is solved with the resultant improvement of UI.

Table 13.3 Acute and correctable causes of urinary incontinence	Delirium
	Infection-urinary
	Atrophic urethritis and vaginitis
	Pharmaceuticals
	Psychologic disorders, especially depression
	Excessive urine output (e.g., from heart failure or hyperglycemia)
	Restricted mobility
	Stool impaction

Table 13.4 Drugs having effects on continence

Medicine	The effect on continence
Alcohol	Frequency, urgency, sedation, and increased immobility
α-Adrenergic agonists	Outflow obstruction (male)
α-Adrenergic blockers	Stress type incontinence (in woman)
ACE inhibitors	Increase in stress UI by causing cough
Anticholinergics	Impaired bladder emptying, retention, delirium, sedation, constipation, fecal plug
Antipsychotics	Anticholinergic effects, rigidity, and immobility
Calcium channel blockers	Impaired detrusor contraction and retention; ankle edema due to dihydropyridine group agents and nocturnal polyuria secondary to it
Cholinesterase inhibitors	UI, interaction with antimuscarinic agents
Estrogen (systemic)	Worsening of stress and mixed-type UI (in woman)
GABAergic agents (gabapentin and pregabalin)	Edema and secondary nocturia, nocturnal UI
Loop diuretics	Polyuria, frequency, urgency
Narcotic analgesics	Urinary retention, fecal plug, sedation, delirium
NSAIDs	Ankle edema and nocturnal polyuria secondary to it
Sedative hypnotics	Sedation, delirium, immobility
Thiazolidinediones	Ankle edema and nocturnal polyuria secondary to it

ACE angiotensin-converting enzyme, *GABA* γ-aminobutyric acid, *NSAID* non-steroidal anti-inflammatory drug

Infection: Urinary tract infections may lead to an increase in physiological sensory stimulation from the bladder mucosa and pathologically to urgency and urge incontinence. Incontinence is also a risk factor for the development of urinary tract infection.

Atrophic vaginitis and urethritis may cause incontinence by simulating or predisposing to urinary tract infection symptoms. Atrophic and inflamed urethral tissue due to estrogen deficiency may result in urgency and urge incontinence due to hypersensitivity.

Drugs that are *pharmacological agents* as diuretics, anticholinergic agents, and opioids may be involved in the etiology of incontinence in different ways. Drugs that cause sedation may also impair the ability of an old individual to access the bathroom. Drugs with effects on continence are shown in Table 13.4 [29].

For *psychological reasons*, serious depression should also be emphasized, which may disrupt the bathroom motivation.

As for endocrinological reasons, hyperglycemia, diabetes insipidus, and hypercalcemia (diabetes mellitus) leading to osmotic diuresis may result in polyuria to produce UI.

Restriction of mobility may be responsible for UI by prolonging access to the bathroom.

Stool impaction: The presence of fecal impaction may cause bladder outlet obstruction due to compression effect, with the consequent urinary retention.

13.8 Chronic and Persistent Causes of Urinary Incontinence

Incontinence due to chronic causes can be divided into five groups: urge (stress), stress, mixed, overflow, and functional [6].

Urge incontinence refers to incontinence resulting from the inability to delay the need for voiding stimulated by filling the bladder sufficiently. Urge incontinence is the most common cause of UI in men and women over 65 years of age. It occurs due to early and sudden contraction of the detrusor muscle through the transmission of non-repressible stimuli [6, 30]. Although the terms overactive bladder (OAB) and urge incontinence are used interchangeably, they refer to different conditions. OAB, a syndrome of the symptoms including frequency, urgency, and nocturia, may or may not be associated with urge incontinence [30, 31]. Although the most common cause of urge incontinence is intractable detrusor muscle contractions, local urinary conditions with mucosal stimulation, such as cystitis, urethritis, tumors, and stones, can also lead to "urgency" and urge incontinence. Bladder neck obstruction may also be presented with urgency and urge incontinence [6, 30]. Stress incontinence is the involuntary incontinence occurring in situations that increase intra-abdominal pressure, such as coughing and laughing. It usually causes a small amount of UI. The main reason is that the output path resistance is reduced, which is due to giving birth, pelvic surgery, and weakening of the pelvic muscle base secondary to menopause, bladder outlet pathway, and urethral sphincter weakness due to previous pelvic surgeries. Sphincter-associated incontinence can also be seen in men who have undergone prostate surgery. Urinary incontinence may occur in such patients with a slight strain because of the loss of effective urethral sphincter function. α-Adrenergic antagonists may cause bladder outlet to remain open, leading to stress incontinence. Obesity is also a risk factor for stress UI [6, 29, 31].

Overflow incontinence is a condition caused by exceeding bladder volume, accompanied by an overstretched detrusor muscle. Patients often suffer frequent but small amounts of leakages, expressing they feel they cannot empty their bladder. There are two possible causes of overflow incontinence: outflow obstruction or less running or denervated detrusor muscle. The common cause of outflow obstruction in men is the enlarged prostate gland. Urethral stricture due to previous infections or catheterization may also lead to obstruction. In women, a large cystocele can prevent urine flow by compressing the urethra. Impaired detrusor muscle activity is often associated with impaired muscle innervation or use of drugs as α-adrenergic agonist [6, 29, 31].

Mixed incontinence is a common condition where urge and stress incontinence coexist. It is important to determine the severity of each component because the patient's symptoms and treatment are particularly directed to the dominant component. In a patient with stress-dominant mixed incontinence, it would be appropriate to treat the stress component first. Functional incontinence occurs when a patient has limited access to the bathroom secondary to a problem other than the urinary system. Causes include dementia, depression, impaired physical functionality, and/or environmental barriers.

13.9 Evaluation of Urinary Incontinence in Older People

13.9.1 Targets

It is crucial to make the diagnosis of UI correctly to provide effective treatment [32]. Nevertheless, only 20–25% of individuals with UI seek medical support [33, 34]. For these reasons, it is important to question each older individual for UI at each visit. Screening questions can be the following: "When you feel you are in need of voiding urgently, do you loss a little bit of urine before you reach the toilet?" "Do you loss a little bit of urine by coughing, sneezing or laughing?" [35].

First of all, the presence of UI is confirmed in a patient describing incontinence. Then it will be appropriate to identify correctable transient factors. If possible, typing should be made in persistent UI cases. It is important to distinguish those that require further examination before starting treatment [6, 34]. In evaluating UI, it is essential to detect how much incontinence affects the functionality and quality of life of the individual. There are over 40 validated questionnaires to assess its impact on quality of life, some of which are "Incontinence Quality of Life Scale" (I-QOL), "International Consultation on Incontinence Questionnaire-Short Form" (ICIQ-SF), and "SEAPI-QMM Incontinence Classification System" [36].

Basic assessment of UI is possible by history, physical examination, coughing test for women who need voiding urgently, determination of the post-voiding residual (PVR) by ultrasonography or catheterization, blood biochemistry (creatinine, potassium, calcium, glucose), and complete urinalysis (CU). If there are signs suggestive of infection in CU, it would be appropriate to study urine culture. A practical approach to UI is shown in Fig. 13.1 [31].

13.9.2 What Should Be Considered in the Anamnesis?

Recurrent urinary tract infections, kidney disease, diabetes, congestive heart failure, and venous insufficiency should be questioned in the history. The presence of multiple sclerosis, Parkinson's disease, stroke, and dementia is crucial among neurological diseases. Other conditions that impair physical functionality should be questioned. Bowel habits should be detailed for constipation and fecal incontinence. Symptoms of depression should be taken into consideration. While taking anamnesis, questions should be asked to elaborate the characteristics of incontinence. The time of onset; timing of incontinence during the day (day and/or night); duration; course of severity over time; benefits from previous treatment interventions, if any; the presence of lower urinary tract symptoms; frequency; urgency; dysuria; and nocturia should be determined. Conditions that trigger and facilitate incontinence should be identified. For example, increased incontinence by coughing, sneezing, or laughing indicates stress incontinence. Urge incontinence is thought to be present in a patient who needs to void urgently and cannot reach the bathroom. A similar complaint may also be observed in overflow-type incontinence. Decreased or interrupted urinary flow, difficulty in urination, dripping, and a feeling of incomplete

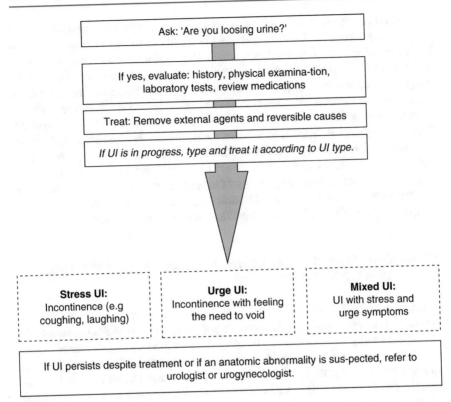

Fig. 13.1 The approach to the UI

emptying signify dysfunctional voiding, suggesting overflow-type incontinence. This is primarily related to an increase in prostate volume in male patients. The presence of hematuria without urinary tract infection always requires further investigation, as it may be due to an underlying bladder or kidney disease.

The determination of the type, amount, and timing of fluid intake is important. Drinks containing caffeine, alcohol consumption, and liquids, especially before bedtime, can facilitate incontinence. Careful examination of prescription and non-prescription drugs is essential. Especially diuretics, sedative agents, anticholinergics, and psychotropic drugs are frequently involved in the etiology. There are many drugs with anticholinergic effects that can disrupt the contraction of the detrusor muscle. While cholinesterase inhibitors can cause "urgency," α-blockers may have adverse effects on urethral sphincter functions. The drugs to be considered are listed in Table 13.4 [29]. In women, symptoms of organ prolapse, history of surgical treatment for incontinence or prolapse treatment, and history of urinary retention or radiotherapy should be questioned. The 3-day urine diary to be kept by the patient or the caregiver is useful in the diagnosis and evaluation of the response to initiated treatment [36].

It would be appropriate for the patient not to change any dietary/beverage habits while keeping the urine diary. To measure the volume of urine, the patient needs to use a measured or known container, which offers information on the urine measured, functional bladder capacity, voiding pattern, and incontinence and can give insight into the possible cause of incontinence. The disadvantage of the urine diary is that it can be difficult for patients to understand and apply it. Therefore, it should be adequately explained to the patient and/or the caregiver how it should be applied. Daily voiding pattern; frequency; volume; the moments, characteristics, and time of the incontinence; and the properties of drinks are specified. The history should also include information about the patient's environment. Whether there are any obstacles in accessing the bathroom, whether the walker fits in the bathroom if any, or whether lighting is sufficient should be detailed, in which case it would be appropriate to obtain sufficient information from the patient or the caregiver.

13.9.3 What Should Be Considered in Physical Examination [8, 29–31, 34, 37]?

Physical examination should be performed holistically, especially in abdominal, genital, pelvic, and neurological aspects. In addition, it will be useful to evaluate the patient's mobility and cognition. The patient's cognition can be examined with a cognitive screening test appropriate to the educational level. The patient's dexterity should be evaluated in terms of being able to unbutton and take off clothes. Gait and balance should be evaluated. A physical examination should be performed in terms of abdominal tenderness, palpable mass, and especially globe vesical. In men, examination of the penis body and glans penis, testes, and skin characteristics should be evaluated. The presence of fecal plugs and masses should be investigated by rectal examination. Since the anal and urethral sphincters innervate the same nerve roots (S2–S4), there are maneuvers that can be used to assess the neurological integrity of the lower urinary tract. Examination of sensory sensation in the hip and perianal region allows the examination of the afferent cycle of the reflex arch. The voluntary contraction of the anal sphincter also indicates that the motor components of nerve roots S2–S4 are intact. Another maneuver in the evaluation of neural innervation is anal reflex. The gentle stimulation of the perianal skin by means of a rod is the expected response to contraction of the external anal sphincter. Bulbocavernosus reflex can also be used to evaluate sensory and motor cycles. An open anus indicates paralysis of the anal sphincter, but distension secondary to chronic constipation and previous rectal surgery may lead to similar findings. Inspection of the vagina in women is necessary for the detection of atrophy findings. Atrophic epithelium is pale, flat, and bright. Patchy erythema and petechiae areas are also frequently accompanied. The presence of pediatric speculum and cystocele, uterine prolapse, vaginal dome prolapse, enterocele, and rectocele should be investigated in elderly women. The provocation test of the filled bladder should be performed as part of the pelvic examination. The patient is made to strain and cough in the supine position when he/she wants to void urgently. UI at the time of the maneuver indicates stress incontinence, and delayed incontinence refers to urge incontinence due to bladder contractions triggered by coughing.

13.9.4 Which Tests Should Be Performed [6, 31, 38]?

Routine blood biochemistry (especially BUN, creatinine, glucose, calcium, potassium) and CUA should be studied in all patients with incontinence. In the case of finding favorable infection in CUA, urine culture should be studied, and appropriate antibiotherapy should be given. It has been shown that the treatment of asymptomatic bacteriuria in patients living in a nursing home has no positive effect on UI [39]. Urinary system ultrasonography and urine cytology should be examined in patients with persistent hematuria without infection. If abnormal findings are detected, they should be referred to the urologist for further examination. Postvoid residual volume can be determined by ultrasonography or catheterization. Postvoid residual volume above 100–150 cc (particularly >200 cc) confirms the presence of urinary retention. In summary, it will be possible to confirm the presence of UI in the patient and to determine the reversible causes by making the abovementioned evaluations. After exclusion of reversible causes, chronic UI typing can be performed in most patients, and the underlying cause can be determined. After these evaluations, cases that require further examination should be referred to a urologist or urogynecologist. Urodynamic tests should be applied to patients who cannot be diagnosed with baseline tests, who do not respond with empirical treatment, or who are scheduled for surgery. Urodynamic tests are not a single procedure but involve five different maneuvers, which include filling and voiding cystometry, non-invasive and invasive uroflowmetry, simultaneous sphincter electromyography, urethral pressure profilometry, and radiographic imaging in indicated cases. Cystoscopy may also be particularly useful in patients with hematuria or recurrent urinary tract infection.

13.9.5 Which Cases Should Be Referred to a Urologist or Urogynecologist?

Such cases are those who have uncertainty in the diagnosis after the abovementioned evaluations and/or fail to provide adequate bladder emptying and/or those without inadequate response to empirical treatments, and/or those who require invasive procedures such as surgery and/or those who have a history of previous surgical intervention for the lower urinary tract, and/or those with hematuria and suspected urine cytology without infection, all presented in Table 13.5 [6, 31].

Table 13.5 Conditions requiring the older patient to be referred to urologist or urogynecologist for further examination

Example	Reason
A history of surgery or radiotherapy for the pelvic region or lower urinary tract in the last 6 months	Suspected structural abnormalities due to the procedure
A history of ≥2–3 symptomatic urinary tract infections in the last 1 year	Suspected structural abnormality that paves the way for infection
Significant pelvic organ prolapses or prostate enlargement	Suspected anatomic abnormalities or exclusion of BPH and prostate cancer
Residual volume over 200 mL	Anatomical or neurological abnormalities suspected
Difficulty passing urethra with 14-F Foley catheter	Suspected anatomic obstruction
Hematuria (≥3–5 RBC/HPF) without known etiology	Lower urinary tract pathologies without inflammatory in TIT
Lack of response to UI despite adequate and appropriate treatment	Urodynamic examination to guide treatment

13.10 Treatment of Chronic Urinary Incontinence

UI treatment is directed to the underlying cause. Treatment for chronic causes after exclusion or removal of reversible causes (DIAPPERS) includes lifestyle changes, behavioral and other non-pharmacological approaches, and pharmacological and surgical interventions. The first step for a patient is to ensure that he/she has sufficient access to the bathroom. For this, adaptive clothing should be used in patients with handicap problems, and improved mobility should be considered in those with limited mobility. Lifestyle changes are among the procedures that should be recommended to all patients [6]. It should be recommended for patients with excessive or low fluid intake to increase fluid intake and to avoid late fluid intake. Avoiding caffeine-containing or carbonated beverages is helpful in improving frequency and urgency symptoms and quality of life. Weight loss of individuals with obesity (especially women) leads to a reduction in UI symptoms. Quitting smoking should be offered to the patient within the scope of general health recommendations, but it is not shown to have a significant effect on UI. In older women, moderate exercise has been shown to be associated with lower UI rates [40]. If diuretic medication is required for another reason, it would be appropriate to avoid taking it in the evening. Pad use is not recommended alone but can be considered as an expert opinion in men and women with mild UI, which may be preferred in refractory patients or in those with motivational loss [40]. To prevent and treat dermatitis due to pad use, regular perineal cleansing, humidification, and incontinence-related barrier against moisture may be considered. Topical antifungal, steroid-based topical anti-inflammatory, and topical antibiotics may be added to treatment in appropriate cases [41].

13.10.1   Urge Incontinence Treatment

Behavioral treatment methods, such as bladder training, are the first choice for treatment of urge incontinence after lifestyle changes. Bladder training requires adequate cognitive and physical function and motivation. Patients are advised to urinate at specified intervals even if they are not in need of any. This is an effective method of reducing the incidence of incontinence but requires that the patient to be cognitively healthy and sufficiently motivated [29, 31]. In another method, the bladder suppression technique, if the patient needs to void, is recommended for him/her to focus attention on something else until he/she reaches the bathroom by contracting his/her pelvic muscles five times in a row. Although behavioral therapies are beneficial in the treatment of UI in women, the benefit disappears when interrupted. There is no consistent evidence that bladder training is better than drug treatments. Combination of bladder training with antimuscarinic agents has not been shown to make a major change in UI healing. Bladder training is superior to the use of pessary alone [40]. Kegel exercises, known as pelvic floor muscle rehabilitation, are used to treat urge and stress UI. The aim is to prevent involuntary detrusor contractions and to improve voluntary external sphincter contraction by repetitive muscle and relaxation movements of pelvic floor muscles. This method has been shown to reduce UTI episodes [29]. The beneficial effect of these exercises persists in older patients in a similar way to young people [40]. Learning and performing these exercises in the presence of a physiotherapist who is interested in UI can increase the effectiveness and patient compliance. Continuing these exercises with bladder training is a more effective treatment strategy.

Scheduled bathroom training (timed voiding) is carried out by a caregiver at regular intervals, usually by placing the patient on the toilet seat every 2 h during the day and every 4 h during the night. It may be preferred in individuals with cognitive impairment, and the aim is to prevent incontinence episodes rather than correct the normal pattern of urination. This method requires a highly motivated caregiver to be successful [42]. Pharmacological methods are used to increase bladder capacity by suppressing detrusor muscle contractions. These agents play a role in the treatment by competitively inhibiting muscarinic receptors with their anticholinergic effects. There are seven anticholinergic agents (oxybutynin, tolterodine, fesoterodine, trospium, propiverine, darifenacin, and solifenacin) that can be used in different doses and formulations. Studies have shown that the effects of these agents on urgency and UI, frequency, nocturia, increase in the volume of urine in each voiding, patient's satisfaction, and quality of life were similar [34, 40]. Dose frequency, drug interactions, potential side effects, and cost should be considered in the selection of these agents with similar efficacy. Antimuscarinic agents, especially oxybutynin, should be used with caution in patients with cognitive impairment or in older patients when it is used together with antihistamines or cytochrome system inhibitors. It is recommended that antimuscarinic agents should be started at the lowest dose and reevaluated after 2–4 weeks although they are generally well tolerated, and the most common side effects are orthostatic hypotension and dizziness [43].

Desmopressin decreases urinary volume by increasing the reabsorption of water from the renal tubule, and when used to reduce urinary frequency at night, it acts for about 6 h, providing symptomatic treatment; however, it should be used carefully as it may cause hyponatremia in older people [44].

Mirabegron, a β3-adrenoceptor agonist that can be used in the treatment of urge UI, improves bladder filling as well as urge symptoms and UI, with relaxation of the detrusor muscle. Similar results have been obtained in studies with solabegron, but data are limited. Increased blood pressure and heart rate, nasopharyngitis, and urinary tract infection are the expected side effects [31, 45, 46]. The use of topical estrogen in the vaginal region has been shown to improve urge UI symptoms in postmenopausal women with vaginal atrophy [40]. In appropriate cases, estrogen-containing ring therapy can be used for long periods [47]. Finally, according to the characteristics and preferences of the patients, advanced treatment methods include percutaneous tibial nerve stimulation, sacral neuromodulation, intravesical botulinum toxin (Botox) application, bladder expansion operation, and urinary diversion operation [31].

The pharmacological and non-pharmacological approaches used in the treatment of urge UI are summarized in Table 13.6.

13.10.2 Stress Incontinence

Some non-surgical interventions may be useful in patients with stress incontinence. Pelvic floor muscle exercises (e.g., Kegel exercises) may reduce incontinence episodes [45]. Devices such as biofeedback and intravaginal electrical stimulators or pessaries may be useful in selected patients with pelvic organ prolapse [34]. Since the use of pessaries requires manual dexterity, they may be limited in older patients as well as in patients with limited dexterity. Pseudoephedrine and duloxetine may be used as a pharmacological treatment option [31]. Pseudoephedrine has a sympathomimetic effect on α and β receptors. Since the risk of side effects rises with increasing doses, it is appropriate to start with a single dose in older patients [48]. Duloxetine, a serotonin and noradrenaline re-uptake inhibitor (SNRI), is an approved agent for the treatment of stress UI in Europe. Pudendal motor neuron, acting by stimulating α-adrenergic and 5HT2 receptors, was shown to improve stress and mixed-type UI at a dose of 80 mg/day in female patients. It has been reported that it also may be beneficial when used in similar doses for stress incontinence in male patients. At the indicated doses, the rate of discontinuation of treatment is high due to duloxetine-induced gastrointestinal and CNS side effects. It should also be kept in mind that there may be an increase in blood pressure due to the use of duloxetine. It is recommended to start at low doses and gradually increase the dose [40]. Imipramine, a tricyclic antidepressant, can be used with α-adrenergic and anticholinergic properties and stress UI, but its use is very limited, especially in older people, due to its anticholinergic side effects [34]. There is limited data that topical estrogen use in the vaginal region reduces stress UI in women. Systemic estrogen use is known to increase UI [31].

Table 13.6 Pharmacological and non-pharmacological approaches used in the treatment of UI (adapted from source [44])

UI type	Medicine	Dose/daily	Non-pharmacological approach
Urge	Oxybutynin	5 mg	Lifestyle change
	Tolterodine	1–2 mg	Clock voiding
	Fesoterodine	4–8 mg	Pelvic floor muscle training
	Trospium	30–45 mg	Vaginal cone exercise
	Propiverine	15 mg	
	Darifenacin	7.5–15 mg	
	Solifenacin	5–10 mg	
	Mirabegron	25–50 mg	
	Topical estrogen	100 µg estradiol or 1 mg estriol[a]	
Stress	Ephedrine	30–60 mg	Lifestyle change
	Pseudoephedrine	30–60 mg	Electrical stimulation
	Estrogen	Topical	Biofeedback
	Imipramine	10–20 mg	Pessary application
	Duloxetine	30–60 mg	
Mixed	*Treatment is planned according to dominant UI type*		*Treatment is planned according to dominant UI type*
Overflow	Prazosin	3–15 mg	Lifestyle change
	Terazosin	1–10 mg	Clean intermittent catheterization
	Doxazoine	1–8 mg	
	Tamsulosin	0.4–0.8 mg	
	Bethanechol	10–50 mg	

[a]In topical estrogen administration, it is recommended to apply the dose indicated daily for 2 weeks followed by administration twice a week [47]

Pharmacological and non-pharmacological approaches used in the treatment of stress UI are summarized in Table 13.6. Surgical treatment may be particularly helpful in patients with stress incontinence secondary to urethral hypermobility and who do not sufficiently benefit from behavioral or pelvic floor muscle exercises [31]. Surgical treatment procedures include:

- Sling (autologous, cadaveric, synthetic).
- Bladder neck support (Burch urethropexy, vaginal support).

13.10.3 Overflow Incontinence

The common cause of BPH in men is obstruction at secondary bladder outlet. Although it is rare in women, a similar picture may develop due to organ prolapse. It should be borne in mind that bladder or prostate-induced malignancies may cause overflow-type UI in patients. Overflow incontinence secondary to obstruction usually requires surgical intervention. For example, in a male case, transurethral resection of the prostate is the treatment option in overflow-type incontinence secondary to benign prostatic hypertrophy (BPH) leading to obstruction [34]. All prescription and over-the-counter (OTC) drugs causing anticholinergic and α-adrenergic agonist effects that may impair detrusor muscle contractility should be questioned in each patient with overflow-type incontinence [34]. For example, common drugs used in the symptomatic treatment of colds may include an anticholinergic agent as antihistamine capable of disrupting detrusor muscle contraction and a decongestant with α-agonistic action which may bring about contractions in bladder neck sphincters. Therefore, the use of this drug combination in an older patient with underlying BPH may lead to urinary retention and overflow-type incontinence. In this case, BPH secondary obstruction may be considered, yet there is a urinary retention triggered by the drugs used, and the treatment is not transurethral resection, but catheter placement and decompression of the bladder and discontinuation of responsible drugs. If urethral catheterization fails in high-risk, unstable patients, adequate urinary drainage can be achieved by placing a suprapubic catheter. During follow-up, the bladder voiding function should be restored with bladder gymnastics.

The use of α-blockers may be preferred to increase urine output in patients who are not suitable for surgical intervention. The use of α-blockers is discussed under the title of "urge UI treatment." If the use of α-blockers is not sufficient in patients with BPH, 5-α reductase inhibitors, finasteride or dutasteride, may be added to the treatment. Inhibition of this enzyme, which converts intracellular testosterone to more potent dihydrotestosterone, reduces androgenic prostate stimulation, minimizing prostate volume. A combination with α-blockers may be considered in patients with BPH, causing severe symptoms, prostate volume 40 mL and above, PSA > 1.5 ng/mL, which is slowly effective and suitable to use for 3–6 months for full efficacy. Side effects such as decrease in the amount of ejaculation, sexual dysfunction, and gynecomastia may be seen in men [34]. Tadalafil, a phosphodiesterase type 5 inhibitor (PDE5), was thought to have an effect on bladder neck and smooth muscle relaxation in the prostate and approved by the FDA in 2011 for the treatment of BPH. The use of concomitant PDE5 inhibitors should be avoided in patients taking nitrate due to hypotension [34, 49]. There is a small study showing that intraprostatic administration of botulinum toxin has positive effects on BPH-related lower urinary tract symptoms [34]. The pharmacological and non-pharmacological approaches used in the treatment of urge UI are summarized in Table 13.6. There is no effective pharmacological agent to stimulate bladder voiding. Using the Credé maneuver (manual compression of the lower abdomen) may be helpful in increasing the volume.

Clean intermittent catheterization (TAC) is performed in patients with overflow-type incontinence due to loss of detrusor muscle contraction function. Transurethral or suprapubic catheterization is the only option if the patient or caregiver cannot perform TAC.

Indications for Transurethral or Suprapubic Catheterization
1. Urinary retention
2. Urinary incontinence

> And open sacral ulcers or perineal wounds
> And palliative care or patient preference

3. Sensitive monitoring of urine output (e.g., monitoring in the ICU or inability of the patient to accumulate urine properly)
4. After general or spinal anesthesia

13.10.4 Functional Incontinence

Cognitive impairment can be the cause of development of UI due to creating difficulty in accessing the bathroom due to limitation of mobility or environmental barriers. Treatment is based on environmental regulations or behavioral approaches in care. In order to facilitate access to the bathroom, an assessment should be made for the use of auxiliary devices such as walking sticks, walkers, wheelchairs, handrails in the bathroom, and bedside bathroom sets [31]. In patients with dementia, other etiologies (stress, urge, or overflow type) should be considered before the UI symptoms can be attributed to cognitive impairment. Some behavioral approaches, the most commonly used of which is timed voiding, should be applied in patients with cognitive impairment or movement limitations. Patients are usually taken to the bathroom every 2–4 h. In this application, the goal is to prevent the episodes in which the patient gets wet and needs care. Guided voiding, which is useful in patients who can express the need to void, is another method in patients with cognitive impairment or limitation of movement. In this technique, the patient is asked every 1–2 h if there is any need to void, and if necessary, the patient is supported to reach the bathroom. Habit education is another behavioral approach that can be preferred in patients with cognitive impairment. Urination is started every 2 h, and the intervals are adjusted according to the patient's incontinence periods and urination pattern. Although it has been shown to be associated with less bacteriuria and symptomatic urinary tract infection compared with transurethral urinary catheters [50], external urine collection devices such as condom catheters should be avoided as much as possible due to the ongoing infection risk, which may also cause cellulite and tissue necrosis.

13.10.5 The Role of the General Practitioner in Managing Urinary Incontinence

General practitioners (GPs) are the most involved specialist, especially in the long-lasting follow-up and in the management of UI. However, it is reported that many of them do not feel confident about managing UI [51]. The first task of GPs is to inform the general population, with particular attention to older people, and to detect any case of UI. In fact, it is estimated that a large number of patients with UI are reluctant to consult a doctor for many reasons. First of all, adults with enuresis may not be aware that treatments are available [52]. Another reason could be due to the stigmatizing nature of the condition, with adults being too embarrassed to seek professional help for their problem. Interestingly, one study found that 20% of adults with persistent enuresis have never consulted a doctor about their problem

[53]. Once UI is diagnosed, it is crucial to start the patient education and treatment that in the first line includes lifestyle advice, pelvic floor muscle training, or pessary placement [54]. Although GPs perform the diagnostic procedure according to available guidelines, it is estimated that only one-third of patients receive optimal treatment [55]. Factors that prevent GPs from providing optimal treatment are a lack of time, a lack of knowledge, and the feeling of not being capable to coach pelvic floor muscle training [56]. Although GPs experience barriers in providing care for UI, they consider optimizing treatment of UI important [56]. Growing evidence suggests a possible solution to improve care for UI is Internet-based therapy, eHealth. Indeed, eHealth interventions have shown to be effective for various health-related topics as substance abuse, mental health, and chronic pain [57]. Recently, also for UI, there is evidence that eHealth interventions are effective [56].

13.11   Conclusion

In conclusion, UI is not a natural result of aging but, rather, a geriatric syndrome that is common in older people and has negative physical, psychological, social, and economic consequences. Despite the fact that it is common in older people, it is underreported by patients and, generally, under-treated by physicians. The most common cause of continuous UI in older people is the urge type, and the most common cause is detrusor overactivity. UI should be questioned and evaluated as part of a detailed geriatric evaluation. In fact, it is important to determine the type of UI, because each type of treatment approach is different. Transient causes should be eliminated in patients with UI (DIAPPERS). Basic evaluation of UI is possible with anamnesis, physical examination, urine diary, determination of PVR volume, blood biochemistry, and TIT. Non-pharmacological therapies should be started and, if necessary, combined with pharmacological therapies.

References

1. Abrams P, Cardozo L, Fall M, Griffiths D, Rosier P, Ulmsten U, et al. The standardisation of terminology of lower urinary tract function: report from the Standardisation Sub-committee of the International Continence Society. Am J Obstet Gynecol. 2002;187(1):116–26.
2. Silva WA, Karram MM. Anatomy and physiology of the pelvic floor. Minerva Ginecol. 2004;56(4):283–302.
3. Andersson K-E. Bladder activation: afferent mechanisms. Urology. 2002;59(5 Suppl 1):43–50.
4. Juenemann KP, Lue TF, Schmidt RA, Tanagho EA. Clinical significance of sacral and pudendal nerve anatomy. J Urol. 1988;139(1):74–80.
5. de Groat WC, Yoshimura N. Mechanisms underlying the recovery of lower urinary tract function following spinal cord injury. Prog Brain Res. 2006;152:59–84.
6. Gibbs CF, Johnson TM II, Ouslander JG. Office management of geriatric urinary incontinence. Am J Med. 2007;120(3):211–20.
7. Al-Mukhtar Othman J, Akervall S, Milsom I, Gyhagen M. Urinary incontinence in nulliparous women aged 25–64 years: a national survey. Am J Obstet Gynecol. 2017;216(2):149. e1–149.e11.

8. Wagg AS. Urinary incontinence. In: Fillit H, Rockwood K, Young J, editors. Brocklehurst's textbook of geriatric medicine and gerontology. 8th ed. Philadelphia, PA: Elsevier Inc; 2017. p. 895–903.
9. Dessole S, Rubattu G, Ambrosini G, Gallo O, Capobianco G, Cherchi PL, et al. Efficacy of low-dose intravaginal estriol on urogenital aging in postmenopausal women. Menopause. 2004;11(1):49–56.
10. Lepor H. Pathophysiology, epidemiology, and natural history of benign prostatic hyperplasia. Rev Urol. 2004;6(Suppl 9):S3–10.
11. Marberger MJ, Andersen JT, Nickel JC, Malice MP, Gabriel M, Pappas F, et al. Prostate volume and serum prostate-specific antigen as predictors of acute urinary retention. Combined experience from three large multinational placebo-controlled trials. Eur Urol. 2000;38(5):563–8.
12. Johnson TM II, Sattin RW, Parmelee P, Fultz NH, Ouslander JG. Evaluating potentially modifiable risk factors for prevalent and incident nocturia in older adults. J Am Geriatr Soc. 2005;53(6):1011–6.
13. Johnson TM, Burgio KL, Redden DT, Wright KC, Goode PS. Effects of behavioral and drug therapy on nocturia in older incontinent women. J Am Geriatr Soc. 2005;53(5):846–50.
14. Resnick NM. Voiding dysfunction in the elderly. In: Yalla S, McGuire E, Elbadawi A, Blaivas JG, editors. Neurourology and urodynamics: principles and practice. New York: MacMillan Publishing Company; 1984. p. 303–30.
15. Marques LPJ, Flores JT, Barros Junior O d O, Rodrigues GB, Mourao C d M, Moreira RMP. Epidemiological and clinical aspects of urinary tract infection in community-dwelling elderly women. Braz J Infect Dis. 2012;16(5):436–41.
16. Irwin DE, Milsom I, Hunskaar S, Reilly K, Kopp Z, Herschorn S, et al. Population-based survey of urinary incontinence, overactive bladder, and other lower urinary tract symptoms in five countries: results of the EPIC study. Eur Urol. 2006;50(6):1305–6.
17. Nygaard I, Barber MD, Burgio KL, Kenton K, Meikle S, Schaffer J, et al. Prevalence of symptomatic pelvic floor disorders in US women. JAMA. 2008;300(11):1311–6.
18. Aggazzotti G, Pesce F, Grassi D, Fantuzzi G, Righi E, De Vita D, et al. Prevalence of urinary incontinence among institutionalized patients: a cross-sectional epidemiologic study in a mid-sized city in northern Italy. Urology. 2000;56(2):245–9.
19. Buckley BS, Lapitan MCM. Prevalence of urinary incontinence in men, women, and children—current evidence: findings of the Fourth International Consultation on Incontinence. Urology. 2010;76(2):265–70.
20. Offermans MPW, Du Moulin MFMT, Hamers JPH, Dassen T, Halfens RJG. Prevalence of urinary incontinence and associated risk factors in nursing home residents: a systematic review. Neurourol Urodyn. 2009;28(4):288–94.
21. Baztan JJ, Arias E, Gonzalez N, Rodriguez de Prada MI. New-onset urinary incontinence and rehabilitation outcomes in frail older patients. Age Ageing. 2005;34:172–5.
22. Ateşkan Ü, Mas M, Doruk H, Kutlu M. Yaşlı Türk popülasyonunda üriner inkontinans: Görülme sıklığı, muhtemel klinik tipleri ve birey açısından öneminin değerlendirilmesi. Geriatri. 2000;3:45–50.
23. Haylen BT, de Ridder D, Freeman RM, Swift SE, Berghmans B, Lee J, et al. An International Urogynecological Association (IUGA)/International Continence Society (ICS) joint report on the terminology for female pelvic floor dysfunction. Neurourol Urodyn. 2010;29(1):4–20.
24. Melville JL, Katon W, Delaney K, Newton K. Urinary incontinence in US women: a population-based study. Arch Intern Med. 2005;165(5):537–42.
25. Shamliyan TA, Wyman JF, Ping R, Wilt TJ, Kane RL. Male urinary incontinence: prevalence, risk factors, and preventive interventions. Rev Urol. 2009;11(3):145–65.
26. Farage MA, Miller KW, Berardesca E, Maibach HI. Psychosocial and societal burden of incontinence in the aged population: a review. Arch Gynecol Obstet. 2008;277(4):285–90.
27. Langa KM, Fultz NH, Saint S, Kabeto MU, Herzog AR. Informal caregiving time and costs for urinary incontinence in older individuals in the United States. J Am Geriatr Soc. 2002;50(4):733–7.

28. Resnick NM, Yalla SV. Management of urinary incontinence in the elderly. N Engl J Med. 1985;313(13):800–5.
29. Cook K, Sobeski L. Urinary incontinence in the older adult [Internet]. Lenexa; 2013.
30. DuBeau CE. Beyond the bladder: management of urinary incontinence in older women. Clin Obstet Gynecol. 2007;50(3):720–34.
31. Kim D. Evaluating and managing urinary incontinence. Boston; 2015.
32. Coyne KS, Kvasz M, Ireland AM, Milsom I, Kopp ZS, Chapple CR. Urinary incontinence and its relationship to mental health and health-related quality of life in men and women in Sweden, the United Kingdom, and the United States. Eur Urol. 2012;61(1):88–95.
33. Minassian VA, Yan X, Lichtenfeld MJ, Sun H, Stewart WF. The iceberg of health care utilization in women with urinary incontinence. Int Urogynecol J. 2012;23(8):1087–93.
34. DeMaagd GA, Davenport TC. Management of urinary incontinence. Pharm Therap. 2012;37:345–361H.
35. Brown JS, Bradley CS, Subak LL, Richter HE, Kraus SR, Brubaker L, et al. The sensitivity and specificity of a simple test to distinguish between urge and stress urinary incontinence. Ann Intern Med. 2006;144(10):715–23.
36. Soysal P, Aydın A. İnkontinans Ölçekleri. In: Işık A, Soysal P, editors. Geriatri Pratiğinde Ölçekler. Istanbul: İstanbul Tıp Kitabevleri; 2016. p. 137–49.
37. Abrams P, Andersson KE, Birder L, Brubaker L, Cardozo L, Chapple C, et al. Fourth International Consultation on Incontinence Recommendations of the International Scientific Committee: evaluation and treatment of urinary incontinence, pelvic organ prolapse, and fecal incontinence. Neurourol Urodyn. 2010;29(1):213–40.
38. Thirugnanasothy S. Managing urinary incontinence in older people. BMJ. 2010;341:c3835.
39. Lucas MG, Bosch RJL, Burkhard FC, Cruz F, Madden TB, Nambiar AK, et al. EAU guidelines on assessment and nonsurgical management of urinary incontinence. Eur Urol. 2012;62(6):1130–42.
40. Lucas M, Bedretdinova D, Bosch J, Burkhard F, Cruz F, Nambiar A, et al. Guidelines on urinary incontinence [Internet]. 2014.
41. Gray M, Beeckman D, Bliss DZ, Fader M, Logan S, Junkin J, et al. Incontinence-associated dermatitis: a comprehensive review and update. J Wound Ostomy Cont Nurs. 2012;39(1):61–74.
42. Üriner OJ. İnkontinansta Davranış Tedavisi. In: Işık A, Bozoğlu E, editors. Geriatrik Olgularda Üriner İnkontinans, vol. 2. Istanbul: SomKitap; 2010. p. 130–7.
43. Kaplan SA, Roehrborn CG, Rovner ES, Carlsson M, Bavendam T, Guan Z. Tolterodine and tamsulosin for treatment of men with lower urinary tract symptoms and overactive bladder: a randomized controlled trial. JAMA. 2006;296(19):2319–28.
44. Okudur S, Soysal P, Mas M, Işık A. İnkontinans. In: Işık A, Soysal P, editors. Geriatri Pratiğinde İlaç Tedavisi, vol. 1. Istanbul: O'tıp Kitabevi; 2015. p. 113–29.
45. Qaseem A, Dallas P, Forciea MA, Starkey M, Denberg TD, Shekelle P. Nonsurgical management of urinary incontinence in women: a clinical practice guideline from the American College of Physicians. Ann Intern Med. 2014;161(6):429–40.
46. Olivera CK, Meriwether K, El-Nashar S, Grimes CL, Chen CCG, Orejuela F, et al. Nonantimuscarinic treatment for overactive bladder: a systematic review. Am J Obstet Gynecol. 2016;215(1):34–57.
47. Bachmann G, Santen R. Treatment of genitourinary syndrome of menopause (vulvovaginal atrophy) [Internet]. UpToDate. 2017 [cited 2017 Jun 3].
48. Işık A. Üriner İnkontinans Tedavisi. In: Işık A, Bozoğlu E, editors. Geriatrik Olgularda Üriner İnkontinans, vol. 2. Istanbul: SomKitap; 2011. p. 143–56.
49. Gibson W, Wagg A. New horizons: urinary incontinence in older people. Age Ageing. 2014;43(2):157–63.
50. Saint S, Kaufman SR, Rogers MAM, Baker PD, Ossenkop K, Lipsky BA. Condom versus indwelling urinary catheters: a randomized trial. J Am Geriatr Soc. 2006;54(7):1055–61.
51. Caldwell PH, Manocha R, Hamilton S, Scott KM, Barnes EH. Australian community health practitioners' knowledge and experience with managing urinary incontinence that begins in childhood. Aust J Gen Pract. 2019;48(1–2):60–5.

52. Wilson GJ. The lived experience of bedwetting in young men living in Western Australia. Aust N Z Continence J. 2014;20(4):188.
53. Nappo S, Del Gado R, Chiozza ML, Biraghi M, Ferrara P, Caione P. Nocturnal enuresis in the adolescent: a neglected problem. BJU Int. 2002;90(9):912–7.
54. Damen-van Beek Z, Teunissen D, Dekker JH, Lagro-Janssen AL, Berghmans LC, Uijen JH, et al. Practice guideline 'Urinary incontinence in women' from the Dutch College of General Practitioners. Ned Tijdschr Geneeskd. 2016;160:D674.
55. Shaw C, Das Gupta R, Williams KS, Assassa RP, McGrother C. A survey of help-seeking and treatment provision in women with stress urinary incontinence. BJU Int. 2006;97(4):752–7.
56. Firet L, de Bree C, Verhoeks CM, Teunissen DAM, Lagro-Janssen ALM. Mixed feelings: general practitioners' attitudes towards eHealth for stress urinary incontinence - a qualitative study. BMC Fam Pract. 2019;20(1):21.
57. Rogers MA, Lemmen K, Kramer R, Mann J, Chopra V. Internet-delivered health interventions that work: systematic review of meta-analyses and evaluation of website availability. J Med Internet Res. 2017;19(3):e90.

Red Flags in Geriatric Medicine: Assessing Risk and Managing It in Primary Care

14

Erik Lagolio, Ilaria Rossiello, Andreas Meer, Vania Noventa, and Alberto Vaona

Abstract

To identify an emergency in older people is often challenging because symptoms are frequently atypical or minimal. Any abnormality in vital parameters could hide a serious and progressive condition. At the same time, it could be related to a physiological change in homeostasis. Any stressor acts as a trigger in frail people with consequent sudden decline in health and functions.

Family doctors have the task to recognize whether any minimal change in patients could lead to critical events or not. The general practitioner should also know if a diagnostic or therapeutic intervention will produce an improvement in patients' condition and quality of life and decide accordingly whether to proceed or not.

Emergencies' treatment and management in palliative care differ when caused by cancer, but even in a palliative setting, the physician should try to recognize and treat reversible illnesses.

E. Lagolio (✉)
Emergency Medicine (A&E) - Hospital Santa Corona, Asl2, Pietra Ligure, Italy
e-mail: erik.lagolio@gmail.com

I. Rossiello
General Practice, AV3, Montecosaro, Italy

A. Meer
General Internal Medicine, Bern, Switzerland

V. Noventa
Primary Care Department, Geriatric Unit, Azienda ULSS 3 "Serenissima", Venice, Italy

A. Vaona
Primary Care Department, ULSS 9 Scaligera, Verona, Italy

© Springer Nature Switzerland AG 2022
J. Demurtas, N. Veronese (eds.), *The Role of Family Physicians in Older People Care*, Practical Issues in Geriatrics, https://doi.org/10.1007/978-3-030-78923-7_14

The aim of this chapter is to provide a list of red flags (i.e., alerts that help doctor to prevent pitfalls) a general practitioner should detect during clinical examinations. These signs and symptoms are not enough to decide whether to refer patients to an emergency department, but they alert about a potential serious condition.

Keywords

Frailty · Emergency · Risk assessment · Primary care · Red flags · Risk management

14.1 Introduction

A medical emergency is an acute, serious, and unexpected injury or illness that put at immediate risk life or long-term health and requires immediate action.

A medical urgency does not lead to immediate danger or threat to life and health, but if not treated, the situation may turn into an emergency.

The common feeling is that emergency/urgency is managed by the emergency department. **In a primary care setting, it is not infrequent to face this kind of situations, and the family doctor has to decide whether to treat the patient at home or refer him to the hospital.** This decision is based on the clinical situation, will/expectation/perception of the patient/family, and needs for further investigation or medical equipment. It is possible to quantify the amount of patients getting in contact with an emergency department/service, but **it is challenging to acknowledge the prevalence of medical emergency/urgency in primary care.**

The acute medical problems of older people are often similar to those of younger adults, but the presentation can be atypical or there can be a number of co-existing problems that make a diagnosis difficult. Furthermore, major illnesses such as serious infections, heart disease, and cancer can also present in a non-specific way [1]. Injury is a growing cause of mortality and morbidity in the geriatric population, with geriatric patients now accounting for one fourth of all trauma admissions in the United States [2]. It is increasingly recognized that significant under-triage exists in the geriatric population [3]. There are nearly 650,000 fall-related attendances to emergency department in the United Kingdom (UK) for older people each year, and about half of them are likely to fall again [4].

Elderly people usually have a fragile health condition and comorbidities, and 40% are under polypharmacological treatments [5] that can lead to negative outcomes [6]. In these patients an apparently minor illness can lead to deterioration in a non-specific way leading to immobility, a fall, or acute confusion [1].

Detection of treatable conditions in frail people is clinically challenging. This clinical syndrome can perplex even experienced physicians. Initial assessments can be imprecise, and a missed diagnosis is associated with an increased risk of poor clinical outcomes [7]. **Practitioners dealing with emergencies in older adults in the community should be able to recognize the atypical presentation of illness in older person and have a high index of suspicion that apparently innocent symptoms can be the presentation of serious underlying pathology.** With an older patient, it is safer to err on the side of caution to avoid denying patients a specialist assessment [1]. On the other hand, acute care settings are stressful for patients and caregivers [8].

Moreover, an unnecessary access to the emergency room or hospitalization with associated diagnostic tests can further decompensate the fragile patient, aggravate or induce a bedridden syndrome, and in some cases diagnose pathologies with a benign course that would not have changed patient's prognosis nor would have needed for therapies or controls. Thus the GP's decision is challenging.

14.1.1 What Do We Mean by Red Flags?

A red flag is an alert that helps doctor to prevent pitfalls, in particular, in those conditions associated with fatalities.

We provide a list of signs and symptoms (red flags) occurring in geriatric patients that should alert a general practitioner (GP). A minimal change in vital signs or non-specific symptoms can hide a critical situation that rapidly evolves into a serious condition and poor prognosis. They are not necessary associated with an emergency/urgency. The GP needs to evaluate the situation in a global assessment of the patient.

General red flags to be considered
- Dyspnea
- Hypoxemia
- Typical chest pain
- Tachycardia/unknown arrhythmia
- Change in mental status/confusion
- Fainting or loss of consciousness
- Sudden dizziness, weakness, or change in vision
- Choking
- Incessant bleeding
- Sudden and severe pain
- Trauma
- Dehydration
- Caregiver reports that the patient "does not seem the same"

Most of the red flags are objective and easily detected by GPs during the consultation. However the absence of evident red flags doesn't exclude an acute disease. Thus unusual behavior or change in everyday status referred by the caregiver deserves attention.

Risk factors associated with patient's general condition
- Diabetes mellitus
- Relevant trauma in the last 14 days
- Surgical or medical intervention (operation, puncture, infiltration) in the last 14 days
- Serious underlying chronic disease:
  - Organ failure (e.g., kidney or liver failure)
  - Tumor diseases and tumor therapy
- Autoimmune disease
- Heart disease, chronic heart failure, generalized arteriosclerosis
- Respiratory disease (e.g., chronic obstructive pulmonopathy/COPD, interstitial pneumopathy)
- Neurological disease (e.g., dementia, multiple sclerosis, Parkinson's disease)
- Chronic infectious disease (e.g., tuberculosis)
- Immunosuppression (e.g., st. n. splenectomy, st. n. organ transplantation, stem cell transplantation, cytostatic drugs, cortisone, radio-chemotherapy, HIV infection/AIDS
- Prosthesis wearer:
  - Joint prosthesis
  - Heart valve or vascular prosthesis

14.2　Chest Pain and Dyspnea

Chest pain and dyspnea can coexist and confound the clinical examination. The main urgencies underlying are pulmonary embolism, ischemic cardiac attack, and pneumonia.

The guidelines currently available on the management of chest pain paradoxically do not define precisely in terms of location and duration of the symptom what should be considered as chest pain. Traditionally, any pain that appears suddenly in the body area between the nose and navel is considered as **chest pain of possible coronary origin** (in any case, it should be remembered that up to 20% of heart attack patients do not have chest pain).

Given this definition, the incidence of the symptom in the general population is around 5.4 cases per 1000 inhabitants per year.

The clinical characteristics of pain at the onset have proven in several studies to be completely unreliable in predicting the origin of pain if taken individually.

So, for example, irradiation to the left arm is a predicatively weaker feature than irradiation to both arms [9].

Since 2010, a clinical prediction rule (Marburg Score) has also been available which combines some pain characteristics and which allows to exclude with reasonable certainty chest pain may have a coronary origin only by the data available in the out-of-hospital phase. It takes into account five one-point clinical characteristics:

- Female ≥65 years or male ≥55 years.
- Known CAD, cerebrovascular disease, or peripheral vascular disease.
- Pain worse with exercise.
- Pain non-reproducible with palpation.
- Patient assumes pain is cardiac.

The best overall discrimination was with a cut-off value of 3 (positive result 3–5 points; negative result ≤2 points), which had a sensitivity of 87.1% (95% CI 79.9–94.2%) and a specificity of 80.8% (77.6–83.9%) [10, 11].

The guidelines currently not available take this rule of clinical prediction into account and recommend that **all patients with chest pain be tested by electrocardiogram as soon as possible, agreeing to have many false positives in order not to lose the true positives.** The recommended speed is dictated by the risk of sudden death at an early stage (60% of deaths happen before the patient reaches the hospital and not less than 28% in the first hour from the onset of the symptoms) [12].

Red flags for thoracic pain
- Acute onset
- Severe pain ("worst ever")
- Respiratory thoracic pain
- Severe abdominal pain (8–10/10)
- Radiation of pain: in the back (between the shoulder blades), neck, chest, groin, or legs
- Dyspnea, respiratory exhaustion/speech dyspnea
- Orthopnea
- Hemoptysis
- Pathological pulse
- Collapse/syncope (shock)
- Cyanosis
- Relevant trauma
- Neurological deficit
- Suspicion of internal bleeding
- Change of consciousness
- Change of mental condition, acute confusion, acute disorientation
- Known aneurysm/aortic aneurysm

In older people, the most common causes of dyspnea are heart failure, chronic obstructive pulmonary disease, asthma, parenchymal lung disease, pulmonary vascular disease, upper airway obstruction, and pneumonia. **Dyspnea should not be attributed to aging without excluding the before-mentioned causes.**

Dyspnea is a common complaint with negative influence on daily functioning and quality of life (QOL) and requires prompt and adequate pharmacological intervention. Chronic dyspnea must first be distinguished from acute dyspnea which requires rapid diagnosis.

Red flags for dyspnea
- Chest pain, including respiratory pain
- Severe pain (8–10/10)
- Pain radiation into both arms, left arm, right shoulder, neck, or jaw
- Persistent severe pain >20 min
- Severe, unusual pectanginous complaints
- Acute onset
- Orthopnea
- Hemoptysis
- Pathological pulse
- Collapse/syncope (shock)
- Cyanosis
- Feeling of suffocation/anxiety
- Persistent palpitations/heart palpitations
- Gastrointestinal symptoms: nausea, vomiting, abdominal pain, diarrhea
- Status after anaphylaxis/allergic reaction/known allergy
- Orthostatic vertigo
- Generalized rash
- Fast expanding skin rash
- Swelling of face, lips, tongue
- Fever

Pulmonary embolism has nuanced presentation symptoms (dyspnea, hypoxemia, chest pain, and tachycardia). This is the reason why pulmonary embolism is still widely under-diagnosed in the geriatric population: autopsy studies have shown that it is the most unrecognized cause of death in this population [13].

The incidence increases with advancing age due to increased tendency to blood coagulability and addition of the risk factors that predispose to venous thrombus-embolism, such as the underlying pathologies and reduced mobility. Mortality is directly related to age and concomitant diseases (e.g., heart failure, acute myocardial infarction, COPD, stroke, femur fracture, neoplasm) [14].

The clinical classification of pulmonary embolism no longer uses the terms massive and non-massive as clinic depends on the size of the embolus and extent of involvement of the pulmonary arterial lung tree in relation to pre-existing cardiopulmonary conditions.

In the older patient, the most common signs and symptoms are dyspnea (range 59–91.5%), tachypnea (46–74%), tachycardia (29–76%), chest pain (26–57%), syncope (8–62%), shock (5–31%), cough (12–43%), and hemoptysis (3–14%). Bed rest was present in 15–67% of patients, while deep vein thrombosis and oncologic disease were found in 15–50% and 4–32%, respectively [15].

Pneumonia is an important cause of morbidity and mortality, representing the fourth cause of death in patients of the decades of advanced age and is often the terminal event of a long and severe disease. Age and comorbidities are the major risk factor for the development of pneumonia; comorbidity also affects the appearance of complications and mortality itself.

The signs and symptoms of pneumonia in elderly are often atypical and nuanced and are characterized, as well as cough with sputum production, confusion, lethargy, and general deterioration without the typical feverish picture of pneumonia. Only about 50% of cases present a particularly high fever.

There are many guidelines for hospital treatment of pneumonia, much less about how to manage community-acquired pneumonia in primary care. As recommended by the NICE guidelines, if the doctor is sure of the diagnosis, the judgment is reliable without the need for a chest X-ray, and empirical therapy should be started as soon as possible [16].

Chest radiography and C-reactive protein (CRP) point-of-care test can be helpful when the doctor is unsure of the diagnosis.

An aspect of great importance is to establish where to treat the patient (home or hospital) by combining the clinical judgment and the level of severity with an assessment of the pre-existing clinical conditions and any conditions that compromise home treatment. According to an observational study in the United Kingdom, 11.9% of patients with community pneumonia treated at home were over 85 years old while 36.3% between 65 and 84 years old. In this regard there are some clinical scores, many of which require laboratory tests [17].

In primary care, CRB-65 is commonly used (confusion; respiratory rate 30 breaths/min or greater; blood pressure—systolic of 90 mmHg or less or a diastolic of 60 mmHg or less; 65 years of age or older), simple and useful in predicting mortality; however it does not consider comorbidities and oxygen saturation, two determining factors as we have seen in conditioning the prognosis. For this reason the DS-CRB65 implements these two factors, underlying disease (malignancy, heart failure, hepatic, renal, and cerebrovascular disease) and pulse oximetry (SpO_2), by increasing the accuracy of the test without needing laboratory tests [18].

14.3 Trauma

Older adults undergo fewer a trauma than younger patients but with higher mortality [19, 20].

The 67% of death from a trauma occurs in older adults. Trauma at older age is more often caused by falls and pedestrian accidents. Older people can fall due to both minor balance and medical reasons (e.g., syncope, stroke, benzodiazepines use). The consequence can result in a major injury such as femoral fracture or intracranial bleeding.

When a GP is confronted with an older traumatized patient, there are some red flags that should be investigated:

- Severe pain
- Inability to move
- Externally rotated foot and shortened leg
- Bruising and swelling

These symptoms suggest a bone fracture. Femoral fracture is particularly worrying at this age, and hospitalization is recommended.

Red flags to be considered
- Fall
- Neurological deficit
- Change of consciousness
- Change of mental state
- Acute confusion
- Acute disorientation
- Strong pain (8–10/10)
- Bruising
- Swelling
- Misalignment
- Inability to move

In the case of a chest trauma, be aware of the possibility of hypoxia and hypercapnia even if there is no dyspnea nor breathing alteration.
Also circulatory features are different in older people. **Heart rate over 90 and systolic blood pressure under 110 mmHg are burdened by higher mortality.** If you decide to treat him/her at home, don't forget to **create a safety net and evaluate again his/her conditions after a while.** Red flags that should be explained for the safety net include confusion, dyspnea, and worsening of symptoms such as pain. The absence of a caregiver can be considered as hospitalization criterion.

In the case of a head trauma, diagnosing an intracranial bleeding is really challenging because of the cerebral atrophy that allows more space for blood collection. Bleeding can be present even if Glasgow Coma Scale is 15 and there are no neurological signs. According to Canadian computerized tomography (CT) scan head rule, CT is recommended in minor head injury in patient >65 years. On the other hand, the risk of intracranial hemorrhage in patients with minimal head injury and no symptoms is very low, and even in patients found to have an intracranial hemorrhage, none had any serious adverse outcome [21].

Ten percent of head trauma occurs in patients under anticoagulant therapy, and 15% of bleeding are symptomless, but a reverse therapy is recommended [22].

Thus **consider a CT head within 1 h in the following scenery:**

- GCS less than 13 on initial assessment
- GCS less than 15 at 2 h after the injury on assessment
- Suspected open or depressed skull fracture
- Any sign of basal skull fracture (hemotympanum, "panda" eyes, cerebrospinal fluid leakage from the ear or nose, Battle's sign)
- More than one episode of vomiting
- Neurological signs or symptoms
- Moderate/severe trauma

- Use of anticoagulants
- Absence of a caregiver who monitors the onset of signs/symptoms in the following 24 h

According to NICE guidelines, **perform a CT head scan within 8 h in patients over 65 who have experienced some loss of consciousness or amnesia since the injury** [23].

14.4   Altered State of Consciousness

An altered state of consciousness is a red flag per se. To identify a worsening in consciousness in older adults is challenging, mostly because mental faculties can be already compromised. In this case caregivers' perception is crucial.

Awareness requires that the cerebral hemispheres are functioning and that the function of the ascending reticular activating system (ARAS) is preserved. Older adults have more often a pre-existing brain disease. Thus a small unilateral lesion can result in change of consciousness. There may be damage to the ARAS due to toxic or metabolic disorders (e.g., hypoglycemia, hypoxia, uremia, focal ischemia, hemorrhage, or overdose).

It is important to remember that **older patient may be more sensitive to coma, impaired consciousness, and delirium** due to many factors, including the following:

- Minor cognitive reserve due to age and/or pre-existing brain disorders.
- Greater risk of drug interactions with central effects due to polytherapy.
- Increased risk of drug accumulation and drug effects on the central nervous system due to decreased function of organs responsible for drug metabolism.
- Increased risk of incorrect drug dosage due to polytherapy with complex dosage regimens.
- Relatively minor problems, such as dehydration and urinary tract infections, can alter consciousness in older individuals.
- In older patients, mental state and communication skills are more likely to be compromised, making lethargy and disorientation more difficult to recognize.

Delirium according to *Diagnostic and Statistical Manual of Mental Disorders* (DSM-5) can be diagnosed if there is a disturbance of attention and awareness associated with another cognitive deficit (memory, disorientation, language, visuospatial abilities, etc.) which cannot be explained by a pre-existing neurocognitive disorder, with acute onset (hours or a few days) and fluctuating course during the day.

Three clinical forms are distinguished:

- Hyperactive form: alert and hyperactive patient, responding to stimuli
- Hypoactive form: torpid patient, with reduced psychomotor activity
- Mixed form: Normal level of psychomotor activity or rapid alternation of forms during on the day or during the episode

It's a common and serious condition in older people, often undiagnosed and therefore not treated, that can have an adverse outcome: patients who develop delirium present a ten times greater risk of death at 6 months (35–40%). It affects 20–30% of hospitalized patients in ordinary hospital wards and between 10% and 50% of patients treated surgically. While the problem of delirium in hospitalized patients is well known, we still know little about the delirium that arises in long-term care (in this setting 20% of prevalence is estimated) or at home. Delirium occurs in nearly one in five patients in the nursing home who suffer from an acute disease and is one of the main risk factors for cognitive decline after the acute episode [24, 25].

Prevalence is influenced by cognitive status ranging from 3.4% in a population with MMSE (Mini-Mental State Examination) greater than 10–33.3% with a lower MMSE value, with an overall incidence of 20.7 per 100 person-years [26, 27]. In an Italian prevalence study, the variables significantly associated with delirium in the nursing home were dementia (OR 3.12, 95% CI 2.38–4.09), functional dependence (OR 6.13, 95% CI 3.08–12.19 for ADL score 0; OR 1.99, 95% CI 1.03–3.84 for ADL score 1–5), malnutrition (OR 4.87, 95% CI 2.68–8.84), antipsychotics (OR 2.40, 95% CI 1.81–3.18), and physical restrictions (OR 2.48, 95% CI 1.71–3.59) [28].

Among the main difficulties encountered by family doctors in treating delirium in the nursing home are the management of behavioral disorders and relationships with the different caregivers of the nursing home [29].

14.5 Oligoanuria

Oliguria is defined as a urine output that is less than 400 mL or 500 mL per 24 h in adults—this equals 17 or 21 mL/h [30].

Anuria is clinically defined as less than 100 mL urine output per day [31]; it occurs quickly and it is usually a sign of obstruction or acute kidney failure.

Apart from patients with urinary catheter, GPs do not know the amount of urine produced during the day. Usually caregivers note dry diaper or the patient refers a low urine output. **Most of the time, diuresis is a parameter that must be investigated in case of minimal changes in patient's status instead of the reason of the visit/contact.**

Oligoanuria can be categorized in three patterns:

- Prerenal: in response to hypoperfusion of the kidney (e.g., dehydration, cardiogenic shock, diarrhea, massive bleeding, or sepsis).
- Renal: due to kidney damage (severe hypoperfusion, rhabdomyolysis, medication).
- Postrenal: as a consequence of obstruction of the urine flow (e.g., enlarged prostate, tumor compression urinary outflow, expanding hematoma, or fluid collection).

Postrenal oligoanuria can be easily detected by POCUS (point-of-care ultrasound) at patient's bed or in practice. **In case of anuria and lack of ultrasound,**

GP can try to insert a catheter to overstep a lower obstruction or flaccid neurogenic bladder.

The incidence of acute kidney injury increases significantly as age advanced. Identification of risk factors might lead to more intensive monitoring and early prevention and might improve acute kidney injury patients' outcomes in very old people [32].

Prerenal oligoanuria in older people is often caused by dehydration and leads to confusion, fainting, fever, and tachycardia. Dehydration can also quickly lead the patient to **acute renal failure** with an increased risk of drug toxicity [33].

Older persons are more easily affected by dehydration because of impaired thirst sensation, age-related renal tubular dysfunction, reduced fluid intake, and effects of diuretics. It has a greater negative outcome in this population than in younger adults and increases mortality, morbidity, and disability.

Among the elderly the increase in adipose tissue and the decrease in lean mass lead to a reduction in total body water from 60% to 45%. The control of fluid intake is fundamental for homeostasis and is managed by the sense of thirst that is activated when the loss of water reaches 2%. The osmolarity that activates the sense of thirst in older people is higher, and the response is therefore slower and less intense. Total body water is controlled by sodium balance which in the older people is altered due to the reduced glomerular filtrate, reduced renal blood flow, reduced ability to concentrate and dilute urine (maximum urinary osmolarity is about 900 mOsm/kg, compared to 1200 in young adults), and therefore the reduced ability to conserve sodium. A loss of homeostasis is revealed by an alteration of natremia (normal range 135–145 mEq/L): a decrease in the concentration of sodium in the extracellular compartment involves a compensatory movement of water toward the intracellular compartment and vice versa. Therefore hyponatremia means cellular hyperhydration; hypernatremia means cellular dehydration.

Dehydration in older people is the most common electrolyte disorder and can be acute or chronic. The first is due to a rapid reduction in total body water without a corresponding reduction in total body sodium, such as in gastroenteritis, intake of diuretics, feverish disease, or hot climate. The second is due to a persistent reduced intake of liquids which leads to hypo-dehydration. Traditional markers for dehydration do not take into consideration many of the physiological differences present in older adults. Clinical assessment of dehydration in older adults poses different findings, yet is not always diagnostic. In older people, there aren't obvious signs or symptoms of dehydration. The dryness of the mucous membranes can be missing, as well as how difficult to evaluate the firmness of the skin, and the difference in body weight is insensitive. An indication of dehydration is the increased heart rate of 10–20 beats per minute, moving from the clinostatic position to the orthostatic, as well as a decrease in systolic blood pressure of 20 or more mmHg due the transition from the clinostatism to orthostatism or of 10 or more mmHg for diastolic blood pressure. These are all signs of mild dehydration (water loss <5% of body weight), but unfortunately in older people, they can also occur in presence of a normal volume. Oliguria or anuria, mental confusion, and hypotension at rest until to hypovolemic shock are instead symptoms of moderate dehydration (water loss about 5% of body weight). Oral rehydration should always be preferred if the patient is stable, but in the event of a gastrointestinal disease or an alteration of state of consciousness (even pre-existing), it may not be feasible. In this case, intravenous infusion therapy can be practiced with saline solution. In the event of acute dehydration, hospitalization for the appropriate treatment is advisable; instead if the clinical situation is subacute and stable, it is also possible in the nursing home setting to provide for the reintroduction of liquids. For this purpose, however, it is necessary to have the sodemia dosage available as soon as possible.

Though it is not possible to provide a proper list of symptoms related to dehydration in older persons, when recognized and treated, it is a good example of home management of acute illness.

Red flags to be considered
Red flags for dehydration:
- Headache
- Thirst, dry mouth, and dry tongue
- Lack of concentration
- Tiredness, weakness
- Dizziness
- Strongly colored to dark urine, decrease in urine volume
- Dry, itchy skin
- Brittle to cracked lips
- Weight loss

Red flags for oligoanuria:
- Fever
- Acute, severe (8–10/10) flank pain
- Severe pain (8–10/10)
- Bloody urine
- Urinary retention
- Relevant trauma
- Collapse/syncope (shock)

14.6 Fever

Fever, the cardinal sign of infection, may be absent or blunted 20–30% of the time in older people. An absent or blunted fever response may in turn contribute to diagnostic delays in older people. On the other hand, the presence of a fever in the geriatric patient is more likely to be associated with a serious viral or bacterial infection than is fever in a younger patient. A diagnosis can be made in the majority of cases of fever of unknown origin (FUO) in older adults and often associated with treatable conditions [34].

Fever is caused not only by infectious diseases:

- Noninfectious inflammatory diseases (e.g., temporal arteritis, polymyalgia rheumatica)
- Tumors
- Pulmonary embolism
- Subacute thyroiditis
- Hyperthyroidism
- Drug (neuroleptic malignant syndrome)

and should be considered as differential diagnosis.

Systemic inflammatory response syndrome (SIRS) is an exaggerated defense response of the body to a noxious stressor (e.g., infection) to localize and then eliminate the endogenous or exogenous source of the insult. Even though the purpose is defensive, the dysregulated cytokine storm has the potential to cause massive inflammatory cascade leading to reversible or irreversible end-organ dysfunction and even death. SIRS with a suspected source of infection is termed sepsis. Sepsis with one or more end-organ failure is called severe sepsis and with hemodynamic instability in spite of intravascular volume repletion is called septic shock [35].

The incidence of **sepsis** is 5/100,000 <65 years, but this number increases up to 26/100,000 >85 years, as it also increases the mortality. The older patients are more likely than younger patients to have nonspecific signs and symptoms of infection, more severe disease, and resistant microorganisms. As a result, **physicians must maintain a high index of suspicion for infection, even in the face of nonspecific symptoms, and should tailor empiric antibiotic therapies to the expected pathogens in this population** [36].

Urinary tract infections, lower respiratory tract infections, skin and soft tissue infections, intra-abdominal infections (cholecystitis, diverticulitis, appendicitis, abscesses), infective endocarditis, bacterial meningitis, tuberculosis, and herpes zoster appear to have a special predilection for older persons [37].

Among visits for severe sepsis, older adults compared with younger adults had modestly higher rates of intensive care unit admission ICU (27% vs. 21%), hospital length of stay LOS (median, 6 vs. 5 days), and in-hospital mortality (24% vs. 16%). Nursing home residents with severe sepsis, compared with non-nursing home residents, had significantly higher rates of ICU admission (40% vs. 21%), hospital LOS (median, 7 vs. 5 days), and in-hospital mortality (37% vs. 15%) [38].

Urinary symptoms at this age can be difficult to investigate due to the concomitance of prostatic hypertrophy, bladder prolapse, urinary catheter, neurogenic bladder, or verbal difficulties. GPs can easily perform a urine stick at patient's home or in their practice; it can be useful to make diagnosis when symptoms are nonspecific. In case of urinary sepsis, hospitalization can be necessary.

Red flags in patient with fever
- High fever (>39 °C)
- Hyperthermia (>40 °C)
- Dyspnea, respiratory exhaustion/speech dyspnea
- Strong pain (8–10/10)
- Chest pain
- Bleeding (purpura, ecchymosis)
- Hemoptysis
- Headache, neck stiffness
- Skin rash (petechiae, exanthema)
- Warm, swollen, painful joint
- Neurological deficit
- Change of consciousness
- Change of mental state, acute confusion, acute disorientation
- Collapse/syncope (shock)
- Cyanosis
- Postoperative condition
- Organ transplantation
- Prosthesis wearer (heart valve, joint, vessel prosthesis)

14.7 Abdominal Pain

In older people (>65 years), abdominal pain is the cause of access to the emergency room in 3–13%. An inaccurate diagnosis leads to a high risk of complications and a high mortality [39].

The difficulties for GP in the diagnosis and treatment of abdominal pain in this population are multifactorial and consist, for example, in the **lack of evident clinical signs and late presentation, baseline alteration of physical findings, pre-existing medical disorders altering clinical manifestations, and the variability of presentation of intra-abdominal disorders** [40].

Even in the presence of mild or apparently harmless symptoms, the older patient may have a severe surgical or extra-abdominal pathology. For example, a frequent presentation of lower myocardial infarction is isolated abdominal pain, especially in diabetic women; therefore it is always prudent to perform an electrocardiogram in the older patient with epigastralgia, even in primary care, in particular in the absence of palpatory tenderness [41].

The physiological changes linked to the aging processes are the cause of both a greater susceptibility to intra-abdominal diseases and atypical presentations. The before mentioned changes involve [42]:

- The immune system: reduced humoral and cellular immunity facilitates infections and infectious recurrences; a lower basal temperature and a lower response to pathogens mean that 30% of the older persons with surgical abdomen are apyretic.

- Genitourinary system: increased urinary stasis and bacterial growth, reduced clearance of both drugs and metabolites.
- Gastrointestinal system: frequent colic diverticulosis, reduced intake of liquids and foods with predisposition to constipation, reduced elasticity of the stomach, and increased gastric acid production due to the reduction of prostaglandins.
- Central and peripheral nervous systems: cognitive decline and dementia can cause symptomatic blurring. Progressive switch from A-delta fibers to C fibers reduces the presence of peritonism.

As suggested by Ragsdale and Southerlan, organizing the differential diagnosis into categories based on the pathological cause (inflammatory, obstructive, vascular, or other causes) provides a method to guide the anamnestic, physical, and diagnostic investigations. **In any case older patients with an acute abdomen should not receive anything by mouth until surgical disease is ruled out** [43].

Red flags for abdominal pain
- Fever
- Icterus
- Severe pain (8–10/10)
- Persistent pain (>12–24 h)
- Localized pain
- Rectal bleeding, melena, bloody diarrhea
- Vomiting blood or coffee grounds
- Chest pain
- Dyspnea
- Muscle weakness
- Fall, abdominal trauma
- Urinary retention
- Bloody urine
- Unusual vaginal bleeding
- Neurological deficit
- Collapse/syncope (shock)
- Suspicion of internal bleeding
- Relevant trauma
- Known aneurysm

14.7.1 Inflammatory Pain

It is necessary to consider that the increasingly frequent use of nonsteroidal anti-inflammatory drugs (NSAIDs), aspirin, steroids, and anticoagulants and higher incidence of *Helicobacter pylori* in older person increase the risk of **peptic ulcer** (PUD) which can occur painlessly directly with secondary complications (perforation, hemorrhage and anemia, discrepancy angina, effort intolerance, gastric outlet obstruction, etc.) [44].

Up to 35% of people over 60 years of age with endoscopically tested PUD had no abdominal pain, unlike only 8% of patients under 60 years of age. Moreover if the diagnosis is delayed for 24 h, the mortality rate increases by eight times. In peptic ulcer the most frequent sign of presentation is melena, vital signs may be normal, and due to the atrophy of the abdominal muscles, the classic symptoms of peritonism are absent in 80% of cases [45–48].

Acute cholecystitis is the most frequent reason for acute abdominal pain in older person and is also the most frequent surgical indication over 70 years. With aging increases the formation of stones because it changes the production of bile, increases the saturation of cholesterol, and decreases the sensitivity of the gallbladder to cholecystokinin. Unlike younger patients, more than 30% of older patients have an nonspecific clinical picture unrelated to the severity of the disease: nausea and vomiting may be lacking, pain can be poorly localized without signs of peritonitis, and in 50% of cases there is no fever. However, complications from acute cholecystitis (perforation, emphysematous cholecystitis), which can be quick and without warning, are more frequent in this segment of the population. It must always be suspected in the patient with a history of gallstones [49–52].

Ultrasound has good sensitivity and specificity in gallbladder stones, and its use in POCUS mode in primary care can significantly improve the management and prognosis of these patients.

Appendicitis is the third indication for surgery in older people. Although the overall incidence is lower in the older population, the mortality rate is four to eight times higher. Compared to the young, the mortality of the appendectomy increases from 1% to 50% depending on the comorbidities. The diagnostic difficulty associated with a more complex differential diagnosis and atypical symptoms (fever rarely present, up to a quarter of patients have no lower right quadrant pain) explains the higher rate of presentations with perforated appendicitis for diagnostic delays. In addition, atherosclerosis alters the vascularization of the appendix, and its wall thickens becoming fibrotic and more vulnerable to perforate for even minimal increases in intraluminal pressure [53–55].

The clinical scores do not have sufficient discriminatory power in this slice of the population; therefore in older adults with abdominal pain and suspected acute appendicitis, it needs hospitalization and study with computed tomography considering the reduced risk of ionizing radiation.

Diverticulosis is present in over 80% of old people. As in all the other situations already described, diverticulitis in older people can have an atypical course: in half of the cases, in fact there is no fever, in 30% there is no abdominal pain, and in many cases being present also urinary symptoms, it is mistaken for colic kidney or urinary infection [56].

If the patient seems to be well, has no comorbidity, and has easy access to treatment, follow-up can be treated at home with oral antibiotic therapy effective against gram-negative organisms and anaerobes for 7–10 days and with a low-residue diet. A month after the resolution of the acute event, a colonoscopy is indicated to exclude the presence of an underlying tumor [57, 58].

14.7.2 Obstructive Pain

The most frequent causes of obstruction in the old person are hernias, adhesions, neoplasm, and rarely gallstone ileus for the **small bowel obstruction** (SBO) while diverticulitis, volvulus, and neoplasms for the **large bowel obstruction** (LBO). SBO is more frequent and is characterized by higher mortality than the young adult, while LBO can occur without vomiting or previous constipation; indeed paradoxical diarrhea may be present.

It is important to underline that even in the absence of dilated bowel or air-fluid levels on the plain film radiography (sensitivity of 66%), the SBO cannot be excluded and at the same time abnormalities on radiography may not be associated with clinical findings. For LBO the abdomen radiography is more accurate [59, 60].

When there is an underlying neoplastic disease, recent and unexplained weight loss and fecal volume changes may be present.

Predisposing factors both by mechanical and paralytic obstruction are previous abdominal surgery and adhesions, chronic constipation, drugs "slowing down" peristalsis, abdominal infections, metabolic alterations (dyselectrolytemia, hypothyroidism), neurological disorders, and tumors.

To keep in mind in debilitated patients who take drugs with anti-peristaltic effects and recent history of non-abdominal surgery is the **Ogilvie syndrome** which has a slow onset and massive distension of the colon.

14.7.3 Vascular Pain

The high prevalence of peripheral atherosclerosis, atrial fibrillation, and hypertension makes abdominal vascular pathologies more frequent in older individuals even if with low overall incidence but with high mortality.

Typically the pain can be related to meals, being visceral and not parietal cannot be reproduced by palpation, and is "out of proportion to exam findings." It can manifest as a history of post-prandial discomfort (angina abdominis) and weight loss with sudden worsening from acute arterial insufficiency. Venous occlusion is less frequent and less lethal and associated with hypercoagulability, portal hypertension, previous surgery, or abdominal trauma.

In the case of clinical suspicion, the patient must be hospitalized urgently, and multidetector CT angiography should be performed, as an alternative to angiography (gold standard), compared to which it is less invasive, faster, and more available with good accuracy.

The other vascular abdominal pain is due to the **rupture of an abdominal aneurysm**, which has a pre-hospital mortality of about 50%. The classic triad of broken AAA presentation (hypotension, abdominal pain, and pulsating mass) is found in less than half of cases. Risk factors are older males, smokers, white people, familiarity with AAA, and presence of obstructive arterial disease and connective disease. Pain can be referred to the back, and if bleeding is retroperitoneal, it can be tamponade without causing hypotension. The symptoms can be very varied, and in fact it is frequently misdiagnosed; for this reason aortic aneurysm should be excluded in any patient with intense abdominal or back pain [61, 62].

Bedside ultrasound (point of care ultrasound, POCUS) allows GP to exclude ruptured AAA easily, quickly, and reliably after a learning curve of a few hours of training with a high level of competence [63].

References

1. Lawson P, Richmond C. 13 Emergency problems in older people. Emerg Med J. 2005;22:370–4.
2. Matsushima K, Schaefer EW, Won EJ, Armen SB, Indeck MC, Soybel DI. Positive and negative volume-outcome relationships in the geriatric trauma population. JAMA Surg. 2014;149:319–26.
3. Chang DC, Bass RR, Cornwell EE, Mackenzie EJ. Undertriage of elderly trauma patients to state-designated trauma centers. Arch Surg. 2008;143:776–781; discussion 782.
4. Scuffham P, Chaplin S, Legood R. Incidence and costs of unintentional falls in older people in the United Kingdom. J Epidemiol Community Health. 2003;57:740–4.
5. Haider SI, Johnell K, Thorslund M, Fastbom J. Trends in polypharmacy and potential drug-drug interactions across educational groups in elderly patients in Sweden for the period 1992–2002. Int J Clin Pharmacol Ther. 2007;45(12):643–53.
6. Haider SI, Ansari Z, Vaughan L, Matters H, Emerson E. Prevalence and factors associated with polypharmacy in Victorian adults with intellectual disability. Res Dev Disabil. 2014;35(11):3071–80.
7. Young J. Red flags in geriatrics: diagnoses not to be missed in acute units. Clin Med. 2007;7:512–4.
8. Terence J, Mooijaart S, Gallacher K, Burton JK. Acute care assessment of older adults living with frailty. BMJ. 2019;364:l13.
9. Al Fanaroff AC, et al. Does this patient with chest pain have acute coronary syndrome?: the rational clinical examination systematic review. JAMA. 2015;314(18):1955–65.
10. Bösner S, Haasenritter J, Becker A, Karatolios K, Vaucher P, Gencer B, Herzig L, Heinzel-Gutenbrunner M, Schaefer JR, Abu Hani M, Keller H, Sönnichsen AC, Baum E, Donner-Banzhoff N. Ruling out coronary artery disease in primary care: development and validation of a simple prediction rule. CMAJ. 2010;182(12):1295–300.
11. Harskamp RE, Laeven SC, Himmelreich JC, Lucassen WAM, van Weert HCPM. Chest pain in general practice: a systematic review of prediction rules. BMJ Open. 2019;9(2):e027081.
12. NICE Clinical Guideline. Recent-onset chest pain of suspected cardiac origin: assessment and diagnosis. 2010 (last evidence check September 2019).
13. Lebovitz A, Blumenfeld O, Baumoehl Y, Segal R, Habot B. Postmortem examinations in patients of a geriatric hospital. Aging (Milano). 2001;13:406–9.
14. Becattini C, Agnelli G. Risk factors for adverse outcome in patients with pulmonary embolism. Thromb Res. 2001;103:V239–44.
15. Ray P, Righini M, Le Gal G, Antonelli F, Landini G, Cappelli R, Prisco D, Rottoli P. Pulmonary embolism in the elderly: a review on clinical, instrumental and laboratory presentation. Vasc Health Risk Manag. 2008;4(3):629–36.
16. Moberg AB, Taléus U, Garvin P, Fransson SG, Falk M. Community-acquired pneumonia in primary care: clinical assessment and the usability of chest radiography. Scand J Prim Health Care. 2016;34(1):21–7.
17. Launders N, Ryan D, Winchester CC, Skinner D, Konduru PR, Price DB. Management of community-acquired pneumonia: an observational study in UK primary care. Pragmat Obs Res. 2019;10:53–65.
18. Dwyer R, Hedlund J, Henriques-Normark B, et al. Improvement of CRB-65 as a prognostic tool in adult patients with community-acquired pneumonia. BMJ Open Respir Res. 2014;1:e000038.

19. Richmond TS, Kauder D, Strumpf N, et al. Characteristics and outcomes of serious traumatic injury in older adults. J Am Geriatr Soc. 2002;50:215–22.
20. Perdue PW, Watts DD, Kaufmann CR, et al. Differences in mortality between elderly and younger adult trauma patients: geriatric status increases risk of delayed death. J Trauma. 1998;45:805–10.
21. Davey K, Saul T, Russel G, Wassermann J, Quaas J. Application of the Canadian computed tomography head rule to patients with minimal head injury. Ann Emerg Med. 2018;72(4):342–50.
22. Alrajhi KN, et al. Intracranial bleeds after minor and minimal head injury in patient on warfarin. J Emerg Med. 2015;48:137.
23. NICE guidelines. Investigation for clinically important brain injuries in patients with head injury injuries in patients with head injury; 2019.
24. Flaherty JH, Morley JE. Delirium in the nursing home. J Am Med Dir Assoc. 2013;14(9):632–4.
25. Boockvar K, Signor D, Ramaswamy R, Hung W. Delirium during acute illness in nursing home residents. Am Med Dir Assoc. 2013;14:656–60.
26. McCusker J, Cole MG, Voyer P, et al. Prevalence and incidence of delirium in long-term care. Int J Geriatr Psychiatry. 2011;26:1152–61.
27. Boorsma M, Joling KJ, Frijters DH, et al. The prevalence, incidence and risk factors for delirium in Dutch nursing homes and residential care homes. Int J Geriatr Psychiatry. 2012;27:709–15.
28. Morichi V, Fedecostante M. A point prevalence study of delirium in Italian nursing homes. Dement Geriatr Cogn Disord. 2018;46(1–2):27–41.
29. Elkouby L, Moulias S. [Delirium in a nursing home: a survey of general practitioners]. Soins Gerontol. 2017;22(128):35–8.
30. Klahr S, Miller S. Acute oliguria. N Engl J Med. 2009;338(10):671–5.
31. Jameson JL, Longo D, Kasper D, Hauser SL, Loscalzo J, Fauci A. Harrison's principles of internal medicine. 19th ed. New York: McGraw Hill; 2015. p. 292.
32. Li Q, Zhao M, Zhou F. Hospital-acquired acute kidney injury in very elderly men: clinical characteristics and short-term outcomes. Aging Clin Exp Res. 2019.
33. Miller HJJ. Dehydration in the older adult. Gerontol Nurs. 2015;41(9):8–13.
34. Norman DC. Fever in the elderly. Clin Infect Dis. 2000;31(1):148–51.
35. Chakraborty B. Systemic inflammatory response syndrome. Treasure Island, FL: StatPearls Publishing; 2020.
36. Caterino JM. Evaluation and management of geriatric infections in the emergency department. Emerg Med Clin N Am. 2008.
37. Yoshikawa TT. Epidemiology and unique aspects of aging and infectious diseases. Clin Infect Dis. 2000;30(6):931–3.
38. Ginde J. Impact of older age and nursing home residence on clinical outcomes of US emergency department visits for severe sepsis. J Crit Care. 2013.
39. Samaras N, Chevalley T, Samaras D, et al. Older patients in the emergency department: a review. Ann Emerg Med. 2010;56:261–9.
40. Kizer KW, Vassar MJ. Emergency department diagnosis of abdominal disorders in the elderly. Am J Emerg Med. 1998;16:357–62.
41. Canto JG, Shlipak MG, Rogers WJ, Malmgren JA, Frederick PD, Lambrew CT, Ornato JP, Barron HV, Kiefe CI. Prevalence, clinical characteristics, and mortality among patients with myocardial infarction presenting without chest pain. JAMA. 2000;283(24):3223–9.
42. Bhutto A, Morley JE. The clinical significance of gastrointestinal changes with aging. Curr Opin Clin Nutr Metab Care. 2008;11(5):651–60.
43. Ragsdale L, Southerland L. Acute abdominal pain in the older adult. Emerg Med Clin North Am. 2011;29(2):429–48, x.
44. Wakayama T. Risk factors influencing the short-term results of gastroduodenal perforation. Surg Today. 1994;24(8):681–7.
45. Martinez JP, Mattu A. Abdominal pain in the elderly. Emerg Med Clin North Am. 2006;24:371–88.

46. Levrat M. Peptic ulcer disease in patients over 60: experience in 287 cases. Am J Dig Dis. 1996;11:279–85.
47. McNamara RM. In: Sanders AB, editor. Acute abdominal pain in emergency care of the elder person. St. Louis: Beverly Cracom Publications; 1996. p. 219–43.
48. Chang CC, Wang SS. Acute abdominal pain in the elderly: review article. Int J Gerontol. 2007;1:77–82.
49. Carrascosa MF, Salcines-Caviedes JR. Emphysematous cholecystitis. CMAJ. 2012;184:E81.
50. Wiggins T, Sheraz R. Evolution in the management of acute cholecystitis in the elderly: population-based cohort study. Surg Endosc. 2018;32(10):4078–86.
51. Laurell H, Hansson LE, Gunnarsson U. Acute abdominal pain among elderly patients. Gerontology. 2006;52(6):339–44. Epub 2006 Aug 11.
52. Bedirli A. Factors effecting the complications in the natural history of acute cholecystitis. Hepatogastroenterology. 2001;48:1275–8.
53. Omari AH, Khammash MR, Qasaimeh GR, Shammari AK, Yaseen MKB, Hammori SK. Acute appendicitis in the elderly: risk factors for perforation. World J Emerg Surg. 2014;9:6.
54. Storm-Dickerson TL, Horratas MC. What have we learned over the past 20 years about appendicitis in the elderly? Am J Surg. 2003;185:198–201.
55. Pitchumoni CS, Dharmarahan TS. Abdominal pain. In: Pitchumoni CS, Dharmarajan TS, editors. Geriatric gastroenterology. New York: Springer; 2012.
56. Ferzoco LB. Acute diverticulitis [review]. N Engl J Med. 1998;338(21):1521–6.
57. Dickinson M, Leo MM. Gastrointestinal emergencies in the elderly. In: Kahn JH, Maguaran Jr BG, Olshaker JS, editors. Geriatric emergency medicine: principles and practice. New York: Cambridge University Press; 2014. p. 207–18.
58. Place RJ, Simmang CL. Diverticular disease. Best Pract Res Clin Gastroenterol. 2002;16:135–48.
59. Thompson WM, Kilani RK, Smith BB, et al. Accuracy of abdominal radiography in acute small bowel obstruction: does reviewer experience matter? AJR Am J Roentgenol. 2007;188(3):W233–8.
60. Al Dean DT, et al. Small-bowel obstruction: state-of-the-art imaging and its role in clinical management. Clin Gastrienterol Hepatol. 2008;6(2):130–9.
61. Lederle FA. In the clinic. Abdominal aortic aneurysm. Ann Intern Med. 2009;150(9):ITC5-1-15; quiz ITC5–16.
62. Banerjee A. Atypical manifestations of ruptured abdominal aortic aneurysms. Postgrad Med J. 1993;69:6–11.
63. Andersen CA, Holden S, Vela J, Rathleff MS, Jensen MB. Point-of-care ultrasound in general practice: a systematic review. Ann Fam Med. 2019;17(1):61–9.

Part IV

The Older Patient in His Context

The Older Patient at Home

15

Peter Konstantin Kurotschka, Maria Stella Padula,
Maria Teresa Zedda, Pietro Gareri, and Alice Serafini

Abstract

Ageing societies and technological achievements are changing dramatically the practice of family medicine/primary care and are leading to new models of care delivery to older patients in their homes.

In the first part of the chapter, we point out how the role of home-based primary care has changed in the last decades, and we discuss the available evidence about the clinical- and cost-effectiveness of home care.

In the second part of the chapter, we describe the types of home visits generally performed by general practitioners, namely, acute illness visits, preventive and periodic visits for homebound and frail patients, follow-up visits after hospitalization, and home-based palliative care. Furthermore, we discuss the home

P. K. Kurotschka (✉)
Department of General Practice, University Hospital Würzburg, Würzburg, Germany
e-mail: kurotschka@hotmail.com

M. S. Padula
Italian College of General Practitioners and Primary Care, Florence, Italy

EduCare Lab, University of Modena and Reggio Emilia, Modena, Italy

Local Health Trust Modena, Modena, Italy

M. T. Zedda
Italian College of General Practitioners and Primary Care, Florence, Italy

Regional Health Trust of Sardinia, Cagliari, Italy

P. Gareri
ASP Catanzaro, Catanzaro, Italy

A. Serafini
EduCare Lab, University of Modena and Reggio Emilia, Modena, Italy

Local Health Trust Modena, Modena, Italy

243

© Springer Nature Switzerland AG 2022
J. Demurtas, N. Veronese (eds.), *The Role of Family Physicians in Older People Care*, Practical Issues in Geriatrics, https://doi.org/10.1007/978-3-030-78923-7_15

visit bag equipment (including the diagnostic possibilities offered by portable technologies) and an outline of the points to be addressed to perform a comprehensive home assessment.

Keywords

Home care · Home visits · General practitioners · Homebound patients · Older people

15.1 Introduction

A scientific approach to home care in older patients needs a premise on some of the epidemiological and societal aspects of ageing.

It is well known that the increase in life expectancy and the reduction of fertility rates are determining that the world population is rapidly ageing. Currently, only in Japan the proportion of people aged 60 years or older exceeds 30%; by 2050 the vast majority of high-income countries will have a similar proportion of older people to that of today's Japan [1]. Unfortunately, the fact that people are living longer lives does not necessarily means that people are living healthier lives. In fact, research shows conflicting results: rising rates of frailty, chronic diseases and multimorbidity are accompanied by slightly decreasing rates of severe disability but stable rates of less severe disability [2, 3].

Not only nowadays older people are expected to live longer than 50 years ago; the world around them has changed deeply.

First of all, the majority of world's population lives in urban areas rather than in the countryside; this could have affected the links between and within communities and extended families, reducing the strength of social safety nets. On the other hand, the better communication and transportation infrastructures could represent an opportunity for older people to live more independent lives.

Moreover, social changes happened within families. If, on the one hand, the number of surviving generations within families increases as life expectancy increases, on the other hand, the rate of older people living alone raised significantly in the last decades in many countries. This trend is fostered by the fall of fertility rates, especially in high-income countries, and the consequent increase of the mean age of family members. Contemporarily, women are participating in new roles in society as active paid workforce. This is leading to more opportunities for women, even if the model in which women were responsible for care of older people is not sustainable anymore [4, 5].

Given the WHO definition of *healthy ageing* as "the process of developing and maintaining the functional ability that enables well-being in older age" [1], all people, even those with some sort of functional limitation, have the right to live and be included in their community [6]. It is therefore not surprising that it is generally encouraged what is known as *ageing in place*, that is, the ability of older people to live in their homes and to be included in their communities [1].

In this epidemiological context of a rapidly ageing population, there is no doubt that the demand for home care is expected to increase significantly [5]. In this chapter we'll discuss about the current evidence of the role of family physicians in caring for older people who live in their homes.

15.2 First Part: A Public Health Perspective of Home-Based Primary Care

15.2.1 How Should Home Care Be Defined?

In this chapter we will refer to home-based medical care (HBMC), as a service that "refers to clinical practices that provide physician or nurse practitioner-led, longitudinal interdisciplinary care to homebound, functionally-impaired and seriously-ill adults who have difficulty accessing traditional primary care; it includes both home-based primary care and home-based palliative care" [7].

According to the American Academy of Home Care Medicine (AAHCM), home-based primary care (HBPC) programs "provide appropriate care (primary, urgent, or palliative) to high-risk, medically vulnerable patients, often suffering multiple chronic conditions, when and where they need it. This patient-centric, continuous care model delivers clinical, economic and human benefits such as:

- Facilitating timely interventions when chronic conditions worsen and preempting avoidable emergency department visits and hospitalizations.
- Alleviating social stressors that contribute to poor health.
- Comforting patients by giving them loving care and letting them know they're not alone".

Home care is defined as expert or professional care delivered to adult people at home with formally assessed requirements and needs. It includes personal care, domestic aid, technical nursing care, supportive and rehabilitative nursing care and respite care performed by informal caregivers. It is possible for home care to range from care for the people who only require occasional help with some simple tasks such as frail adults and elderly people with a handicap to care for individuals with complex needs such as support for the whole day. It even includes both short-term and long-term care for people [8].

Home care tends to vary with providers. Therefore, in this chapter we'll focus on home care for elderly people delivered by primary care teams, intended as a type of care delivered by a physician that deals with home-based medical care for elderly people and is directed in a primary care setting by general practitioners (GPs). Keeping this in mind, readers should be advised that different terms such as home visits, house calls and home calls can minimize the value, quality and efforts that generally stay underneath the whole system and assistance that is offered to people. While using also these terms, in this chapter we will prefer terms such as home-based medical care (HBMC) and home-based primary care (HBPC), terms that imply a care model that possesses systems' characteristics such as community-based and team-based care, comprehensiveness and longitudinality.

15.2.2 The Past, Present and Future of Home Visits: Current Trends in Home Visits

Until the first decades of the twentieth century, physician's house calls were the primary mode in which healthcare was delivered. Almost everything a physician needed to diagnose a disease could easily find its place in the doctor's bag, and doctors, rather than patients, were more likely to have access to transportation to reach their patient's home. This is true especially in family medicine. The traditional image of a family physician is that of a man, walking, with his leather bag, through the door to bring medical care at the patient's bed [9].

With the growing advances of technologies to diagnose and treat diseases and the bettering of private and public transport systems that allowed patients to reach care more easily, a dramatic shift of the way in which healthcare was delivered could be observed: medical practice came to be based in institutions, such as hospitals or practices. Sub-specialization of medicine, urbanization and the spread of an efficiency-driven approach to clinical practice (alongside with a change of payment systems) contributed to this phenomenon, exemplified by the falling trend of home visits in the past decades: in 1930 40% of physician encounters were house calls, in 1980 less than 1% [10].

Moreover, across and within countries and among individual GPs, there is a high variability of home visiting rates. A study performed across 18 European countries shows the extent of this variability: the number of house calls performed by each GP in 1 week ranged from an average of 2 home visits per normal week in Portugal to 44 home visits per normal week in Belgium. The same study shows that this variability is closely associated to factors related to the health system but, at the same time, the observed differences at a GP level are explained by patient-related factors such as the age of the patients of each GP [11].

Apparently, this could mean that house calls are declining as a way in which primary care is delivered. Should therefore doctors, patients and healthcare systems definitely abandon the romantic image of the family physician with his leather bag at the patient's bed and embrace the fresh one of a high-technology and high-efficiency ambulatory care model?

In fact, home visits have surprisingly started to make a comeback. Looking at data provided by the American Academy of Home Care Medicine (AAHCM), Medicare-reimbursed house calls are rising in the United States since 1995 [12]. It must be recognized that technological advancements in healthcare such as ultrasounds and X-ray machines that are specifically available in hospitals are no longer a hurdle to home visits because portable devices have been developed in modern times (portable respirator pumps, electronic medical records, lab instruments, portable ultrasound, ECG and X-ray consoles). This makes the delivery of high-quality medical care easier. In addition, it should be considered that the home setting could provide home care teams and physicians with useful and reliable informations about different health hazards including environmental risk factors or structural deficiencies [13].

In the past few years, various mobile application-based services have been developed in the model of house calls including whether a nurse practitioner or doctor is sent to the home and whether prime complaints are analysed and assessed through a telemedicine-based visit or whether insurance is accepted. Typically, these services operate within one to a few large cities. Medicast was one of the first applications as it was launched in 2013 in Miami. It was followed by another service, Pager, in 2014 that served Manhattan. New York City is also served by FRND, and it employs nurses for house calls with video conferencing when necessary. In addition to it, Dispatch Health that is Denver-based provides urgent care services and solutions through either a triage of local calls to 911 or through a patient mobile request. Similarly, Ped-specific PediaQ and Mend provide urgent care services through simple house calls. Circle Medical, similar to Heal, has the aim of extending the platform of house calls including chronic disease management, vaccinations, and wellness exams in San Francisco [9].

Up until these platforms for on-demand house calls became accessible in the major markets of the United States, physicians who tended to perform house calls would be older, and they worked in rural settings. They would often be working together with a model of multidisciplinary medical care that is generally targeted to a geriatric high-risk population. In general, patients who are served in this capacity include the ones who are recently discharged with several medical co-morbidities and have limitations in their access to normal care or patients who are generally enrolled in palliative care. Moreover, younger patients generally requested and required house calls through an application, which might indicate new model's limited reach. Still, further studies are required for determining if mobile health applications are capable of addressing the requirement of continuity for care in different primary care settings [9].

15.2.3 Clinical Outcomes and Cost-Effectiveness of Home Care

Given that technology isn't a barrier to home visits (and home-based medical care in general), what is the clinical effectiveness of home-based medical/primary care? And is home-based medical/primary care cost-effective?

It is common sense that home visits tend to provide access to healthcare services and could improve health in many ways for homebound older patients. In fact, it has to be considered that, because of the often complex social and medical comorbidities of homebound older people, office-based medical care sometimes does not appropriately address the needs of these individuals. HBPC tends to offer a number of benefits for people in the modern healthcare paradigm where patients need to travel to reach the doctor. Chronic medical conditions tend to increase with time and age, and they often lead to functional impairments that reduce the capability of accessing medical care. The ability of seeking medical care is diminished further when a person does not have social support or lacks in terms of financial or social resources like family members who can take them to various appointments or the funds that they need to reach primary care. Generally, these barriers to access lead to poor control of different chronic conditions, fragmented care and missed appointments. Recognizing this barrier to access to care, many programs were developed worldwide with the aim to provide homebound elderly people with primary care at their homes. HBPC is effective in providing a way for patients with function-limiting, complex conditions and cost complications for receiving longitudinal and comprehensive medical care in their homes. Thus, they are able to avoid acute hospitalizations, visits to emergency rooms and even lengthy institutionalizations [13].

Other than filling a comprehensive access gap, when primary care is provided to patients in their homes, it was found to affect patients positively. For instance, the provider who might be a physician assistant, nurse practitioner or a physician is visiting patients in their living context. It could serve to change the power dynamic of meeting or encounter and facilitates relationship building. In fact, providers, caregivers and patients often feel easier and connected with each other. Operating in the environment of home also offers an opportunity to the provider to learn things that could never be discovered in a normal or typical clinic like the way in which patients generally store their medications, the empty refrigerator that might be contributing to weight loss or the fall hazards that are faced by [13].

Several studies have been conducted to gain an understanding of the health and economic benefits of home-based medical/primary care programs. A review of HBPC interventions for community-dwelling older adults from 2014 tried to identify the successful operational components of HBPC programs [14]. Authors found that these programs could have positive effects on important health outcomes, namely, emergency department visits, hospital admissions, long-term care admissions, bed days of care, costs, quality of life and level of satisfaction of patients and caregivers. In all programs, a fully integrated interprofessional care team was responsible for the home care program, and in four of nine of the described interventions, an after-hour urgent telephone service was available. These findings are in line with the report by Yang et al. who enumerate, among the "key facts about HBPC that every geriatrician should know", team-based home visits and after-hour support [15].

Regarding the cost-effectiveness of HBMC/HBPC, a study aimed at analysing the cost reductions due to HBPC determined that the model of HBPC led to 17% lower Medicare costs over a period of 2 years [16]. The study also compared the costs of Medicare and 722 patients' survival in a Medical House Call program with the use of Medicare claims data. This house call program ensured hospice and palliative services, urgent house calls for preventing avoidable hospitalizations, social workers who coordinated supportive and psychological services and an interdisciplinary team of nurse practitioners and physicians who offered telephone coverage all day and often made visits to patients. HBPC showed to be effective in saving more than 4000 dollars per patient on year basis, and patients had 27% fewer visits to specialists, 27% fewer nursing facility stays, 20% fewer visits to emergency department and 9% fewer hospitalizations. Payers and providers agree that the fundamental tenets of these programs are capable of driving value in the modern healthcare environment and that HBPC interventions and services are more cost-effective than emergency care visits and hospitalizations [16].

It should be noted that HBPC serves not only to reduce emergency visits and hospital readmissions, but it also controls the high costs for chronic care through the establishment of trust with patients. This trust makes patients follow instructions for care and they self-treat more effectively [17].

More in general, HBPC aims to prevent hospitalization by ensuring that necessary systems can be implemented right at home. Thus, it serves to bring care to patients and not patients to care. It serves to reduce the physical burden on all those patients who are unable to reach out to ambulatory care. Home visits help in the identification of problems before they become worse and adversely affect patients. Seeing a person regularly enables a higher standard of proactivity. In addition to it, for frail people, home provides a safer environment than hospitals [16, 18].

It is also important to note that HBPC programs make use of multidisciplinary teams. Although formulas might be different, a typical team consists of a care coordinator, a nurse practitioner, an occupational therapist and a social worker, and all of them are coordinated by a primary care physician. This team-based approach serves to reduce the workload on every team member and enhances continuity of care. With an evolution in the medical situation of a patient, care can be adjusted in a timely manner [19].

15.2.4 How Is Home Care Organized?

Despite the fact that different home-based medical care programs showed to be effective in improving health for older people while reducing healthcare-related costs, it should be recognized that the generalizability of current published studies is limited.

Scientific literature offers limited information and data on home care service organization in European countries. A recent review included 74 studies, and only a few of them actually compared home care programs of different nations [8]. It is worth noting that no information was present on over one-third of nations, and the available information was unevenly distributed across countries. Information on Eastern and Central Europe was scarce, and many studies concentrated on only one of the four selected domains including policy regulation, informal carers and clients, financing and service delivery and organization. Moreover, the majority of studies were small scaled. Insufficient detail was offered on home care financing. Overall, the information obtained from literature does not really enable a proper understanding of home care organization's core aspects in European nations. Highlighted aspects of variability in home care organization among European countries were found to be the following:

Table 15.1 Fields of variability of home care organization in Europe (adapted from [20])

Organizational aspect	Variability
Financial	Profit
	Non for-profit
Integration with the HC service	Integrated in the public healthcare system
	Private initiative
Relationship with other HC services	Dedicated service
	Extension of service of HC Centre-based activity
	Hospital-led
	Primary care based
	Integrated with the social services
	Not integrated
Type of illness addressed	Long-term service
	Short-term service (acute illnesses)
Leadership	Physician-led service (geriatrician or family physicians)
	Nurse-led service
Collaboration	Multidisciplinary and team-based work
	Single-doctor

- Service eligibility: several nations considered availability and financial situation of informal caregivers.
- Targeted population groups: in several Mediterranean nations, poor population was focused on by governments, while this targeting was not considered in other nations.
- Organizational and financial competence of central government vs. decentralized competence to regional/local level.
- Connected/integrated policy and vision on cure and care at home was considered in some nations, whereas in other nations, policies on social services and home health were separate.
- Funding mechanisms: there was a contrast in the public funding level among different nations (private for-profit, private non-profit, pubic, combination of private/public) [8] (Table 15.1).

15.2.5 What Physicians and Patient Think About Home Care?

As we previously pointed out, the rate of house calls performed by physicians is generally declining in different parts of the world, despite the diverse organization of the various health-care systems. However, it could be useful to better understand why this is happening, to know what physicians and patients think about the house calls.

The physician's view *Ling Ling Soh* et al. performed an extensive literature review looking for articles that investigate primary care physicians' attitudes and perceptions towards house calls [21]. Despite the evidence that there is a declining interest in house calls also in the research community, with a few articles being suitable for this research question, their findings illustrate that GPs generally recognized house calls to be important. Another interesting issue is that this attitude seems to be relatively stable along the time: findings reported in recent articles, in fact, do not seem to differ from the ones of papers from 30 years ago. This could suggest that barriers to the delivery of home care have grown, while physician's attitudes seem to be stable. The reasons for which physicians chose to perform or not to perform house calls are summarized in the Table 15.2.

Table 15.2 Physicians' attitudes towards house calls (adapted from [21])

Dimensions	Why GPs perform house calls	Why GPs do not perform house calls
Responsibility/ necessity	– Part of the job – Obligation – Pressure from patient's family – Important for providing good, comprehensive care – Elderly, homebound or bedbound patients, especially those with transport issues – Patient who needs end-of-life care	– Unnecessary – Patients can come to the practice – Can be made by other professionals such as nurses – Doubt additional value
Rewards	– Job and life satisfaction – Please and satisfy patients – Enhance practice's market value – More time spent with patients	– Unsatisfactory/inadequate reimbursement for house calls – Not cost-effective for practitioners – Too expensive for patients
Organizational aspects	– Diversion from daily routine – Patients' comfort and convenience/avoid travel – Patients' avoidance of the waiting room	– Time-consuming – Busy practices – Inefficient – Poor/inefficient use of physician's time
Doctor-patient relationship	– Long-term patient – Enhances doctor-patient relationship – Psycho-emotional support for patients and caregivers – Reassurance (especially for the elderly) that reduces feelings of isolation for those who live alone	
Clinical aspects	– Gathering information about patient and family, especially non-medical aspects – Opportunity to assess patient's function and safety – Preventing hospitalization and hospital-acquired infections – Reducing institutionalization of geriatric patients – Better compliance with medical treatment plan	– Clinical inadequacy in home setting – Restricted diagnostic options/support (laboratory/X-rays) – Lack/unavailability of equipment and/or personnel to assist – Providing inadequate or substandard care as compared to clinic setting – Poor control of consultations in the patient's homes

(continued)

Table 15.2 (continued)

Dimensions	Why GPs perform house calls	Why GPs do not perform house calls
Training		– Inadequate or lack of training in the area of house calls
		– Lack of professional role models
		– Difficulty performing minor procedures
Other		– Medical liability issues - personal safety
		– Not enjoyable
		– Inconvenient to travel
		– Displeasure about abuse or misuse of service

Nevertheless, despite the fact that in the field of house calls there is a large influence of subjective attitudes, there are some fields in which these attitudes could be addressed and, eventually, changed. This is especially true for the training issues, with some research highlighting how the exposure of students during medical school to home visits was a factor associated to a positive attitude towards house calls in their practice [22].

Patients' views A study that focused on the opinion of the elderly towards preventive home visits pointed out that 83% of patients were satisfied with the service and 90% stated that patient home visits (PHVs) are important for older people [23]. The main reasons for being satisfied reported were that PHVs added to their feelings a sense of safety and support for their ability to live at home and for having a good life. A sense of support and safety was perceived especially by older patients, by patients with poor physical health and by those without children. In fact, assessing the meaning and importance of home visits only through measuring heavy outcomes like hospitalization rates and increased life expectancy could be misleading as it could fail to understand the extent of the effects of HBMC on frail and older patients. For this reason, this topic has been addressed also through qualitative studies to better understand views, needs and preferences of community-dwelling and frail older people and their informal caregivers on home visits conducted by primary care providers. For example, a Dutch qualitative study found that the issues patients generally want to address during home visit are their psycho-social context and well-being, rather than health problems, disability or dependence. Other interesting aspects raised by patients and caregivers have been the importance of home visits in building the trust needed to a good patient-professional relationship and the acceptability of home visits performed by nurse practitioners, in continuity of care with the GP [24].

15.3 Second Part: Performing a House Call

15.3.1 Who Is Eligible for a House Call?

As mentioned in the first part of this chapter, the frequency of house calls performed by family physicians is highly variable among countries and individual physicians, depending more on organizational aspects of the healthcare sector than on substantial patients' needs. However, the main reasons and needs that drive physicians to perform home visits could be grouped into four different categories [25]:

- *Acute illness visits.* Unless these types of visits are becoming less frequent due to the diffusion of public and private transport that made it easier for the patient to reach the doctor's office, they are still performed, mostly in rural settings. An acute illness could temporarily make patients homebound (e.g. acute pain, high fever, breathlessness) and, thus, could justify the need for a home visit, above all in that patients in which hospitalization should be avoided with every effort. In the last decade, there has been a growing demand for this type of home visits. Despite this, physicians tend to perform fewer home visits as they used to do in the past, tendency that is more evident in publicly funded health systems. Therefore, this leaves space to private companies that perform on-demand house calls to meet this patient's/consumers' needs, mainly through digital platforms (app, websites) [9]. A study that profiled the consumer's demographics and the reasons for the encounter of one of these companies found that patients that queried on-demand house calls were mainly young adults and parents of newborns with a self-reported health status defined good to excellent. This means that the demand of this type of services could grow with the increase of the purchase power of this new generation of patients. Patients requested on-demand house calls mainly for upper-respiratory-tract infections (cough, fever, sore throat, ear infection, flu-like symptoms, sinus infection or pink eye), and the first two most-prescribed medications were antibiotics [9].
- *Preventive and periodic visits for homebound or frail patients.* Actually, the assessment home visit can be defined as an investigational visit during which a physician generally evaluates the role that is played by the home environment on the health status of the patient. Often, an assessment visit is made when a frail patient is suspected for incompliance or is using healthcare resources excessively. Several elements could be better evaluated through a home visit than through an ambulatory consultation, such as the use of medications in the patient who is taking several drugs due to different medical problems, hygienic conditions and environmental or socio-economic hazards. Indeed, when the home environment is analysed, it can reveal some important evidence of social isolation, neglect or abuse. Moreover, family members and patients who are attempting to cope with different chronic problems including incontinence or cognitive impairment might benefit particularly from this evaluation. In addition to it, a

joint assessment at the patient's home is capable of facilitating the coordination of efforts of different healthcare professionals and home health agencies.

In addition, a home visit could be important in the assessment of needs for a frail elderly patient's nursing home placement with uncertain and undetermined social support [25]. In fact, for frail patients, home visits are capable of leading to improved medical care through the assessment and identification of unmet needs in the context of healthcare. Home assessment of frail and elderly patients was described to lead to the identification of new medical issues and intervention recommendations if compared to ambulatory care [26, 27]. This implies that periodic and preventive visits for frail and homebound patients have the potential of revealing information about their conditions that might not be identified at first. Other than just identifying the issues and problems that might be faced by elderly people, it also determines that the current interventions can be adjusted and modified [26].

An important role is played by the home environment in influencing the status of a patient. For instance, there might be some factors that are hindering the recovery of a patient, and they are not generally revealed. These factors can be identified through periodic and preventive visits. Other than the identification of these factors, possible interventions can also be devised for resolving the issues that are being faced by patients. Moreover, periodic home visits could identify areas of incompliance or they could help in determining if the patient is consuming something unhealthy or a substance that can adversely influence health [25].

- *Home-based palliative care*. Most people desire to die at their own home [28], but the proportion of people who die at home vary consistently among countries. The experience of death has been increasingly institutionalized in the last decades, but in the last years, this trend seems to have changed: in 2017 in the United States, home surpassed hospital as "the most common place to death for the first time since the early twentieth century" [29], testimony of a changed receptivity of the healthcare sector on this needs. The provision of home-based palliative care service increases the chance of dying at home for patients with end-stage diseases, and it also reduces the symptoms' burden without worsening the grief of family and caregivers [30]. GPs are ideally positioned to deliver home-based palliative care, as the provision of person and family-centred, longitudinal and holistic care is part of their professional core competences [31]. However, some barriers still exist in the provision of palliative care provided by general practitioners and specialized nurses. A qualitative study highlighted the following as barriers for the delivery of home-based palliative care to end-stage cancer patients: poor coordination and discharge planning, difficulty in arranging necessary equipment and services and inadequate out-of-hour medical provision [32]. Regarding the elements required for the delivery of end-of-life care at home, in another qualitative study, healthcare professionals reported several elements as of pivotal importance: (1) the importance of a "good start" among all the professionals involved in the care team, the family and the patient (in this sense, the first home visit performed by the GP plays an important role); (2) the collaboration among different levels of the healthcare system (acute hospital care, GPs, hospital palliative care, home care agencies); and (3) the need of competences and collaboration within the primary care sector to avoid new hospitalizations [33]. In conclusion, the three key essential clinical processes that enable high-quality home-based palliative care could be identified in (1) the correct and early identification of patients at risk of dying or deteriorating; (2) the formulation of a clear *medical patient care plan* (a communication tool to be shared with all the healthcare professionals that translate a person's advance care plan in medical instructions to be followed in case of deterioration); and (3) the development of a *terminal care management plan* (a document that contains specific measures to be taken to face the most common and predictable terminal symptoms to relief terminal sufferance). In addition, the three essential elements for the delivery of high-quality primary palliative care are identified to be (1) a compassionate GP wishing to help the patient to achieve a good, worthy death; (2) a palliative care team (GP, nurses, social workers, occupational therapists, other healthcare professionals if the patient has complex needs and the caregivers); and (3) available resources to support the GP in the delivery of high-quality home-based palliative care [34].

- *Follow-up visits after hospitalization.* In general, follow-up visits after hospitalization are useful when there are major life changes for patients. For instance, a home visit after a surgery or a major illness can be helpful in the evaluation of coping behaviours of family members and the patient. It also helps in the evaluation of the effectiveness and success of a home healthcare plan [35]. It is important to recognize that one of the goals here is to ensure a safe hospital discharge. A follow-up visit can help in the evaluation of the patient, and it can reveal if the patient is recovering or not. A home visit after hospitalization helps in the prevention of complications that could cause the patient to be readmitted to the hospital. In addition to it, some tests might have been conducted in the hospital, but the necessary results have not been released by the time of discharge. Actually, it is quite important that all the results have been reviewed, and it is determined if the issue is managed properly or not [35].
  A follow-up visit can prove to be beneficial in the evaluation and monitoring of possible medical changes. In the case of a person with acute illness, follow-up visits can not only help in determining if the treatment has positively affected the patient, but it can also help in ensuring the right preventive measures in place so that the patient does not relapse.
  It should be noted that added or new medications that are generally prescribed at discharge from the hospital, e.g. hypertension medications or antidiabetic drugs, are often needed to be monitored [36]. A follow-up visit can help in monitoring and determining whether medications are being taken properly and not accidentally underdosed or doubled up. Therefore, follow-up visits facilitate the process of medication reconciliation.

In general, follow-up visits can help in determining if patients are moving forward with the recommended treatment plan. Other than increasing the possibility of a positive outcome, these visits are quite helpful in minimizing hospital visits, liability concerns and safety concerns [35] (Box 15.1).

Box 15.1 Hospital at Home Programs

The definition of hospital at home (HaH) services is still controversial, leading to the potential misunderstanding about its potential efficacy. The literature describes different types of HaH services [37]:

1. Infusion centres in which patients can receive intravenous therapies.
2. Home care delivered by the hospital in the postoperative period in order to early discharge patients.
3. Services that deliver the same intensity level of care of the hospital setting but at the patient's home.

Potential benefits of HaH programs are [37, 38] the following:

- Avoiding hospitalization and demand for acute hospital beds
- Lowering the risk of cognitive impairment and decline secondary to hospitalization
- Avoiding in older or frail patients the use of sedative medications to treat delirium or behavioural and psychological symptoms of dementia (BPSD)
- Avoiding the risk of a hospital-acquired infection (often caused by antimicrobial-resistant microorganisms)

Hospitals at home programs enable patients to benefit from acute care at their homes and are aimed to improve health status while reducing the economic and societal cost of hospital care. These programs could enable patients to obtain the required healthcare in the manner that they wish (e.g. patients do not have to leave their family or their home).

According to a Cochrane review updated in 2016, HaH programs are likely to increase patient's satisfaction, while the effect of HaH programs on reducing the hospital length of stay or the hospital readmission rates of elderly people with a mix of medical conditions is still insufficient to draw conclusions on efficacy and cost-effectiveness [38].

15.3.2 How Should I Plan a House Call? What Should I Bring with Me During a House Call?

In general, one of the keys for performing effective home care is concerned with clarifying the reasons for the visit and carefully planning the agenda. Preparation enables the physician to collect necessary patient education materials and equipment before departure. Physicians should be carrying a map, the directions to the home of the patient and telephone number of the patient. The home care team, the patient and the physician should set a specific formal time for the visit. Additionally, coordinating the house call for enabling the presence of important family members and other key members can enhance satisfaction and communication. Lastly, confirming the time of appointment with all the involved parties before departure from the clinic or office is a time management strategy and a common courtesy to the family [25].

When it comes to the determination of the equipment used by general practitioners, a sphygmomanometer, a stethoscope, an otoscope and sterile injection syringes were found to be carried by all the interviewed general practitioners for their utilization on house calls [39]. These findings were consistent with that of another study from Israel, which found that the only equipment used in more than 1/3 of home visits were sphygmomanometers, stethoscopes and prescription pads [40]. Less carried equipment were blood glucose sensors, and only one in four of the interviewed GPs took the medical records effectively on home visits. Fifty percent of the practitioners carried all of the common emergency medicines and drugs with them. As it was determined, most practitioners were equipped sufficiently for meeting most situations that might occur during emergency calls and home visits [39].

In Table 15.3 there is listed the suggested equipment for a home visit in general practice [25].

Actually, the application and implementation of portable technology in home care are evolving, and it is recognized as an emerging field. For example, suppose that a diagnostic test normally performed in the emergency department but fundamental to decide the proper management of the patient's needs was performed during a house call, with an effective dispatch system and triage for protecting emergently ill patients from unnecessary hospital admissions. In this scenario, growing interest is emerging around so-called point-of-care diagnostic tests, performed with instruments such as portable ultrasound machines or electrocardiographs. For example, a simple 1-lead portable ECG device, small as a credit card, is able to detect atrial fibrillation with a specificity of 96.5% and a sensitivity of 93.9% if compared to manual pulse palpation followed by a 12-lead ECG [41]. In the last decades, ultrasound technology improved in diagnostic accuracy and portability to reasonable costs to such an extent that point-of-care ultrasonography (POCUS) is claimed to be formally introduced in the training curricula of general practitioners [42]. Beside the fact that the use of such technologies is growing to respond to society's expectation for higher standards of care [42, 43], POCUS has shown to be a useful diagnostic procedure for general practitioners when dealing with elderly patients (e.g. in the diagnosis pneumonia or cardiopulmonar conditions such as pleural and pericardial effusion, left ventricular failure, gallstones, hydronephrosis etc.) [42, 44].

In conclusion, despite the fact that more evidence is needed in the use of portable diagnostic devices in home care settings, the broad utilization of point-of-care testing in ambulatory and hospital settings, where these technologies are indubitably the standard of care, should drive physicians to consider their use in their everyday home practice [45].

Table 15.3 Suggested equipment for home visits in general practice (adapted from [25])

Suggested equipment for home visits
Physician-supplied equipment
Essential
Sphygmomanometer (with various cuff sizes)
Stethoscope
Otoscope and ophthalmoscope
Electronic medical records
Prescription pad
Lubricant
Gloves
Disinfectant solution
Thermometer
Tongue depressors
Urine dipsticks
Optional
Sterile specimen cups
Stool guaiac cards
Glucometer
Measuring tape
Laptop computer or tablet
Diagnostic, prognostic and/or psychometric scales (visual analogue scale, GP-cog, PHQ-9, etc.)
Patient education materials
Other supplies as dictated by patient need
Patient-supplied equipment (as needed)
Portable point-of-care diagnostic instruments (ECG, ultrasound, peak flow metre, spirometer)

15.3.3 What Should I Look at to Perform a Comprehensive Home-Assessment?

As stated above, home visits for frail and homebound patients have the potential of revealing relevant informations that might not be identified during ambulatory consultations. As general practitioners, to have the most of a home visit, especially if we are performing a first assessment of the person, it is useful to focus in a structured manner on following domains that, consistently with the bio-psycho-social model, are identifiable as important determinants of health and well-being of the older patient [25, 26, 46]:

1. *Nutrition.* An observation of kitchen cupboards and refrigerator will let you know about relevant informations about nutrition status or neglect. For example, are there hidden alcohol bottles? Is the fridge empty?
2. *Medications.* In general, a home visit might be the only method of determining how medications are taken by the patient. Therefore, looking around for all the medications that might not have been prescribed or mentioned. It should also be determined whether there are prescriptions from different doctors or not. In addition to it, it could be useful to look over the bottle labels for determining whether

patients are taking the necessary medications or not and whether the patient requires a pillbox for facilitating compliance or not.

3. *Social and community support.* It should be determined with whom the patient is living, if the patient is alone and who is normally available to assist with regular activities. It should also be analysed if outside assistance is needed and how the caregiver(s) are coping and if there is evidence of neglect or abuse.

4. *Mobility.* An observation of the house's condition will tell you how a particular patient is actually managing the daily activities. It should be determined whether the house is clean and whether bathroom and kitchen appear to be used. This type of information can be helpful in making recommendations for the right home care services. It should be determined whether a patient can move safely or not. Are adaptions needed? The footwear of the patient should also be considered. For instance, backless slippers can be dangerous.

5. *Home environmental hazards and safety.* In general, several hazards can be presented by the home to frail elderly people. For instance, lighting should be observed, and it should be kept in mind that the patient might not have proper vision. Long cords, scatter rugs and clutter are all important to note. Other than that, it should be observed if there are any burn marks and whether bedrooms can be accessed easily or not. It should be observed whether the house has handrails.

6. *Physical examination.* Generally, physical examinations are performed in the same way at home as they are done in offices. Generally, if a patient is incontinent or bedridden, it should be kept in mind to examine the skin in a proper and careful manner.

7. *Finance.* It is important to analyse whether the patient is able to purchase the medications and whether he has the necessary financial resources or not. This can be identified by observing the home environment of the patient. Social support could be offered.

8. *Spiritual health and needs.* In addition to finance, the spiritual needs and health of a patient should be assessed properly. Again, the home environment of the person and the condition of the person should be observed. Other than that, if possible, the patient should be consulted about it as it can reveal more in-depth information.

9. *Caregiver situation.* It should be analysed whether the caregiver is capable of meeting the needs of patients and whether he has the necessary understanding and expertise for delivering the required solutions or not. Professional help could be offered.

References

1. World Health Organization, WHO. World Report on ageing and health. 2015.
2. Hung WW, Ross JS, Boockvar KS, Siu AL. Recent trends in chronic disease, impairment and disability among older adults in the United States. BMC Geriatr. 2011;11(1):47.
3. Chatterji S, Byles J, Cutler D, Seeman T, Verdes E. Health, functioning, and disability in older adults—present status and future implications. Lancet. 2015;385(9967):563–75.

4. OECD. Employment Rate. OECD; 2020 [updated 2020].
5. World Health Organization Europe. In: Tarricone R, Tsouros AD, editors. The solid facts: home care in Europe. Europe: WHO; 2008.
6. UN General Assembly. Convention on the rights of persons with disabilities, 13 December 2006, A/RES/61/106, Annex I.
7. Ritchie CS, Leff B, Garrigues SK, Perissinotto C, Sheehan OC, Harrison KL. A quality of care framework for home-based medical care. J Am Med Dir Assoc. 2018;19(10):818–23.
8. Genet N, Boerma WG, Kringos DS, Bouman A, Francke AL, Fagerström C, et al. Home care in Europe: a systematic literature review. BMC Health Serv Res. 2011;11:207.
9. Fortin Ensign S, Baca-Motes K, Steinhubl SR, Topol EJ. Characteristics of the modern-day physician house call. Medicine. 2019;98(8):e14671.
10. Kao H, Conant R, Soriano T, McCormick W. The past, present, and future of house calls. Clin Geriatr Med. 2009;25(1):19–34.
11. Boerma WGW, Groenewegen PP. GP home visiting in 18 European countries adding the role of health system features. Eur J Gen Pract. 2001;7(4):132–7.
12. American Academy of Home Care Medicine. Number of house calls paid by Medicare Part B. AAHCM; 2020 [updated 2020].
13. Schuchman M, Fain M, Cornwell T. The resurgence of home-based primary care models in the United States. Geriatrics (Basel). 2018;3(3):41.
14. Stall N, Nowaczynski M, Sinha SK. Systematic review of outcomes from home-based primary care programs for homebound older adults. J Am Geriatr Soc. 2014;62(12):2243–51.
15. Yang M, Thomas J, Zimmer R, Cleveland M, Hayashi JL, Colburn JL. Ten things every geriatrician should know about house calls. J Am Geriatr Soc. 2019;67(1):139–44.
16. Eric De Jonge K, Jamshed N, Gilden D, Kubisiak J, Bruce SR, Taler G. Effects of home-based primary care on Medicare costs in high-risk elders. J Am Geriatr Soc. 2014;62(10):1825–31.
17. Muntinga ME, van Leeuwen KM, Jansen APD, Nijpels G, Schellevis FG, Abma TA. The importance of trust in successful home visit programs for older people. Global Qual Nurs Res. 2016.
18. Maru S, Byrnes JM, Carrington MJ, Stewart S, Scuffham PA. Long-term cost-effectiveness of home versus clinic-based management of chronic heart failure: the WHICH? study. J Med Econ. 2016;2016:1–25.
19. Leff B, Lasher A, Ritchie CS. Can home-based primary care drive integration of medical and social care for complex older adults? J Am Geriatr Soc. 2019.
20. Hayashi JL, Leff B. Geriatric home-based medical care: principles and practice. Cham: Springer International Publishing; 2015.
21. Soh LL, Low LL. Attitudes, perceptions and practice patterns of primary care practitioners towards house calls. J Prim Health Care. 2018;10(3):237–47.
22. Knight AL, Adelman AM, Sobal J. The house call in residency training and its relationship to future practice. Fam Med. 1991;23(1):57–9.
23. Tøien M, Bjørk IT, Fagerström L. An exploration of factors associated with older persons' perceptions of the benefits of and satisfaction with a preventive home visit service. Scand J Caring Sci. 2018;32(3):1093–107.
24. van Kempen JAL, Robben SHM, Zuidema SU, Olde Rikkert MGM, Melis RJF, Schers HJ. Home visits for frail older people: a qualitative study on the needs and preferences of frail older people and their informal caregivers. Br J Gen Pract. 2012;62(601):e554–e60.
25. Unwin BK, Jerant AF. The home visit. Am Fam Physician. 1999;60(5):1481–8.
26. Ferrier C, Lysy P. Home assessment and care. Can Fam Physician. 2000;46:2053–8.
27. Ramsdell JW, Jackson JE, Guy HJB, Renvall MJ. Comparison of clinic-based home assessment to a home visit in demented elderly patients. Alzheimer Dis Assoc Disord. 2004;18(3):145–53.
28. Barclay S, Case-Upton S. Knowing patients' preferences for place of death: how possible or desirable? Br J Gen Pract. 2009;59(566):642–3.
29. Cross SH, Warraich HJ. Changes in the place of death in the United States. N Engl J Med. 2019;381(24):2369–70.

30. Gomes B, Calanzani N, Curiale V, McCrone P, Higginson IJ. Effectiveness and cost-effectiveness of home palliative care services for adults with advanced illness and their caregivers. Cochrane Database Syst Rev. 2013;(6):Cd007760.
31. Jamoulle M, Resnick M, Vander Stichele R, Ittoo A, Cardillo E, Vanmeerbeek M. Analysis of definitions of general practice, family medicine, and primary health care: a terminological analysis. BJGP Open. 2017;1(3):bjgpopen17X101049-bjgpopen17X.
32. O'Brien M, Jack B. Barriers to dying at home: the impact of poor co-ordination of community service provision for patients with cancer. Health Soc Care Community. 2010;18(4):337–45.
33. Danielsen BV, Sand AM, Rosland JH, Førland O. Experiences and challenges of home care nurses and general practitioners in home-based palliative care – a qualitative study. BMC Palliat Care. 2018;17(1):95.
34. Reymond L, Parker G, Gilles L, Cooper K. Home-based palliative care. Aust J Gen Pract. 2018;47(11):747–52.
35. Gonçalves-Bradley DC, Iliffe S, Doll HA, Broad J, Gladman J, Langhorne P, et al. Early discharge hospital at home. Cochrane Database Syst Rev. 2017;6(6):Cd000356.
36. Lembeck MA, Thygesen LC, Sørensen BD, Rasmussen LL, Holm EA. Effect of single follow-up home visit on readmission in a group of frail elderly patients - a Danish randomized clinical trial. BMC Health Serv Res. 2019;19(1):751.
37. Shepperd S, Iliffe S. Hospital at home versus in-patient hospital care. Cochrane Database Syst Rev. 2005;(3):Cd000356.
38. Shepperd S, Iliffe S, Doll HA, Clarke MJ, Kalra L, Wilson AD, et al. Admission avoidance hospital at home. Cochrane Database Syst Rev. 2016;(9):CD007491.
39. Devroey D, Cogge M, Betz W. Do general practitioners use what's in their doctor's bag? Scand J Prim Health Care. 2002;20(4):242–3.
40. Nakar S, Vinker S, Weingarten MA. What family physicians need in their doctor's bag. Fam Pract. 1995;12(4):430–2.
41. Duarte R, Stainthorpe A, Mahon J, Greenhalgh J, Richardson M, Nevitt S, et al. Lead-I ECG for detecting atrial fibrillation in patients attending primary care with an irregular pulse using single-time point testing: a systematic review and economic evaluation. PLoS One. 2019;14(12):e0226671.
42. Bhagra A, Tierney DM, Sekiguchi H, Soni NJ. Point-of-care ultrasonography for primary care physicians and general internists. Mayo Clin Proc. 2016;91(12):1811–27.
43. Laurence CO, Gialamas A, Bubner T, Yelland L, Willson K, Ryan P, et al. Patient satisfaction with point-of-care testing in general practice. Br J Gen Pract. 2010;60(572):e98–e104.
44. Chavez MA, Shams N, Ellington LE, Naithani N, Gilman RH, Steinhoff MC, et al. Lung ultrasound for the diagnosis of pneumonia in adults: a systematic review and meta-analysis. Respir Res. 2014;15(1):50.
45. Bayne CG, Boling PA. New diagnostic and information technology for mobile medical care. Clin Geriatr Med. 2009;25(1):93–107, vii.
46. Borrell-Carrió F, Suchman AL, Epstein RM. The biopsychosocial model 25 years later: principles, practice, and scientific inquiry. Ann Fam Med. 2004;2(6):576–82.

The Older Person in Nursing Home and in the Intermediate Care Structures: What's the Role of the GPs?

16

Nicola Veronese, Federica Pascale, Alessandro Menin, Stefano Celotto, Simone Cernesi, Paolo Schianchi, and Jacopo Demurtas

Abstract

Hospitals are the main scenario in which the health problems of older people are managed. The transition of hospital-territory is one of the most important health-care problems worldwide now requiring new solutions. In this regard, intermediate care structures seem to be important for this transition. One of the solutions after hospital and intermediate care transitions is nursing home placement, often due to familial or social choices. Apparently, the case mix in nursing homes is changing, with more patients with advanced cognitive disorders and frail or multimorbid older patients, often affected by severe disability. In both intermediate

N. Veronese
Department of Internal Medicine and Geriatrics, University of Palermo, Palermo, Italy

F. Pascale (✉) · P. Schianchi
Primary Care Department, Azienda Unità Sanitaria Locale di Parma,
Parma, Emilia-Romagna, Italy
e-mail: federicapascale89@gmail.com

A. Menin
Vicenza, Italy

S. Celotto
Primary Care Department, ASUFC—Azienda Sanitaria Universitaria Friuli Centrale,
Udine, Italy

S. Cernesi
AUSL, Modena, Italy

J. Demurtas
Primary Care Department, USL Toscana Sud Est, Grosseto, Italy

© Springer Nature Switzerland AG 2022
J. Demurtas, N. Veronese (eds.), *The Role of Family Physicians in Older People Care*, Practical Issues in Geriatrics, https://doi.org/10.1007/978-3-030-78923-7_16

and long-term care structures, the general practitioner (GP) faces acute conditions in complex patients, being this situation similar to what happens in a hospital. In this chapter, we will discuss the role of the GP in nursing homes and in the intermediate care settings highlighting the most important problems encountered in daily clinical practice.

Keywords

Nursing home · Intermediate care · Hospital transition

16.1 Introduction and Definition of Nursing Home and Intermediate Care

Nursing homes are residential care centers that provide care for people requiring a certain level of medical care that can't be met through home or other community services. The residential care model usually includes nursing care, dietary needs, environmental and maintenance services, as well as activities to ensure active and engaged residents. Typically, nursing homes, or skilled nursing facilities (SNFs) as they are called today in some countries, take care of older people or those facing end-of-life care. However, the definition of nursing home is highly variable across countries and, often even in the same country, can slightly change in terms of health and non-health personnel and in terms of services. Moreover, another important distinction is if these structures may as well be private (i.e., paid by the residents or by their relatives) or public. In some countries, there is a mixed model in which a part is paid by the state and a part by the families.

Nursing homes can be the destiny of a limited part of people accessing to hospitals. Since nursing homes are commonly expensive [1], more recently intermediate care units arose. To define what is intermediate care is still difficult today, and there is still no certified definition [2]. We can define these structures as services provided to patients, usually older people, after leaving the hospital or when they are at risk of being sent to the hospital [3].

The role of general practitioners (GPs) in these settings is still not univocal, but in this chapter we will discuss the most common issues encountered by GPs in their daily clinical practice in intermediate and long-term care units.

16.2 Nursing Home Setting

16.2.1 The Relationship with the Guest

The relationship with the guest, specifically the one residing in the nursing home, is a fundamental element for obtaining the best care and management. In this context, the GP is often faced with critical aspects, some typical of old age and others closely related to the home environment. In fact, with the older person, there may be communication and understanding difficulties related to the language, lack of collaboration due to the presence of cognitive impairment or psychiatric disorders, dysphagia problems, and erroneous beliefs that limit the intake of drugs. Generally, the older person presents himself as a fairly collaborative individual towards the GP. In general, we can say that a serious but friendly approach, sometimes even facetious within the limits of lawfulness and respect for the individual, which is comforting and shifts the patient's attention from his health problems, allows you to tune in to the older patient and to be able to establish a very profitable professional relationship.

In the nursing home patient, it is often evident (as in most people who are hospitalized) not only the "disease" aspect but also the "illness" aspect. The patient can be worried about all aspects related to his illness and his stay in the nursing home: the spatial and social limitation, the lack of privacy, the reduced time with family members, and the expenses that the family has to bear. These concerns affect his psychophysical well-being, especially in the first period of hospitalization, and must be taken into account. The patient in the nursing home is therefore a "frail" subject due to his loss of autonomy in the activities of daily life, a characteristic that depends on multiple factors and is linked to the comorbidities that develop in the older subject.

16.2.2 Communication Problems

Nowadays, the older residents generally have a low educational level. They do not always master the language perfectly, sometimes they express themselves in dialect and obviously do not know the technical language of medicine. In some cases, they are illiterate, or at least unable to write or read correctly. Added to these, vision and hearing problems are often present. For these reasons, the GP should avoid the technicalities and use simple language to deal with the patient in many situations. The use of a figurative language can help to explain more complex concepts. If the patient uses dialect or a language other than the one commonly used (if he/she is a foreigner), the doctor must try to enter the same communication channel, using the same language or using communication tools such as paraphrasing the concepts expressed by the patient or using the support of a dialect-speaking mediator. A very useful tool, especially in the demented patient, can be the capacitive approach, an interpersonal communication system based on the word and which has as its objective, "a sufficiently happy coexistence between frail and/or demented older person" [4].

The older patient, especially if affected by dementia, has a reduced and sometimes inadequate vocabulary to really express his needs. The communicative approach attempts to identify and revive elementary skills (competence to speak, competence to communicate, emotional competence, competence to negotiate, competence to decide). The ability to speak gives value to the word regardless of its meaning (it is a communicative act; however, it expresses a need, and it is an expressive ability even when its meaning is null or incorrect). The competence to communicate concerns the methods of communication, i.e., verbal, paraverbal, and nonverbal. Emotional competence is the one that allows you to experience emotions, to identify those in front of you, and to share them. The competence to negotiate, that is, to negotiate the topics of the conversation with the interlocutor, is an act that is incentivized to stimulate the older to become an active part during the dialogue. The competence to decide is that which shows us the will of the subject and which can be expressed in an evident and clear way, as well as with simple behavior (e.g., of relational closure, with arms folded and the gaze turned by another part). As the psychologist Paul Watzlawick argued, "one cannot not communicate": the doctor must therefore be attentive to even the most subtle and apparently insignificant signals because the patient, and in this case the older in the nursing home, communicates continuously his problems, his needs, and his fears [5].

16.2.3 Problems Due to Cognitive Impairment or Psychiatric Disorders

Cognitive impairment or the presence of psychiatric disorders can further undermine communication between doctor and patient. If the cognitive impairment has advanced, very often the patient is unable to express himself adequately, expresses disconnected and meaningless sentences, or repeats meaningless words or sounds. In this case, however, the paraverbal and nonverbal channels remain active, helping us to identify the patient's needs. The capacitive approach can be useful to stimulate residual capacities in patients with not too advanced dementia.

Another common problem is to face the health problems of the older patients affected by psychiatric conditions. The older psychiatric patient, on the other hand, can refuse to collaborate and be difficult to manage, communication can be limited, and he can shut himself up in his world and refuse therapy. In this case, we believe that it is important to speak the patient's language and try to go along with it, so as to enter his "world": this allows us to gain trust and to make sure that he gradually also satisfies our requests.

16.2.4 Dysphagia Problems

In the nursing home, dysphagia is a frequent problem that can complicate taking care of the patient. It is important, first of all, to catch the first signs of dysphagia, and for this reason it is useful to deal with the social health workers who are most in contact with the patients and who follow them during meals. Once the problem has been identified, we must visit the patient and talk to him about this question and possible solutions, if he is still capable of understanding and willing.

Obviously, there must be a comparison and an evaluation also by the speech therapist who can give useful indications in this regard. Also, in this case it is necessary to have a good relationship with the patient since dysphagia often requires a change of diet and in particular of the consistencies of foods and liquids. The same applies to drugs which, in the nursing home, fall within a limited standard form, and often, due to cost issues, the formulations most suitable for dysphagic subjects are lacking. The guest may not like these new settings, and for this reason it is important to inform him and share the path he intends to take with him. Sometimes it is necessary to mediate, looking for the solution that brings the least damage, in order to come up against even the patient's requests to aim at his complete psychophysical well-being.

16.2.5 Problems Related to Wrong Beliefs

The problem of wrong beliefs can be found across all ages. As mentioned above, the older patient has a medium-low level of education, and there may also be some cognitive impairment. This can sometimes lead to some difficulties in prescribing and administering therapy. For example, there may be those who are against the flu vaccine, those who believe that taking drugs is harmful, and those who rely only on products brought from home and do not want the nurse to administer them [6]. In these cases, it is essential to be clear from the start: we must make the patient aware that he is now in a structure that has rules and that the ultimate goal of our work is the patient's well-being. He should therefore be informed of the reduced risks of the flu vaccination and the benefits for him and for the other guests who get it. In those who do not want to take drugs or who bring products from home, the GP will have to talk to the patient and his family: we must make them understand that there are equal rules for everyone and that, looking at the patient's well-being, certain therapies are undertaken on the basis of the clinical picture. The use of other products (e.g., nutritional supplements) must be agreed a priori with the doctor, because some substances may interact with the drugs in use or alter the state of health. Finally, it should be reiterated that any product in use must be delivered to the nursing staff who will be the only one in charge of the administration. This is important both to make the guest participate in the rules of the structure and standardize it to the new environment and to avoid risks related to autonomous administration or relatives (drug interactions, side effects, ab-ingestis, etc.).

16.2.6 End of Life and Nutritional Support Measures

The older resident is aware that his life has already run its course but rarely has it very clear how the last moments of his life will have to be. If the patient is capable of understanding and willing, it is useful to ask immediately if he/she has any particular requests and what the last wishes are on this issue. Clearly, any therapeutic obstinacy must be avoided, but the decision for the doctor is always rather difficult. Sometimes we are faced with cases in which the patient still has a certain potential for recovery and the correction of some factors could thus prolong his life (e.g., a dysionemia in a decompensated subject). The question to ask is whether such treatment would bring real benefit, that is, if it prolongs life by bringing the guest back to the status quo ante or if, instead, it only prolongs the suffering. The most important goal is in fact to minimize suffering by applying appropriate measures (e.g., morphine therapy if pain is present). In cases of severe dysphagia or poor nutritional status, it must be determined whether it is worth feeding the patient artificially or whether to apply only moisturizing therapy. Here too it is important to respect the patient's wishes, both when expressed verbally and when expressed nonverbally (e.g., when the patient repeatedly takes off the needle-cannula or the nasogastric tube) [7]. In cases where the patient is unable to express his own will, family members must be heard, who may be aware of the patient's presumed will, but the final decision must always be made by the doctor, aware that the treatment must be clinically adequate and proportionate, and that the final objective is to improve the quality of life, not "add days" to life. The choice of the type of food route must be made on the basis of the overall clinical picture and what life prospect the patient will have.

In the patient with advanced dementia, the scientific literature does not recommend the use of artificial nutrition, because it does not bring benefits in terms of quality of life [8]. In such cases instead, as far as possible, oral feeding, even if partial, to encourage human contact and social participation should be encouraged.

16.2.7 The Relationship with Family Members

As soon as the guest enters the nursing home, the GP must introduce himself to the family members. They must be explained the rules of the structure and the objectives they intend to achieve and must be comforted immediately. Often, in fact, there is an ambivalent aspect in family members. On the one hand, they are refreshed by having placed their relative in a nursing home because home management was difficult, stressful, and sometimes the cause of conflict. On the other hand, they feel guilty for having removed their loved one from their home and for having "abandoned" it in some way. Especially in the first few weeks, social health workers should be asked to monitor visits. It happens with some frequency that, even if learned about the internal rules, the family members administer drugs or meals to the patient who perhaps has dysphagia problems. In order to avoid medical-legal problems, these behaviors must be firmly blocked, making relatives aware of the risks of such practices. The doctor must inform family members on a frequent basis about changes in the clinical picture, the results obtained (e.g., motor recovery), and the problems that arise (e.g., appearance of dysphagia, poor nutrition, behavioral disorders, etc.). It is essential to inform them ahead of time about the possible application of restraint or artificial feeding measures. In such cases it is also a good thing to evaluate their opinion which, even if not binding, must be taken into account by the doctor to make the best decision. As already mentioned, in the case of a patient who is capable of understanding and willing, relatives should be asked if their family member had previously expressed specific wishes regarding the end of life or artificial feeding. In the nursing home, financial problems may also arise: in fact, in order to pay the tuition, family members must sell some of the patient's properties or use his funds. In the case of a demented patient, we must advise relatives to ask the judge to appoint a legal guardian. If the patient is unable capable of understanding and willing and has no relatives, to decide on the end of life, on particular therapies not present in the manual and on the possible application of artificial nutrition, the doctor himself must first deal with the legal guardian appointed by the judge.

Relatives must be involved in the social activities of the rest home, in the moments of celebration of the guests, and in the recreational activities to stimulate the emotional part and strengthen the guest's intellectual capacities. Specific time limits must be set, which can be agreed upon in particular cases (e.g., in the last days of the patient's life) to avoid that relatives disturb other patients or interfere with the activities of the various professional figures. Let us remember that the patient always feels homesick for his home, and an excessive presence of relatives, especially in the first phase, makes it difficult for the guest to accept his new reality.

16.2.8 Multi-professional Team Case Management

Generally, in the nursing home, there are other professional figures in addition to the GP and nursing staff. These figures are extremely important having competencies that complete and improve GP work. In Table 16.1 we briefly report the role of these important figures.

The older resident frequently needs the evaluation and the work from all these figures. A dysphagia problem, for example, can be firstly detected by all these figures and reported to the doctor, who will give preliminary indications to the social health worker about nutrition and will warn the speech therapist to evaluate the swallowing ability of the patient and give the specific indications of the case.

Although each professional figure works in his or her specific field, teamwork helps the doctor above all in managing complex issues. Take, for example, the case of a patient who is still able to capable of understanding and willing but who refuses to express himself verbally and to take food. The comparison of the doctor with the various figures will lead to a better assessment of the picture as a whole: the nurse will tell us if the guest is collaborating and takes therapy, the social health worker may report if and how much the patient manages to feed himself, the speech therapist will evaluate the degree of dysphagia possibly present, the psychologist will be able to tell us if the patient is depressed and if his cognitive skills allow him to understand what he is doing, the educator and the physiotherapist will give us news about his social participation and motor skills (and therefore on his life project in general). This may allow the doctor to deal with various problems and more efficiently take care of the older patient who lives in a nursing home. It is of utter importance to have a medical record shared with all professionals, being able to update the others about the needs of the patients and to share and clearly define the responsibility in the various aspects of the management of the patient.

Table 16.1 Multi-professional team case management roles and competencies

Figure	Role and competency
Nurse	The nurse is the professional figure with whom the GP has probably the most collaborative relationship. He is a very precious and indispensable reference in administering the therapy, managing any emergencies, and feeding the dysphagia; he personally collects a lot of clinical information from the continuous contact with the guests
Department coordinator	He is the first point of contact for the other professional figures, able to collect information from the various figures and then report it to the doctor who can later deepen directly with the specific operator. Frequently this figure also has greater contact with family members from whom he receives any appreciations and complaints, manages convivial moments with relatives, takes care of monitoring the work of the SDGs, and monitors the availability of the principals, food, and consumables
Social health worker	Probably he is the professional figure closest to the older patient who is in the nursing home. He can grasp even the smallest changes in behavior, detects the presence of any skin lesions, reports on the appearance of any swallowing and/or walking difficulties, signals the appearance of alterations of the hollow and possible urinary infections, and informs the nurse about sudden changes in the patient's psychophysical picture. The doctor therefore receives valuable information from the socio-health operator and, in turn, can give indications on the methods of feeding, walking (with or without operator), hygiene (in case of urinary or genital infections, protocol in the presence of multiresistant infections), and restraint (spatial/environmental or with devices)
Physiotherapist	This figure reports to the GP motor problems or new disorders highlighted during physiotherapy sessions. In turn, he receives from the doctor a report of any motor dysfunction to promptly start a rehabilitation program. The same applies when a patient tends to fall with a certain frequency or gets up from the wheelchair, in order to identify the aid (e.g., walker, stick, wheelchair) or the most suitable means of restraint (e.g., a table in a wheelchair)
Speech therapist	This figure takes care of the patients' swallowing, phonetic, and hearing skills. Therefore the doctor can receive indications to change a diet in the presence of dysphagia, the signaling of the presence of oral thrush that needs medical treatment, and the presence of earwax plugs to be eliminated with ear washing or sensorineural hearing loss that requires hearing aids. The doctor can ask the speech therapist to evaluate a guest when a certain difficulty in swallowing has been detected, he can request that a diet with the right consistencies be set, and he can indicate to the speech therapist a guest who needs speech therapy treatment to safeguard the residual abilities
Psychologist	Psychologist evaluates the presence and the severity of the cognitive impairment of the patients reporting to the doctor if there have been any deteriorations that require any pharmacological treatments. This figure also deals with providing psychological support to anxious and depressed patients, who may or may not need drug therapy. Moreover, the psychologist can also be very useful to support family members who are excessively worried about their family member or those suffering from the sudden loss of their loved one, to be helpful in responding to the complaints of relatives more difficult to manage and to alleviate any internal tensions between the guests of the structure who have moved to live in a social reality that is new to them

(continued)

Table 16.1 (continued)

Figure	Role and competency
Educator	The educator takes care of keeping older patients active, both physically and psychically with outdoor activities, manual activities, and group games. It can detect sudden changes in the guest's psychophysical picture and then report them to the doctor. The latter may suggest the educator to stimulate a specific patient with a specific activity (e.g., with manual activities in those who are losing these skills, music, and singing in the subjects who are more reactive in those moments, reading in those individuals who tend to remain solitary, etc.), in order to allow the maintenance of residual capacities and stimulate the patient who is in the context of the rest home
Social worker	The social worker takes care of some structural problems, e.g., when the patient needs an additional period of stay in the structure, when there are extra expenses to be addressed (e.g., specialist visits for a fee, request for off-the-shelf drugs), or when the guest from self-sufficient becomes non-self-sufficient (with consequent change of the tuition and the treatments that are due to him)

16.3 Intermediate Care Setting

16.3.1 A General Perspective

The resulting pressures on acute services have been instrumental in the development of intermediate care as a new healthcare model, which has its origins in the National Health Service in the United Kingdom around 20 years ago [2].

Intermediate care is thus an emerging concept, which may offer attractive alternatives to hospital care for older patients [2]. The main recognized objectives of intermediate care are to promote timely discharge from hospital, to prevent unnecessary hospital admissions, and to reduce the need for long-term residential care by optimizing functional independence [2], even if intermediate care units can also be summarized as a set of services designed to facilitate the transition from hospital to home and from medical dependence to functional independence [9].

Some countries have already tried different ways to implement intermediate care in their health systems. Examples include the United Kingdom, New Zealand, Canada, the United States, and Australia, although each in a different and peculiar way [10].

16.3.2 Intermediate Care Unit Aims

The multidisciplinary approach for the older patient aims to enhance his functional abilities, reduce the risk of rehospitalization, and progress his frailty status [11].

Therefore, intermediate care is the desirable care setting for the following types of patients:

- Patients discharged from the acute care hospital, in the clinical stabilization stage, whose health and/or social conditions do not guarantee adequate care at home.
- Patients who are dischargeable at home but with fragile or inadequate social contexts that do not allow them to return, except after a period of treatment aimed at acquiring and/or recovering the residual autonomy.
- Patients with recrudescence of chronic diseases or for whom the family physician requires a protected environment to implement/continue their therapies in order to prevent hospitalization.
- Patients needing continuous nursing care.
- Oncological patients not suitable for hospitalization in palliative care facilities.

Intermediate care unit commonly incorporates an integrated care model, based on teamwork between the case manager nurse and the social worker, as well as the caregiver, in a therapeutic alliance whose objectives are:

- To guarantee continuity of hospital-community care through joint work between the GP and the community multi-professional team.
- To reduce hospital readmissions by temporarily managing diseases with a high level of health care, thus avoiding admissions of an inappropriate nature.
- To bring the patient back to its home or in the community settings most suitable to his/her needs.
- To ensure the implementation of the reactivation plan, rehabilitation, and maintenance of residual autonomy through patient-centered interventions in a more personalized environment.
- To promote the therapeutic education of the patient and/or caregiver.

These services are provided on the basis of a patient multidimensional assessment, supported by an integrated and individualized care plan.

Intermediate care is an easy and intuitive way for community health care to achieve recovery and stabilization of a fragile patient before returning home or in another structure with a lower health capacity. Intermediate care should offer a service based on a holistic approach, coordinated by different professionals who interact with each other in drafting an individual care plan, aimed at taking care of the whole patient. Intermediate care can therefore be the reference for care continuity in the community setting, prior to a final discharge or instead of an improper hospitalization. In addition, admissions to intermediate care are characterized by significantly reduced hospitalization costs compared to high-intensity care.

Intermediate care services such as community hospitals constitute an appropriate response to the demands of fragile users, favoring not only the reduction of long hospital stays, but also act by preventing the often significant post-hospitalization disability and therefore promote a reduction in health costs on a long-term care for family members and for the society as a whole.

16.3.3 What's the Role of the GP in Intermediate Care Units?

Family physicians' role in intermediate care is multifaceted and can be acted in several different settings. First of all, the GP's role could be in the safe return to home of an hospitalized patient, through a *protected discharge*, which thus requires also coordination between the hospital setting and territorial setting. In this case the GP could act either as a manager in primary care departments, leading and coordinating the operations to allow the patient to come back to his home or nursing home setting, or as the patient's personal physician, managing with other health professional patient's needs in the home setting. Moreover, the role of family physicians could also be acted in community hospital structures for patients still having a complex need but which can be managed by family doctors and nurses.

The important social role the GP has in the society, the social net he is inserted in, makes it important for him to be a patient's advocate with local institutions. The need for a social support, for activities being able to maintain older people's autonomy, to improve rehabilitation after a long hospital stay may be identified by the GP and, if lacking, asked to local politicians and associations. Changing the environment and institutions to better fit the patients' needs, especially the most fragile ones, should be taken into consideration, since it may have a long-term positive impact.

16.4   Conclusion

In both intermediate or long-term care structures, the GP faces complex conditions in complex patients, being this situation often similar to what happens in a hospital, but without the resources that we have in a hospital. This chapter reported the most important problems that are faced by the GP suggesting that specific preparation for older persons living in a nursing home or accessing intermediate care structures is needed.

References

1. Mor V. Cost of nursing home regulation: building a research agenda. Med Care. 2011; 49(6):535.
2. Melis RJ, Rikkert MGO, Parker SG, van Eijken MI. What is intermediate care? London: British Medical Journal Publishing Group; 2004.
3. MacInnes J, Jaswal S, Mikelyte R, Billings J. Implementing an integrated acute response service: professional perceptions of intermediate care. J Integr Care. 2020;29(1):48–60.
4. Dawson A, Bowes A, Kelly F, Velzke K, Ward R. Evidence of what works to support and sustain care at home for people with dementia: a literature review with a systematic approach. BMC Geriatr. 2015;15(1):59.
5. Watzlawick P, Beavin JH, Jackson DD. Pragmatica della comunicazione umana, vol. 35. Roma: Astrolabio; 1971.
6. Bond L, Nolan T. Making sense of perceptions of risk of diseases and vaccinations: a qualitative study combining models of health beliefs, decision-making and risk perception. BMC Public Health. 2011;11(1):943.

7. Veronese N. Artificial feeding in older people; 2019.
8. Veronese N, Minto S, Bonso O, Merlo A. Importance of quality of life in people with dementia treated with enteral nutrition: the role of the nurse. Geriatric Care. 2019;5(2).
9. Salsi A, Calogero P. Intermediate care. Italian J Med. 2010;4:57–62.
10. Griffiths PD, Edwards ME, Forbes A, Harris RG, Ritchie G. Effectiveness of intermediate care in nursing-led in-patient units. Cochrane Database Syst Rev. 2007;2:CD002214.
11. Akpan A, Roberts C, Bandeen-Roche K, Batty B, Bausewein C, Bell D, et al. Standard set of health outcome measures for older persons. BMC Geriatr. 2018;18(1):36.

The Role of Caregivers in the Care of Older People

17

Pinar Soysal, Francesca Rossi, Donatella Portera,
Lee Smith, Lin Yang, and Ahmet Turan Isik

Abstract

In this chapter, caregivers' roles in the care of older people are discussed in detail. With older people having multiple comorbid diseases, such as osteoarthritis, cancer, chronic obstructive pulmonary disease, heart failure, stroke, and chronic kidney disease, and numerous geriatric syndromes such as

P. Soysal (✉)
Department of Geriatric Medicine, Faculty of Medicine, Bezmialem Vakif University,
Istanbul, Turkey
e-mail: psoysal@bezmialem.edu.tr, dr.pinarsoysal@hotmail.com

F. Rossi
Expert Patient, TANDEM Association, Modena, Italy

D. Portera
Expert Patient, TANDEM Association, Modena, Italy

Primary Care Department of Modena, Modena, Italy

L. Smith
The Cambridge Centre for Sport and Exercise Sciences, Anglia Ruskin University,
Cambridge, UK

L. Yang
Department of Oncology, Cumming School of Medicine, University of Calgary,
Calgary, AB, Canada

Department of Community Health Sciences, Cumming School of Medicine, University of
Calgary, Calgary, AB, Canada

A. T. Isik
Unit for Aging Brain and Dementia, Department of Geriatric Medicine, Faculty of Medicine,
Dokuz Eylul University, Izmir, Turkey

© Springer Nature Switzerland AG 2022
J. Demurtas, N. Veronese (eds.), *The Role of Family Physicians in Older People
Care*, Practical Issues in Geriatrics, https://doi.org/10.1007/978-3-030-78923-7_17

polypharmacy, urinary incontinence, malnutrition, depression, dementia, falls, and frailty, their increased dependence on daily living activities causes them to have difficulty maintaining their lives independently, and so they need a caregiver. Caregiving involves various tasks ranging from helping the older people in basic and instrumental activities of daily livings to providing complex health care. Caregiving domains can be grouped as follows: (1) assisting with daily living activities; (2) emotional and social support; (3) health and medical care; (4) care coordination; and (5) decision-making. Each of these areas includes a number of separate tasks. In performing these roles, caregivers face stress in physical, psychological, social, and financial terms, which causes caregiver burden. To reduce caregiver burden, it is very important to provide caregivers with systematic training about older people's care and to develop supportive health strategies while they perform caregiving tasks.

Keywords

Caregiver · Older · Dependence · Decision-making · Caregiver burden

17.1   Introduction

While aging is defined as a period when an individual experience declines in terms of physical appearance, power, role, and position and with increased disability and physical diseases, the individual becomes increasingly dependent on the social environment. It is emphasized that the approach towards the mental and physical conditions of older people should be different from the approach to other age groups. According to the World Health Organization (WHO) report, the number of people aged 60 and over, which was 600 million in 2000, will increase to 1.2 billion in 2025 and 2 billion in 2050 [1]. In addition, WHO emphasizes that all countries in the world should be prepared for the negative consequences of the demographic process (i.e., an increase in frequency of people living longer), stating that industrialized countries are prospered before aging whereas developing countries will grow older before prosperity [1, 2]. Life expectancy increases over time. In the twenty-first century, it is predicted that 20% of the world's population will be aged by the increase in the life expectancy and the increase in the number of older people over 85 years of age. It is obvious that with the increase in the older population, not only the health problems of older people, but also their caregivers' and caregiver-related problems will surge. According to the 2014 nationally representative caregiver report, there are an estimated 18 million caregivers in the United States that care for 9 million older people. Moreover, the fact that the average age of caregivers is 69.4 years and that almost half of the caregivers care for 75 years or older reveals the importance of older people's care [2, 3].

Today, the majority of older people's care is provided by informal caregivers (family caregivers and unpaid caregivers) [4]. However, the latest report from the National Academies of Sciences, Engineering, and Medicine shows that changes in social and structural factors (such as reduced fertility, increased life expectancy, increased caregivers) will transform care from informal to professional in the future [5]. The fact that the older population in need of increased care cannot be met by the number of formal and qualified caregivers is a remarkable problem for older people's care in the years to come. The increase in the number of care-dependent older people poses an economic burden for most health systems. Institutional care is the primary factor in increasing costs in long-term care of older people. Expenses of long-term health care in nursing homes are much higher than those of home care [6]. This is, therefore, an effective cost reduction strategy for funders to ensure that dependent people remain in the home-based care environment as long as possible. Moreover, many older people prefer to stay in their homes until the end of their lives. All these factors increase the importance and responsibility of family caregivers.

Older age increases multimorbidity and consequently dependence on care [7, 8]. For example, in a large European prevalence study in which more than 80,000 patients aged over 65 years were questioned for ten chronic comorbid diseases (hypertension, lipid metabolism, diabetes, coronary heart disease, cancer, chronic obstructive pulmonary disease, heart failure, stroke, chronic kidney disease, and osteoporosis), it was found that all comorbid diseases increased with age, that at least one comorbid disease was present in one out of two people, and that almost one out of four persons had comorbidity of four or more [9]. On the other hand, not only comorbid diseases are increased with advancing age, but geriatric syndromes occur as well [7]. It was reported that the frequency of polypharmacy was 54.5%, urinary incontinence 47.6%, malnutrition 9.6%, depression 35.1%, dementia 21.6%, falls 33.6%, sarcopenia 31.7%, and frailty 28.3% and that all syndromes were significantly increased with age. Although 20% of cases in the 60–69 age group did not have any syndrome, 48% of cases over ≥80 years had more than four syndromes at the same time [7] (Fig. 17.1). The combination of comorbid diseases and geriatric syndromes increases disability, institutionalization, and hospitalization, which makes it difficult for both clinicians and caregivers [10]. As chronic conditions

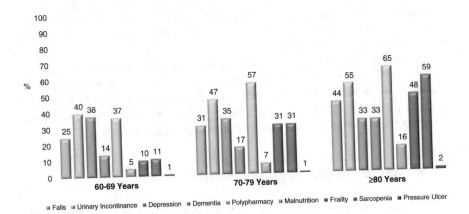

Fig. 17.1 The prevalence of geriatric syndromes

persist for a lifetime, a long-term care plan is needed where active caregivers, particularly family caregivers, are required.

17.2 Care Process

Caregivers are individuals who provide free or formal care to sick, disabled, and/or cognitive impaired older adults, usually family members or friends. As there are many different aspects of long-term older adults' care, the starting form of caregiving may change [11, 12]. The care process, which initially begins with the provision of medical care, such as monitoring of clinical symptoms or supply of medicines, may continue over time as the care recipient becomes more frail or contracts a chronic illness such as dementia, Parkinson's disease, and cancer, resulting in the importance of this role of the caregiver to increase dramatically. Sometimes the need for assistance from a care recipient increases over time (such as increased mobilization limitation due to osteoarthritis), and sometimes an unexpected life-threatening event, such as hip fracture, stroke, and myocardial infarction, may cause a person to assume the role of caregiver.

While 15% of the caregiving process lasts less than 1 year, it takes 2–10 years in 70% and more than 10 years in the remaining 15%. As the whole process continues, after a while the caregiver may begin to play a more effective role than even the care recipient. Studies show that caregivers ask healthcare professionals more questions during visits than do patients and that those questions change direction in time towards care-related procedures and care costs, rather than the disease itself [13].

17.3 Multiple Roles of Caregivers

Caregiving involves various tasks ranging from helping the older patient in basic and instrumental life activities to providing complex health care.

Caregiving domains can be grouped as follows: (1) assisting with daily living activities; (2) emotional and social support; (3) health and medical care; (4) advocacy and care coordination; and (5) decision-making. Each of these areas includes a number of separate tasks (Fig. 17.2).

The two diseases that lead to the most caregiver burden in older adults are cancer and dementia. Although the burden of caregivers associated with both diseases is similar, specific tasks differ from each other. For example, caregivers for cancer patients mostly provide help with getting up and sitting, while incontinence and neuropsychiatric symptoms are managed in dementia patients [14].

17.3.1 Assisting with Daily Living Activities (ADL)

Daily living activities are divided into basic and instrumental activities. Basic daily living activities include feeding, grooming, bathing, dressing, bowel and bladder

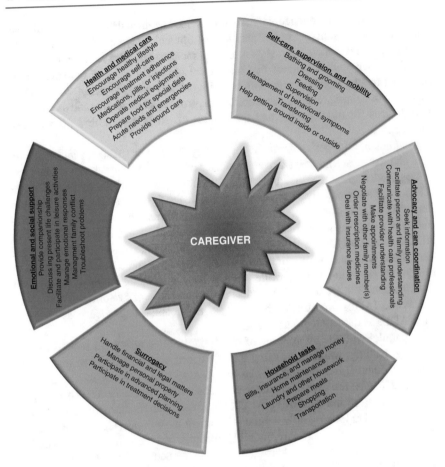

Fig. 17.2 The role of caregivers in the care of older people

care (toilet use), and mobility (ambulation, transfers, and stair climbing), whereas instrumental activities of daily living (IADLs) that are used to describe more advanced activities include those such as using the telephone, housekeeping, managing money, shopping, laundry, responsibility for own medications, ability to handle finances, transportation, and preparing meals. Independence of all these daily activities indicates the functional capacity and disability of the individual [14–16].

Each year, disability develops in 10% of older people without any disability before, which is more common in instrumental ADLs [14, 16]. Besides, more than 30% of people 65 years and older lose their independence in mobilization over a 4-year period [17]. However, some studies demonstrated that the prevalence of ADL and IADL disability has declined in recent years, often with a stronger decline in IADL than in ADL. This can be attributed to improvements in healthcare supports and technological devices to support independent living. From this perspective, it appears important to determine and prevent risk factors for disability. Therefore, the role of caregivers in older people's care may indeed begin at this stage. For example, pain, falls, depression, the use of ancillary equipment, polypharmacy, and multiple comorbid diseases have been shown to be associated with the restriction of ADLs [18–20]. Such studies suggest that one of the important roles of caregivers is to carry out regular health checks (contact with primary care physician) for the early detection of hearing, vision, and mobilization problems that require the use of assistive devices for older people and the control of existing comorbid diseases and medications.

As known, all types of dementia, especially Alzheimer's disease, increase with age, and the most important diagnostic factor of dementia is to determine the level of cognitive impairment that affects the daily life activities of the patients [21]. At this point, family caregivers are very responsible for the correct diagnosis. Because dementia patients often cannot provide accurate information about their daily activities, the caregiver's observations are very important. It has been shown that in ADLs, particularly those with three or more limitations require much more care than those with one or two limitations [22]. Men have more problems managing drugs and preparing meals, while women have disabilities about traveling and mobilization [20]. Dementia is the most important cause of disability in older people. While IADLs are affected by early stage dementia, dependence develops in basic ADLs as dementia progresses [23].

In parallel with the progression of dementia, in basic activities, such as eating, dressing, bathing, walking, or using the toilet, deterioration occurs as much as to require guidance and support. When the disease progresses to intermediate or advanced stages, the care of a caregiver is absolutely necessary for self-care [21, 23]. According to the data from the 2011 US National Health and Aging Trends Study, caregivers looking after a dementia patient have to provide more care in all basic ADLs, including self-care, mobility, feeding, and incontinence, compared to caregivers looking after an older adult without dementia. Only 20% of patients without dementia and 77.7% of older people with dementia receive help for at least one ADL. In three or more ADLs, the proportion of receiving help was 40% in those with dementia and 14% in those without dementia [24]. Caregivers cope with neuropsychiatric problems such as sleep disturbances, anxiety, wandering, and hallucinations in dementia patients, while at the same time trying to care for ADLs; therefore, it is not surprising that caregiver exhaustion is remarkably common in caregivers for those living with dementia [25].

17.3.2 Emotional and Social Support

Older people begin to be in need of emotional support as well as physical support immediately after disability and frailty develop, because there is a mutual relationship between frailty and depression [26]. While the prevalence of emotional problems such as depressive symptoms, anxiety, irritability, and anger is 10–20% among older people living in the community, this rate increases to almost 50% as disability increases [27]. Frailty is a multifactorial geriatric syndrome that may be affected by some important factors such as fragility, pain, mobility and balance problems, weakness, and poor endurance. All of these risk factors may give rise to disability, or functional dependence, and so to depression [28]. On the other hand, depression may predict indicators of frailty caused by a decline in social ties, gait speed and less physical activity, or increased immobility, risk of falling, weight loss, and malnutrition that may raise the continuity of affective symptoms, typical of depression, including sadness, anhedonia, and helplessness [29]. Moreover, depression may be related not only to physical frailty but also to cognitive impairment that can be long-lasting and persist even in emotional remission [30]. Cognitive impairment related to depression may contribute to the emergence of frailty. Therefore, the current estimates on the potential beneficial effects of the approaches to preventing fragility or depression may be conservative. For example, the successful treatment of the depression itself may result in increased behavioral and social activation, thereby increasing physical and social activity levels and improving muscle mass and strength and the elder's overall energy levels, thereby reducing frailty [31]. Likewise, increasing physical activity is an effective intervention for frailty in older adults and can preserve and manage depressive symptoms via potential neurobiological changes and as a result of social and physical engagement [32].

It is important for caregivers to recognize depressive symptoms early in the older individuals and to pass them on to their doctors; thus, the caregiver provides emotional support, consequentially preventing the risk of disability and increased mortality from depression. Emotional support (affection, a sense of belonging, a sense of usefulness, trust, and empathy) is an important part of social support [33]. Other parts of social support include the tools necessary for instrumental support (e.g., mobilization), providing money and informational support (to provide the knowledge or skills necessary to deal with a problem [34]. In the studies conducted, the usefulness of the components of social support was investigated, and it was found that emotional support was the most important one to increase the life satisfaction among older people [33].

Inadequate emotional support is associated with loneliness, anxiety, uncertainty, and a sense of worthlessness [35]. However, unfortunately, social support does not always work, and sometimes it can cause a person to feel guilty due to seeing him(her)self as a burden on others and may even lead to suicidal ideation [36]. On the other hand, it is also known that caregivers are more positively affected than care recipients while providing social support, which positively affects the health and longevity of caregivers [35].

17.3.3 Health and Medical Care

Health and medical care tasks of caregivers are not new, but they have become more complex than in those the past. Older and frail adults' homes have become clinical care settings where caregivers perform a series of care or medical tasks previously provided by licensed or certified professionals only in hospitals and nursing homes [2].

The results of the "Home Alone" study by the AARP Public Policy Institute and the United Hospital Fund are striking [37]. The roles and frequency of the patient's relatives in medical care are summarized as follows:

- Managing medications, including injections and intravenous therapy (78%)
- Helping with assistive devices (canes and walkers) for mobility (43%)
- Preparing food for special diets (41%)
- Doing wound care, such as ostomy care, treatment of pressure sores, and application of ointments and prescription drugs and bandages for skin care (35%)
- Using meters or monitors with glucometers to test blood sugar levels, oxygen, and blood pressure monitors, test kits, and telehealth equipment (32%)
- Administering enemas and managing incontinence equipment and supplies (25%)
- Operating durable medical equipment such as elevators to get people out of bed, hospital beds, and chairs (21%)
- Operating medical equipment, including mechanical ventilators, tube feeding equipment, home dialysis, and suctioning (14%)
- Providing ADL or IADL (more than 96%)

Most caregivers stated that they did not receive the necessary training in performing such tasks and that they were afraid to do wrong or damage the care recipient during the practices [38]. Since the hospital stay of the older patient is limited in order to cut down health expenditures, caregivers, however, will often have to provide home health and medical care services and will try to overcome the numerous equipment and technical procedures such as feeding tube, urinary catheter, and tracheostomy. On the other hand, family caregivers have to interact with almost all components of the health system (physicians, physician assistants, nurses, nurse practitioners, social workers, psychologists, pharmacists, physical and occupational therapists, certified nursing assistants, home health, and personal care aides). Caregivers are also responsible for providing the doctor with medical information about the older patients (e.g., habits, smoking, and alcohol use) and family history (illnesses in other members of the family), illnesses he/she has been diagnosed, and medications he/she has used. If the patient suffers from dementia, caregivers are responsible for communicating the patient's possible complaints (such as pain, incontinence, fever, cough, neuropsychiatric symptoms) to healthcare professionals. Considering all this, it is shown how important the role caregivers play in the medical care of disabled older patients [2, 38].

17.3.4 Care Coordination

Family and informal caregivers (spouse, adult, children, parents, other relatives, partners, co-workers, or friends) are a critical source of support for individuals with chronic or disabling conditions. Family caregivers contribute to increased continuity of care and better outcomes for those in need of care. Caregivers provide valuable information about the patient's medical condition, administer medicines, make complex treatment plans, and make important medical decisions. The presence of a family caregiver can improve medical availability, reduce hospital stay, and prevent hospitalization, unnecessary emergency room and doctor visits, and early care facilities. Therefore, the caregiver is an important member of the healthcare team [3, 12, 25]. One of the most important steps of care coordination is to develop a care strategy for caregivers after care recipients are discharged from a hospital or institution. Caregivers are responsible for deciding whether to continue care at home, nursing home, or another institution after their older patients are discharged from the hospital. In the United States, 40% of older hospitalized patients over the age of 85 are transferred to a skilled nursing facility; thus, inappropriate readmission to the hospital can be avoided [39]. In a study involving 11,855,702 Medicare beneficiaries, 1 out of 5 people applied to the hospital within 30 days of discharge, and 34.0% were rehospitalized within 90 days [40]: (1) transient and general clinical vulnerability after discharge; (2) exposure to a wide range of stressors such as pain, sleep disturbances, catheter applications such as protein-energy malnutrition, bladder catheter, and pain during hospitalization; (3) deterioration of neuro-coordination as a result of prolonged bed rest and hypomobilization; and (4) the development of surgical wound infection or decubitus ulcer, especially in patients discharged from surgical clinics, complicates the care of older individuals [41]. In addition, (1) inadequate information and inadequate training of the caregiver, (2) lack of communication with care providers that will continue to care for the older people, (3) failure of the clinician to continue follow-up after discharge, and (4) poor social support increase the dilemmas in the care plan. For all these reasons, the older people are forced to return to hospital after discharge [39, 40].

In all this process, caregivers should arrange the physician visits to be made again after discharge from the hospital, provide the necessary equipment for home care, (e.g., to provide the handles to prevent the older persons from falling down while taking a bath or to remove the door sills), find the necessary allowance for this, and coordinate not only the care of the older people but the rest of their lives.

17.3.5 Decision-Making

Caregivers make decisions on many issues on behalf of recipients, especially the older patients with cognitive deficiencies. The types of decision-making roles are quite various: there may be some kinds of decision-making, such as guiding and supporting, trying to help the older patient to make decisions or the caregivers making the decision as a surrogate [42]. Although older people can sometimes decide for themselves, they still need help from caregivers to implement them. Caregivers and recipients can face many types of decisions, including decisions about treatment options, place of care, and end-of-life care [42, 43]. Decisions can be affected by religious beliefs, family dynamics, and financial problems [42].

Many people with advanced diseases lack the capacity to make decisions and therefore have to rely on their surrogates. Research shows that for about half (47%) of older adults in hospital, family members are involved in decision-making, while the remaining 23% need additional surrogates' decisions [44, 45]. Most individuals prefer to involve family members in medical decisions, and when the individual loses his/her decision-making ability, his/her family members act as decision-makers by attorney [46]. Some persons are appointed by a court by power of attorney, while others may play a role by default because they are close family members or friends. Family surrogates are not only required to make health-related decisions but also to manage the financial, legal, and insurance issues of the care recipient. In summary, the role of family care is extensive and often requires significant time commitment. The complexity of the caregiving role has increased in recent years.

17.4 Caregiver Burden

Caregiver burden is a multidimensional response to physical, psychological, social, and financial stressors associated with the caregiving experience. There are several factors that determine the burden of the caregiver, which include demographic characteristics such as gender, age, and ethnic identity, as well as patient characteristics and behavioral problems [25]. It has been shown that female caregivers experience higher psychological distress and are at higher risk for psychiatric morbidity. Measures related to burden, conflict and relationship difficulties, anxiety, depression, and quality of life were found to be negative for women [47]. It has been shown that compared to caregivers who are male, female caregivers were aged 65 and over, from black race, married, more educated, unemployed, the primary owners of responsibility, could provide more intensive and complex care, could not maintain the balance for family or professional responsibilities, have health problems, and have increased tendencies to engage in religious activities [2, 24, 47]. When social roles are considered, the majority of caregivers are spouses, who perceive higher levels of stress. In the overall care process, spouses feel more vulnerable, lonely, and isolated. In addition, caregivers of older individuals may be reluctant to express their mental strain and dissatisfaction with the situation, because social and communal values characterize caregiving as an ordinary process of the older age and a duty of the spouses. While women establish more identification with the role of caregiver, men tend to see it as a task to be completed.

Care for dementia patients is an even more challenging process, requiring intensive caring demands for 3–15 years [25]. Behavioral problems, including global destruction of cognitive functions, agitation and psychosis, and inability to maintain daily living activities put a heavy burden on caregivers. The burden of caregivers is closely related to the severity of dementia-related neuropsychiatric symptoms. Neuropsychiatric symptoms, such as anxiety, agitation, disinhibition, aggressive behavior, and sleep disturbances, are more closely related to caregiver burden and negative outcomes such as decline in their general health, quality of life, and social isolation [25].

The burden of caregiver is manifested by negative objective and subjective results such as psychological problems, physical health problems, economic problems, social problems, deterioration of family relations, and lack of control.

Caregivers may feel guilty due to the failure to meet the recipient's ongoing expectations and may feel powerless because they lose control of their own lives. Other emotional problems include frustration, anger towards other family members and the older person, guilt for not being honest, loss of privacy if living with the older person, self-condemnation, coercion, grief, thinking of lack of social support, despair, and so on. Restlessness, insomnia, decrease in self-esteem, social isolation, increase in alcohol and drug use, and troubles in problem solving lead to an increase in stress and anxiety levels of caregivers and often bring about symptoms of depression in the caregiver [25, 47, 48]. Primary care of the patient by the caregiver also negatively affects the relationships between other members of the family and friends and restrains resting and leisure activities, which increases the likelihood that the caregiver will feel left alone in the care role, have a decrease in social support, and experience social isolation over time.

The problems experienced by the caregivers, some unmet needs, the burden resulting from the care itself, cause the caregiver to not be able to help the patient at an appropriate level and not feel psychologically sufficient, which induces the support to be compromised and increases the rate of hospitalization of the patient [49, 50]. Health professionals need to be able to determine the level of burden felt by the caregiver before they can plan appropriate interventions to support caregivers and evaluate the results of these interventions. Knowing the burden and performing the necessary intervention contribute to improving the quality of life of both recipients and caregivers.

With their validity and reliability tested, there are many scales developed to measure both the burden experienced by caregivers and its level [51]. Depending on clinical observations and using the tools developed, healthcare professionals can take suitable approaches in a timely manner to determine the degree and/or risk of care disability.

17.4.1 What's the Role of Family Physicians

Family physicians have a "privileged" position, and the longitudinal care process allows them to follow the progression of diseases and counteract eventual impairing situations, even in case of older patients assisted in difficult social conditions or in vulnerable contexts step by step.

Two important aspects to keep in mind when dealing with older patients and entering their domestic settings are:

– Time of acceptance and adaptation
– Adaptation in space

The time of acceptance and adaptation: acceptance regards the integration of the concept of irreversible change in one's daily life after the diagnosis of a disease that does not heal. Adaptation is about being able to accept the fact that the balance achieved is a balance in constant evolution, depending on the progression of the disease. And this, for caregivers, is the hardest part.

Adaptation in space: the body and mind of the healthy person recognize their environment as familiar. When a disease such as dementia or a physical disability takes over, in general, the space-home becomes an unknown and potentially hostile space. In the rearrangement of spaces, the caregiver must be supported.

Doctors have to evaluate and reassess eventually these two aspects, providing support and counseling if possible.

Doctors can propose the caregiver to reorganize patient's living spaces in order to make them more comfortable and safe, especially for frail persons.

On the other hand, it is important to remind that both patient and caregiver may need help from their family doctor also in coping with the disease affecting the older individual.

References

1. Beard JR, Officer A, de Carvalho IA, Sadana R, Pot AM, Michel J-P, et al. The World report on ageing and health: a policy framework for healthy ageing. Lancet (London, England). 2016;387(10033):2145–54.
2. Committee on Family Caregiving for Older Adults; Board on Health Care Services; Health and Medicine Division; National Academies of Sciences, Engineering, and Medicine. In: Schulz R, Eden J, editors. FC for an AA. Families caring for an aging America. Washington, DC: National Academies Press; 2016.
3. National Alliance for Caregiving PPI. Caregivers of older adults: a focused look at those caring for someone age 50+; 2015.
4. Plothner M, Schmidt K, de Jong L, Zeidler J, Damm K. Needs and preferences of informal caregivers regarding outpatient care for the elderly: a systematic literature review. BMC Geriatr. 2019;19(1):82.
5. Schulz R, Eden J. Families caring for an aging America. Washington, DC: National Academies Press; 2016.
6. Kok L, Berden C, Sadiraj K. Costs and benefits of home care for the elderly versus residential care: a comparison using propensity scores. Eur J Health Econ. 2015;16(2):119–31.
7. Ates Bulut E, Soysal P, Isik AT. Frequency and coincidence of geriatric syndromes according to age groups: single-center experience in Turkey between 2013 and 2017. Clin Interv Aging. 2018;13:1899–905.
8. Koller D, Schon G, Schafer I, Glaeske G, van den Bussche H, Hansen H. Multimorbidity and long-term care dependency—a five-year follow-up. BMC Geriatr. 2014;14:70.
9. Jacob L, Breuer J, Kostev K. Prevalence of chronic diseases among older patients in German general practices. Geriatr Med Sci. 2016;14:Doc03.
10. Lee PG, Cigolle C, Blaum C. The co-occurrence of chronic diseases and geriatric syndromes: the health and retirement study. J Am Geriatr Soc. 2009;57(3):511–6.
11. Gitlin LN, Wolff J. Family involvement in care transitions of older adults: what do we know and where do we go from here? Annu Rev Gerontol Geriatr. 2011;31(1):31–4.
12. Lopez-Anuarbe M, Kohli P. Understanding male caregivers' emotional, financial, and physical burden in the United States. Healthcare (Basel, Switzerland). 2019;7(2):72.
13. Serena Barello, Mariarosaria Savarese GG. The role of caregivers in the elderly health-care journey: insights for sustaining elderly patient engagement. In: Patient engagement: a consumer-centered model to innovate healthcare; 2015.

14. Kim Y, Schulz R. Family caregivers' strains: comparative analysis of cancer caregiving with dementia, diabetes, and frail elderly caregiving. J Aging Health. 2008;20(5):483–503.
15. Gill TM, Hardy SE, Williams CS. Underestimation of disability in community-living older persons. J Am Geriatr Soc. 2002;50(9):1492–7.
16. Guralnik JM, LaCroix AZ, Abbott RD, Berkman LF, Satterfield S, Evans DA, et al. Maintaining mobility in late life. I. Demographic characteristics and chronic conditions. Am J Epidemiol. 1993;137(8):845–57.
17. Lin S-F, Beck AN, Finch BK, Hummer RA, Masters RK. Trends in US older adult disability: exploring age, period, and cohort effects. Am J Public Health. 2012;102(11):2157–63.
18. Connolly D, Garvey J, McKee G. Factors associated with ADL/IADL disability in community dwelling older adults in the Irish longitudinal study on ageing (TILDA). Disabil Rehabil. 2017;39(8):809–16.
19. Cwirlej-Sozanska AB, Sozanski B, Wisniowska-Szurlej A, Wilmowska-Pietruszynska A. An assessment of factors related to disability in ADL and IADL in elderly inhabitants of rural areas of South-Eastern Poland. Ann Agric Environ Med. 2018;25(3):504–11.
20. Bleijenberg N, Zuithoff NPA, Smith AK, de Wit NJ, Schuurmans MJ. Disability in the individual ADL, IADL, and mobility among older adults: a prospective cohort study. J Nutr Health Aging. 2017;21(8):897–903.
21. Isik AT. Late onset Alzheimer's disease in older people. Clin Interv Aging. 2010;5:307–11.
22. Kurichi JE, Streim JE, Xie D, Hennessy S, Na L, Saliba D, et al. The association between activity limitation stages and admission to facilities providing long-term care among older Medicare beneficiaries. Am J Phys Med Rehabil. 2017;96(7):464–72.
23. Huang H-L, Shyu Y-IL, Chen M-C, Huang C-C, Kuo H-C, Chen S-T, et al. Family caregivers' role implementation at different stages of dementia. Clin Interv Aging. 2015;10:135–46.
24. Kasper JD, Freedman VA, Spillman BC, Wolff JL. The disproportionate impact of dementia on family and unpaid caregiving to older adults. Health Aff (Millwood). 2015;34(10):1642–9.
25. Isik AT, Soysal P, Solmi M, Veronese N. Bidirectional relationship between caregiver burden and neuropsychiatric symptoms in patients with Alzheimer's disease: a narrative review. Int J Geriatr Psychiatry. 2019;34(9):1326–34.
26. Soysal P, Veronese N, Thompson T, Kahl KG, Fernandes BS, Prina AM, et al. Relationship between depression and frailty in older adults: a systematic review and meta-analysis. Ageing Res Rev. 2017;36:78–87.
27. Buigues C, Padilla-Sanchez C, Garrido JF, Navarro-Martinez R, Ruiz-Ros V, Cauli O. The relationship between depression and frailty syndrome: a systematic review. Aging Ment Health. 2015;19(9):762–72.
28. Woods NF, LaCroix AZ, Gray SL, Aragaki A, Cochrane BB, Brunner RL, et al. Frailty: emergence and consequences in women aged 65 and older in the Women's Health Initiative Observational Study. J Am Geriatr Soc. 2005;53(8):1321–30.
29. Hajek A, Brettschneider C, Posselt T, Lange C, Mamone S, Wiese B, et al. Predictors of frailty in old age - results of a longitudinal study. J Nutr Health Aging. 2016;20(9):952–7.
30. Bortolato B, Miskowiak KW, Kohler CA, Maes M, Fernandes BS, Berk M, et al. Cognitive remission: a novel objective for the treatment of major depression? BMC Med. 2016;14:9.
31. Lakey SL, LaCroix AZ, Gray SL, Borson S, Williams CD, Calhoun D, et al. Antidepressant use, depressive symptoms, and incident frailty in women aged 65 and older from the Women's Health Initiative Observational Study. J Am Geriatr Soc. 2012;60(5):854–61.
32. Brown PJ, Roose SP, Fieo R, Liu X, Rantanen T, Sneed JR, et al. Frailty and depression in older adults: a high-risk clinical population. Am J Geriatr Psychiatry. 2014;22(11):1083–95.
33. Peng C, Kwok CL, Law YW, Yip PSF, Cheng Q. Intergenerational support, satisfaction with parent-child relationship and elderly parents' life satisfaction in Hong Kong. Aging Ment Health. 2019;23(4):428–38.
34. Tough H, Siegrist J, Fekete C. Social relationships, mental health and wellbeing in physical disability: a systematic review. BMC Public Health. 2017;17(1):414.
35. Sener A. Emotional support exchange and life satisfaction. Int J Humanit Soc Sci. 2011;1(2):79–88.

36. Brown SL, Nesse RM, Vinokur AD, Smith DM. Providing social support may be more beneficial than receiving it: results from a prospective study of mortality. Psychol Sci. 2003;14(4):320–7.
37. Reinhard SC, Levine C, Samis S. Home alone: family caregivers providing complex chronic care. Washington, DC: AARP Public Policy Institute; 2012.
38. Forster AJ, Murff HJ, Peterson JF, Gandhi TK, Bates DW. The incidence and severity of adverse events affecting patients after discharge from the hospital. Ann Intern Med. 2003;138(3):161–7.
39. Zurlo A, Zuliani G. Management of care transition and hospital discharge. Aging Clin Exp Res. 2018;30(3):263–70.
40. Jencks SF, Williams MV, Coleman EA. Rehospitalizations among patients in the Medicare fee-for-service program. N Engl J Med. 2009;360(14):1418–28.
41. Ellis G, Whitehead MA, O'Neill D, Langhorne P, Robinson D. Comprehensive geriatric assessment for older adults admitted to hospital. Cochrane Database Syst Rev. 2011;7:CD006211.
42. Garvelink MM, Ngangue PAG, Adekpedjou R, Diouf NT, Goh L, Blair L, et al. A synthesis of knowledge about caregiver decision making finds gaps in support for those who care for aging loved ones. Health Aff (Millwood). 2016;35(4):619–26.
43. Edwards SB, Olson K, Koop PM, Northcott HC. Patient and family caregiver decision making in the context of advanced cancer. Cancer Nurs. 2012;35(3):178–86.
44. Torke AM, Siegler M, Abalos A, Moloney RM, Alexander GC. Physicians' experience with surrogate decision making for hospitalized adults. J Gen Intern Med. 2009;24(9):1023–8.
45. Torke AM, Sachs GA, Helft PR, Montz K, Hui SL, Slaven JE, et al. Scope and outcomes of surrogate decision making among hospitalized older adults. JAMA Intern Med. 2014;174(3):370–7.
46. Kelly B, Rid A, Wendler D. Systematic review: individuals' goals for surrogate decision-making. J Am Geriatr Soc. 2012;60(5):884–95.
47. Covinsky KE, Newcomer R, Fox P, Wood J, Sands L, Dane K, et al. Patient and caregiver characteristics associated with depression in caregivers of patients with dementia. J Gen Intern Med. 2003;18(12):1006–14.
48. Farcnik K, Persyko MS. Assessment, measures and approaches to easing caregiver burden in Alzheimer's disease. Drugs Aging. 2002;19(3):203–15.
49. Williams A-L, McCorkle R. Cancer family caregivers during the palliative, hospice, and bereavement phases: a review of the descriptive psychosocial literature. Palliat Support Care. 2011;9(3):315–25.
50. Kinsella G, Cooper B, Picton C, Murtagh D. A review of the measurement of caregiver and family burden in palliative care. J Palliat Care. 1998;14(2):37–45.
51. Van Durme T, Macq J, Jeanmart C, Gobert M. Tools for measuring the impact of informal caregiving of the elderly: a literature review. Int J Nurs Stud. 2012;49(4):490–504.

Elder Abuse and Neglect

18

Sara Rigon, Hagit Dascal-Weichhendler, Shelly Rothschild-Meir, and Raquel Gomez Bravo

Abstract

Elder maltreatment was first mentioned in a scientific publication in 1975; nowadays elder abuse has gained the necessary visibility to become internationally recognised as a global public health and social matter. However data and studies on this specific form of violence and the understanding of the phenomenon are still quite limited; recent meta-analysis tried to estimate the scale of the problem and indicated a combined prevalence for overall elder abuse in the past year between 14.3% and 15.7%, psychological abuse being the most common form of elder abuse both in community and residential settings.

Scientific reviewed by Professor Tan Maw Pin.

S. Rigon (✉)
Special Interest Group on Family Violence, WONCA, World Organization of Family Doctors, Penitentiary Primary Health Care, C.C. San Vittore, Milano, Italy
e-mail: sararigon7@gmail.com

H. Dascal-Weichhendler · S. Rothschild-Meir
Special Interest Group on Family Violence, WONCA, World Organization of Family Doctors, Department of Family Medicine, Clalit Health Services, Haifa and West Galillee District and The Ruth and Bruce Rappaport Faculty of Medicine, Technion, Israel

R. Gomez Bravo
Special Interest Group on Family Violence, WONCA, World Organization of Family Doctors, Research Group Self-Regulation and Health, Institute for Health and Behaviour, Department of Behavioural and Cognitive Sciences, Faculty of Humanities, Education, and Social Sciences, University of Luxembourg, Esch-sur-Alzette, Luxembourg

© Springer Nature Switzerland AG 2022
J. Demurtas, N. Veronese (eds.), *The Role of Family Physicians in Older People Care*, Practical Issues in Geriatrics, https://doi.org/10.1007/978-3-030-78923-7_18

Elder abuse and neglect (EAN) has extensive effects on the quality of life, morbidity and mortality of older adults, and health workers are in a unique position to identify it.

The global elderly population is increasing dramatically worldwide, from 900 million in 2015 to nearly 2 billion in 2050, so the incidence and prevalence of EAN will increase as well concomitantly. Identification and management of elder abuse need to be a priority of healthcare providers. At the same time, urgent steps should be taken by policymakers around the globe targeting the population changes and risk factors for EAN comprehensively, from every possible aspect.

Keywords

Elder abuse and neglect · Self-neglect · Elder maltreatment · Primary health care (PHC) · Family medicine

18.1 Introduction

Elder maltreatment was first mentioned in a scientific publication in 1975 when a health professional from the United Kingdom wrote a letter to the BMJ calling for action on "granny battery": "just another manifestation of the inadequate care we as a profession give to elderly population and their relatives who are left to cope with them unaided and supported by us" [1].

It took more than 40 years before elder abuse gained the necessary visibility to become internationally recognised as a global public health and social matter [2–5]. Nowadays elder abuse is also considered a violation of human rights by organisations such as the World Health Organization (WHO) [6] and the United Nations (UN) as stated in the principles for older persons [7]. The European Union in the Charter of Fundamental Rights (Art. 25) [8] also "recognises and respects the rights of older people to lead lives of dignity and independence, and to participate in social and cultural life" [2].

Despite the increased awareness and call for urgent action by major international agencies such as WHO [9], data and studies on this specific form of violence and the understanding of the phenomenon, beginning with terminology and definition, remain limited [3–5, 9].

18.2 Definition and Subtypes

18.2.1 Elder Abuse and Neglect Definitions

Elder abuse was first described as "granny battering" in BMJ in 1975 and is today known as elder mistreatment, abuse of older adults or senior abuse [1–3]. Recently "elder abuse and neglect" and its acronym EAN have gained scientific acceptance and validation as a more comprehensive and all-inclusive denomination will also be used in this text.

Table 18.1 Widely accepted EAN definitions

UK's Action on Elder Abuse, 1995	The US National Academy of Sciences, 2003
Elder abuse is a single or repeated act or lack of appropriate action, occurring within any relationship where there is an expectation of trust which causes harm or distress to an older person [12]	*Elder mistreatment*: (a) intentional actions that cause harm or create a serious risk of harm (whether or not harm is intended) to a vulnerable elder by a caregiver or other person who stands in a trust relationship or (b) failure by a caregiver to satisfy the elder's basic needs or to protect the elder from harm [13]

In addition to terminology, also the definition varies among international agencies, academics and researchers as well as across countries and cultures indicating the complexity of the concept and the philosophical and cultural believes entailed [3, 9–11]. The definition adopted by the WHO and other agencies such as the International Network for Prevention of Elder Abuse (INPEA) [2, 6, 10] was developed by the "UK's Action on Elder Abuse" organisation in 1995 [12]. The US National Academy of Sciences proposed another widely accepted definition presented in Table 18.1, which includes intention and inadvertent [13].

Both definitions present some limitations being based on relationships or at least an expectation of trust between victim and offender. Such definitions exclude any criminal actions performed by strangers [10].

The lack of a standardised, unanimous definition results in ramifications at numerous levels. It affects different disciplines including academia and policymakers, as well as the development and evaluation of various interventions [5, 9, 10, 14]. The WHO along with many scientific experts are now urging for a consensus on definitions, subtypes, and categorisation as well as research methods on the topic [9].

18.2.2 Subtypes

Elder abuse and neglect can take many different forms, as shown in Table 18.2. Although specific subtypes are subjected to cultural differences and vary from country to country, the five widely accepted types of EAN are psychological/emotional or verbal abuse, physical abuse, sexual abuse, financial/material abuse and neglect/abandonment [2–4, 10, 15].

Some studies also include more specific kinds of violence, namely, violence of personal rights [2]. Moreover, some experts debate whether self-neglect should be classified as a specific form of elder abuse or not. Some interpretations consider self-neglect related to elder mistreatment; however recently experts have been questioning such categorisation, just as suicide is not considered a form of murder [15]. Self-neglect is an extreme deficiency of self-care, and it can be associated with hoarding and other mental health disorders such as additions or health conditions and disability. It can occur at any age, although it is most common among the elderly; the signs of self-neglect are presented in Table 18.2 and may include, for example, malnutrition, dehydration, poor hygiene, noncompliance to medical prescriptions or medication misuse [10].

Table 18.2 Subtypes of EAN and related examples

Subtype	Definition	Examples
Physical abuse	The infliction of pain or injury, physical coercion or physical or drug-induced restraint	• Being pushed • Being grabbed • Being slapped • Hit with an object
Psychological/verbal abuse	All actions inflicting mental pain, anguish, or distress on a person through verbal or nonverbal acts	• The use of abusive language • Manipulation • Bullying • Blackmailing • Shouting at • Threatening • Humiliating • Isolating the older person • Infantilising the person
Sexual abuse	Non-consensual sexual contact of any kind or sexual exposure; terror in intimate relations that has the intention to control the partner or a person and is only one-sided	• Unwanted intimacy • Touching in a sexual way • Rape • Undressing in front of the victim • Sexually slanted approaches
Financial abuse or exploitation	All actions of illegal or improper use of an elder's funds, property or assets	• Swindling • Disappearance of money or goods • Obstruction in managing one's own money • Legacy hunting and extortion
Neglect	The refusal (active neglect) or failure (passive neglect) of a designated caregiver to meet the needs of a dependent older person	• Malnutrition • Inappropriate clothing • Decubitus ulcers • Deterioration of health • Poor Hygiene • Lack of needed aids or medical equipment
Violation of personal rights	A violation of an individual's civil or human rights by any other person or persons	• Violation of privacy • Violation of the right to autonomy and/or freedom • Refusing access to visitors/isolating the elder • Reading or withdrawing personal mail
Self-neglect	Adults not willing or not able to perform essential everyday self-care tasks such as providing food, clothing, adequate shelter or obtaining adequate medical care and services necessary to maintain physical and mental health, well-being, personal hygiene and managing financial affairs	• Poor overall self-care • Unsafe or unclean living conditions • Inadequate or inappropriate clothing • Absence of needed eyeglasses, hearing aids, dentures, etc. • Unexpected or unexplained deterioration of health • Drug misuse, etc.

As abuse of older people can be an act of commission or omission (neglect), it is of great importance to clarify that abuse can be deliberate and intended as opposed to accidental or unintended. This, however, may be related to sociocultural contexts and varies from county to county. Scientifically and for research purposes, abuse can be categorised as intentional or unintentional, although it is worth noticing that for various reasons, intentional injuries may be misclassified as unintentional or of undetermined intent which makes analysis and interpretations complicated and speculative [9].

18.3 Epidemiology

Estimating the scale of the problem presents methodological limitations starting from the scarcity of studies and scientific data to the lack of shared indicators and a consensus on definitions which results in difficulties in comparing data [2, 3, 9–11, 14]. Data on prevalence is substantially affected by under-reporting [2–4, 9, 10], which is calculated to be as high as 80%, and may be caused by social norms, fear of retaliation or inability to communicate [2, 11].

18.3.1 Prevalence of EAN

Recent systematic reviews estimate the combined prevalence for all types of EAN in the past year to around 15% [3, 5]. The most common forms of maltreatment appear to be psychological abuse (11.6%), followed by financial exploitation (6.8%) and neglect (4.2%) while physical (2.6%) and sexual abuse (0.9%) proved to be less prevalent [3, 11]. Due to cultural differences and lack of consensus on definitions, national and regional prevalence rates differ significantly [2, 3, 5, 10, 11, 16]. Examples of prevalence in different countries worldwide can be seen in Table 18.3.

Table 18.3 Examples of EAN prevalence in different countries

Region or country	Elder abuse prevalence (%)
Canada	4
China	36.6
Croatia	61.1
India	14
Ireland	2.2
Israel	18.4
Peru	79.7
United States	10
United Kingdom	2.6
Overall elder abuse prevalence 14.3–15.7%	

18.3.2 Prevalence of EAN in Residential Settings

The few available studies on EAN in residential settings depict a critical and pervasive situation [11, 17]. Compared to the community settings, maltreatment prevalence rates in institutions appear to be higher for all types of violence with psychological violence being the most common followed by physical maltreatment; specific percentages are reported in Table 18.4.

A meta-analysis reveals that 64% of residential workers reported abusing older residents in the past year, while more studies are needed to calculate the overall prevalence of older residents disclosing EAN in residential settings [11].

The prevalence of EAN in institutional settings varies substantially from country to country. In several studies, it was found to be more common in residential settings compared to the community setting, ranging from 31% in Israel to 78.8% in Germany [11].

Potential explanations for such variations are complex as shown. While further research is needed, it is already clear that an association can be noticed between the increasing dependency of older people and EAN prevalence both in community and institutional settings [11]. In residential homes, a significant correlation was found between abuse and a high ratio of residents per registered nurse [9]. Moreover, time pressure, shortage of staff and emotional exhaustion have been reported in most cases of abuse [11, 18], as shown in Fig. 18.1.

Table 18.4 Prevalence of EAN per subtype in community and residential settings

Type of violence	Community setting (%)	Residential setting (%)
Psychological abuse	11.6	38.4
Physical violence	2.6	14.1
Financial exploitation	6.8	14
Sexual abuse	0.9	1.9
Neglect	4.2	11.6

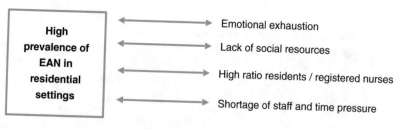

Fig. 18.1 Causes and correlations of EAN high prevalence in residential settings

18.4 Aetiology and Risk Factors

18.4.1 Social-Ecological Model

EAN is a complex and multidimensional phenomenon that involves many factors at the individual, relationship, community and societal level [10, 14] as per the socio-cultural context conceptual model suggested by the US National Research Council, shown in Fig. 18.2 [13]. The model explores the interaction of different factors while considering the sociocultural context in which EAN takes place [4, 5, 10].

Current literature indicates that maltreatment can be triggered by many different factors, their combination and interaction, yet more studies are needed to better understand the complex and specific dynamics [3, 9]. Nevertheless, researchers have shown evidence of some risk factors at individual levels relating to the offender (stress, insufficient training), to the victim (high dependency, mental disorders), to the relationship level (co-dependency, financial needs), to the community level (social isolation) and to the societal level (ageism, poverty) [4, 5, 9, 10].

18.4.2 Risk Factors at Individual Level: Victim

Health: Poor health has been consistently associated with EAN across countries [5]. Evidence shows the main health risk factors for EAN are physical disability and mental impairment [9].

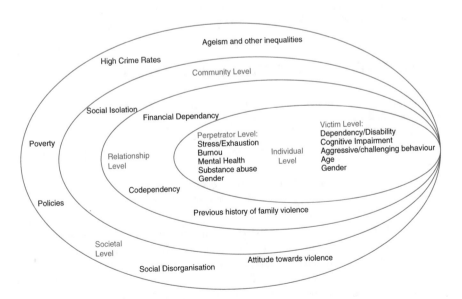

Fig. 18.2 Risk factors for EAN: the sociocultural model

Dependency and Disability: EAN is consistently associated with dependency or physical disability [3, 5, 9]. Some studies show the risk of abuse can increase up to four times in cases of a high level of dependency [9].

Cognitive Impairment: Dementia is believed to be a specific risk factor for EAN [2, 5, 9]. Data across countries shows higher rates of elder maltreatment among older people with Alzheimer's disease and other forms of dementia (up to 14%) compared to the general population. Similarly, family caregivers of people with dementia report higher levels of perpetration (12%) than those of caregivers of relatives without dementia (4%) [9].

Aggressive or Challenging Behaviour: Studies suggest that disruptive patients' behaviours can play a role in EAN and should not be ignored as risk factors, especially in institutional settings [5, 9, 19]. Caregivers often report nocturnal agitation, wandering and aggression may trigger verbal and physical maltreatment [9]. Challenging behaviour is common among patients suffering from all types of dementia as well as other health conditions, and caretakers should be specifically trained on how to respond [9, 19].

Age: Literature shows the risk of EAN increases with age, especially among people 74 years and older [5, 9, 20]. Specifically, the risk for each type of abuse varies across age groups and countries [9].

Gender: Some studies indicate that women are at higher risk for EAN [5, 9, 15, 20]. Moreover, women seem to experience most of the most severe cases of physical and emotional abuse, and a recent WHO study revealed more women than men were reported to be victims of sexual abuse and physical injuries [9]. Recent literature reviews on EAN prevalence show similar rates for men and women [3], but some researchers believe this may be due to under-reporting by women as a consequence of gender roles, norms and level of education [20].

18.4.3 Risk Factors at Individual Level: Perpetrator

Generally abuse of old people can be the result of the offender's lack of knowledge and competence; it can be secondary to a pre-existing difficult family relationship or to a form of dependency, as well as the result of stress and frustration in a household lacking support or in a residential institution in shortage of staff [9, 10, 19].

Stress: Taking care of older people can be stressful, especially if the person is highly dependent or aggressive. Studies show that high levels of stress and the magnitude of care burden involved in caring for older people with behavioural problems are precipitating factors for EAN. Specific training, implementation of appropriate protocols and organisation of the work lower the risk of burnout and exhaustion of caretakers. Moreover, families caring for high dependency people need to be adequately supported [9].

Mental Health and Substance Misuse: Caregivers who perpetrate maltreatment against older people are more likely to present substance misuse issues than the caregivers with no abusive behaviour [5, 9, 14, 16]. Care staff who reported using alcohol to cope with work-related stress were more likely to report being involved in abusive situations, as were family caregivers who used alcohol to relieve stress [9].

EAN perpetrators are also more likely to present mental health problems, most commonly depression [3, 5, 9, 14]. Parents caring for their grown up offspring who suffer from mental disorders are at high risk for EAN. Another study found that the majority of patients admitted to a locked psychiatric unit for assault had attacked a family member, either a spouse or a parent [21, 22].

Gender: Literature shows that both men and women are capable of EAN; the difference lays in the type of abuse. Women appear more likely to be involved in neglect while men are more likely to be responsible for severe physical abuse and sexual abuse [9].

18.4.4 Risk Factors at Relationship Level

Social relationships, such as relations with peers, intimate partners, parents or children and family members in general, are also considered important factors in EAN causality within the sociocultural model, including:

Codependency: Some researchers report relationship dynamics as a major factor in the maltreatment of older people [5, 9, 21]. In this context "Codependency refers to a relationship in which a person is controlled or manipulated by another who is affected with a pathological condition" [21]. Abuse may thus be the result of a strong mutual reliance between the victim and the perpetrator. Studies also suggest that codependent individuals also have greater difficulties leaving stressful relationships and are less likely to seek medical attention [21].

Financial Dependency: Depending on the victim for accommodation and financial support appears to increase the risk of EAN [5, 10]. A European study found that almost 50% of perpetrators were living on the pension and welfare benefits of the older victim as their only source of income [9].

Family Violence: Family relationships, both present and past, play a significant role as risk factors for EAN. Intimate partner violence may be lifelong and persist to old age [23], when it may be regarded as a form of elder abuse. Children who have witnessed intimate partner violence all their lives, once adults may feel ambivalent about caring for their ageing parents [24].

18.4.5 Community Level

The community may also play a role in EAN, increasing as well as mitigating the risk of abuse [5]. Strong evidence indicates that at this level of the sociocultural model, the key risk factor is social isolation.

Social Isolation: In institutional settings, lacking family members and having few visitors are associated with a high prevalence of maltreatment. In community settings living with someone does not necessarily prevent isolation. Low social support, loneliness and lack of social networks among the older persons seem to further perpetuate maltreatment [14], while having a social network reduces the risk [9].

18.4.6 Risk Factors at Societal Level

At the society level, recent studies indicate that EAN is influenced by high crime rates, social disorganisation and lack of social resources and poverty [14]. Moreover, maltreatment is affected by other societal factors such as culture, ethnicity and policies [5, 14]. Ageism, inequality and permissive attitudes towards violence could also be associated with EAN. However, more research is needed to fully understand such potential relationships [5, 9].

18.5 Consequences of EAN

All types of EAN are associated with severe individual consequences and great societal costs as shown in details in Table 18.5 [5]. These include not only negative health outcomes but also economic ramifications. Financial abuse can seriously affect every aspect of the older person's life, including housing and self-sufficiency, as they often survive on limited resources [9, 14]. In Queensland, Australia, the financial exploitation of older people was estimated to range from 1.8 to 5.8 billion A$ for the 2007/2008 fiscal year [9].

18.5.1 Health Costs: Physical

At the individual level, EAN may lead to short- and long-lasting physical and mental outcomes, including psychological distress, morbidity and mortality. Health consequences range from worsened quality of life, bodily pain and disability to invasive medical procedures and hospitalisation. Moreover, longitudinal cohort studies have demonstrated an association between EAN and premature mortality, especially in black populations. Due to the under-diagnosis and under-reporting of EAN, data on its health consequences and costs are lacking. More studies are needed to gain a better understanding of the scale of the problem, including information on mortality, since comparisons of mortality data often challenge as a result of lack of accuracy and incomplete information [9, 16].

18.5.2 Health Costs: Mental Health

With respect to mental well-being, abuse among older people can result in loss of self-confidence and self-esteem, helplessness, anxiety and fear, sleep disturbances and posttraumatic stress disorder. Victims also tend to develop emotional distress

Table 18.5 Consequences of EAN [9]

EAN Consequences				
Human Costs	Health	Physical		Bodily Pain
				Disability
				Hospitalisation
				Morbidity
				Mortality
		Mental Health		Loss of self-esteem and confidence
				Anxiety and fear
				Sleep deprivation
				Emotional distress
				Anger
				Isolation from friend and family
				depression
				PTSD
				Thoughts of self-arm and suicide
Financial Costs	Direct Costs	Healthcare Costs		ER
				Increased Hospitalisation
				Increased 30 days readmission rate
				Rehabilitation
		Protection Services	Police	
		Social Assistance		
		Legal Assistance		
	Indirect Costs	Loss of productivity		

and anger; isolation from family and friends is also common. Longer-term and more severe EAN may result in worse mental effects, such as depression and thoughts of suicide or self-harm. Studies indicate the lasting effects of maltreatment on older people: Some described their experiences as "devastating", something they feel they will never fully recover from [9].

18.5.3 Financial Costs

The overall disease burden of EAN is very high. In addition to the human costs, emerging evidence also shows that EAN has great economic costs, direct as well as indirect [9]. The direct cost arising from maltreatment is attributed to increased healthcare costs to treat and rehabilitate the maltreated elderly. Older adults who suffered maltreatment were found to have longer hospital stays and higher rates of utilisation of emergency services compared to their non-maltreated counterparts as well as higher 30-day readmission rates [14, 16].

In the United States, it was estimated that injuries due to EAN have contributed more than US$ 5.3 billion to the annual healthcare expenditure while in Australia hospital admissions for EAN were estimated to cost between AUD 9.9 million and AUD 30.7 million for 2007/2008 [9].

Other direct costs include social and legal assistance as well as police and protection services [9, 14]. In institutional care settings, costs would also involve maltreatment prevention (staff training and adequate staffing) as well as identification and management (developing specific protocols, staff training) [9].

18.5.4 Indirect Costs

Indirect costs as a consequence of EAN include loss of productivity of caregivers and family members, inability to continue with activities of daily life, diminished quality of life and lost investment in social capital [14]. Estimates on the economic burden for such indirect cost for EAN are not available worldwide but similar to other forms of violence are likely to be substantial [9].

18.6 Identification and Management of EAN

Elder abuse and neglect (EAN) has extensive effects on the quality of life, morbidity and mortality of older adults. Health workers are in a unique position to identify it and have, at least, a moral obligation to do so [9, 14, 15].

Much of the current information on interventions in healthcare settings is focused on hospital-based programs and relies mostly on publications from North America [25]. The availability of professions and professionals differs significantly in a hospital versus community setting and across countries. Roles and tasks of each profession in the management of EAN cases may also differ accordingly [26].

Most recommendations in the literature have not been evaluated thoroughly [26]. As Baker et al. point out, some interventions may have negative consequences and even endanger elders (e.g. breaching patient confidentiality), and thus care should be taken not to harm [14]. Taking all this into consideration, we propose a simplified yet comprehensive approach for the identification and management of elder abuse, presented in Table 18.6, which may be useful in primary and other healthcare settings. *It is important to highlight that not all tasks are necessarily the physicians',*

Table 18.6 Assessment and management of EAN[a]

I. Suspect

Disclosure by patient	Third party Raises suspicion	Screening (see Sect. 18.7.2)	Indicators? Risk factors or "red flags" (see Table 18.7)	Indicators + If risk factors/"red flags" are positive seek additional information, e.g. past medical records

II. Evaluate cognition, competence and functional ability

Cognition and mental status	Function	What is the legal status of the patient?	
	Assess ADL, IADL	If incompetence or physical disability causing dependency is suspected, consider legal obligations and additional clinical evaluation to guide further assessment and management	
Evaluate for dementia, depression, delusions, impaired judgment, etc.			

III. Obtain bio-psycho-social history

From patient	In private	Other causes?	Ask questions about abuse	Collateral history From family,
If capable of giving information	Separate patient from caretaker/ family, etc. Address confidentiality issues	Ask questions to assess for possible differential diagnoses which explain findings	For example, EASI© (Table 18.8)	caretaker or others without breaching confidentiality or compromising safety

IV. Perform physical examination

In private	General	Complete physical examination including:	Injuries	Specialists
After obtaining consent	Vital signs Appearance	Mental status	Inspection	Arrange examination by specific specialists in case of relevant findings, e.g. procto/genital examination
If abnormal findings: ask for more details (e.g. explanation to bruises)	Hygiene Nutritional status Hydration status	Neurological exam Fundus oculi in case of suspected head injury	Palpation	

(continued)

Table 18.6 (continued)

V. Order laboratory and imaging

General	Injuries	Head	Other	Consent
Laboratory tests and imaging to assess general condition, control and evaluation of chronic diseases, nutritional state and possible differential diagnoses	Imaging to evaluate potential acute and past injuries	Consider head imaging (e.g. CT) if a head injury is suspected or if there is any mental deterioration	Specific tests according to suspected abuse type (e.g. check STDs if sexual abuse is suspected, perform toxicological screening if poisoning is suspected)	Should be obtained from the patient, or if incapacitated, act according to local laws

VI. Primary management

Summarise	Treat and plan treatment	Document	Home visit	Difficulties
Available information and findings and consider differential diagnoses, including self-neglect	For all problems on the list (including injuries/medical and mental health/functional issues)	History, physical exam, laboratory tests and imaging results	Consider	With treatment plan: address
Form a biopsychosocial problem list		Use text, body charts, photographs		

VII. Consult/refer/report: multidisciplinary team

Competent and independent patient:	Incompetent patient:	Unclear competence or physical dependence:	Address:	Report or refer
Discuss options with the patient; address patient barriers to action; discuss safety plan; refer; report according to local laws	Consult multidisciplinary team; report according to local laws, and act according to guidance (e.g. by protective services)	Consult multidisciplinary team; report according to local laws, and act according to guidance (e.g. by protective services)	– Context – EAN risk factors – Caretaker burden – Cultural issues	To community services Community and/or legal interventions as required

(continued)

Table 18.6 (continued)

VIII. Follow-up Injuries	Problem list	Patient	EAN—competent patient	EAN—incompetent patient
Healing	Examples: Chronic conditions-compliance/control	Mental health, cognition, psychosocial support	Discuss with patient	Discuss with APS/multidisciplinary team/guardian/other
New	Follow-up after sexual assault	ADL, IADL		
Function Rehabilitation Pain management	Home visit to follow up on living conditions			

Table adapted and reprinted with permission from Dr. Hagit Dascal-Weichhendler and Dr. Shelly Rothschild-Meir (hagitdw@yahoo.com)

ADL activities of daily living, *IADL* instrumental activities of daily living, *APS* adult protective services

ᵃPlease note that the order of actions (for I to VIII) and specific team members' roles may differ according to circumstances, clinical judgment, local laws and services

and some tasks could be done by other team members according to local possibilities. It is very important to appoint a team member to serve as a case manager to coordinate efforts and tasks. Our outline, for simplification, groups actions to be taken in different steps. Yet it is important to note that some of the actions are intertwined, and changes in the order of actions may be suitable. *Because the laws and services may differ among countries and states, this chapter is not intended to replace the need to seek local information and advice on specific cases.*

18.6.1 Suspect

The most important task of healthcare providers (HCPs) who acknowledge the high prevalence and serious impacts of EAN is to have a high index of suspicion. Since older adults may be relatively isolated with few social contacts, any contact with HCPs may serve as a window of opportunity to assess "red flags", risk factors and possible EAN. Raising suspicion and beginning the evaluation process are some of our most important roles, which cannot be underestimated [27].

So when should HCPs suspect EAN? When an older patient discloses any type of abuse or neglect spontaneously or after screening; when a third party (e.g. neighbour) raises a suspicion; and when there are major risk factors or "red flags" linked to EAN as shown in Table 18.7. Behavioural or mental health changes, clinical, laboratory or imaging abnormal findings should also be considered as "red flags". Whenever EAN is suspected, other risk factors and or "red flags" should be investigated (e.g. looking for past information in the medical records) [5, 16, 28].

Table 18.7 Risk factors and "red flags" for EAN

Risk factors

Patient:	Caretaker or perpetrator:	Relationship:	Environment:
• Dementia	• Social factors, e.g.:	• Previous family violence	• Living with perpetrator
• Physical disability	– Unemployment	• Family conflicts	• Physical isolation
• Dependence	– Divorce	• Codependency	• Social isolation
• Chronic disease	– Criminal activity	• Financial dependency	• Unsuitable/unsafe living conditions
• Age >75 years	• Physical health issues or disability		• Lack of medications
• Gender F > M	• Mental health issues		• Lack/inappropriate aids or necessary medical equipment
	• Addiction		• Lack or inappropriate food
	• Caretaker burden		• Signs of possible violence (e.g. marks on furniture; internal locks; objects used for restraining)
	• Lack of knowledge/training		

Symptoms/signs/behaviour

Patient's symptoms:	Patient's behaviour:	Patient's mental health:	Caretaker's behaviour:
• Pain	• Fear, anger	• Depression	• Delays/prevents access to care
• Disability	• Helplessness	• Anxiety	• Avoidance
• Functional decline	• Loss of confidence	• PTSD	• Blames patient
• Hospitalisation	• Noncompliance	• Sleep disorders	• Body language
	• Delayed access to care	• Self-harm	• Physical/verbal abuse in presence of staff
	• Missed appointments	• Self-neglect	• Tries to manipulate patient/staff
	• Multiple or insufficient visits	• Substance abuse	• Leaves incompetent patient unattended (abandonment)
	• Reported behavioural problems	• Suicidal thoughts or attempts	
	• Avoids making decisions	• Delusions	

Physical/laboratory tests/imaging

Physical findings—injury:	Physical findings—neglect:	Lab findings:	Imaging findings:
• ll types of injuries: hematomas, cuts, bruises, burns, fractures, scars, etc.	• Malnutrition	• Nutritional deficits	• Fractures in various healing stages

(continued)

Table 18.7 (continued)

• Different stages of healing	• Dehydration	• Dehydration	• Intracranial bleeding
• Location suggesting nonaccidental aetiology (e.g. in axillae; inner aspects of arms; maxillofacial)	• Poor hygiene	• Uncontrolled chronic diseases	• Other internal organ injuries visible in imaging
• Inconsistent with the reported mechanism	• Inappropriate clothing	• Positive toxic screen	• Findings inconsistent with the reported mechanism
• Uncommon patterns • Broken teeth • Object impressions: ligature marks, belt/finger impressions, object shaped burns, etc.	• Pressure sores • Rashes • Infestations	• Positive STDs • Low levels of prescribed medications	
• Recurrent/unexplained falls • Palpation: tenderness (deeper injuries) • Unusual hair loss patterns • Genital/perianal findings • Bleeding • Hemotympanum	• Uncontrolled medical conditions		

18.6.2 Evaluate Cognition, Competence and Functional Ability

All medical actions should be guided by the legal status of the patient. This will determine whether the patient can consent to further examination and whether there is a duty to report and act according to official guidance, e.g. by adult protective services. Furthermore, in some countries any additional questioning and workup, after the establishment of a reasonable suspicion, may be considered as interfering with formal investigations and should be avoided. Therefore, one of the earliest steps should be the evaluation of the patient's competence, cognition, mental health and functional ability.

There is a tendency to consider patients either capable or incapable of making their own decisions. However *decision-making capacity* (DMC) is rather a spectrum, a gradual correlation between a specific issue and the older adult's ability to make a decision about it.

Cases at the extreme of the cognitive spectrum can be easily appraised with the help of brief assessment tools (e.g. MMSE); in unclear cases, patients that present "grey area" scores on the cognitive spectrum may require additional evaluation [16]. In such cases the Hopkins Competency Assessment Test may be useful [16, 29]. It is important to note that in many countries, this evaluation should be performed by specific consultants (e.g. geriatrician, psychiatrist, neurologist) in order to be valid in legal proceedings. Whenever the patient's DMC is impaired or questionable, further consultation and or reporting is required (Sect. 18.6.7).

Functional status (ADL, IADL) should be evaluated since many elders may be functionally dependent due to physical impairment despite having full DMC. In such cases, the person may not be able to care for himself which could imply a duty to report as well. All HCPs should be aware of local laws on EAN reporting. Always consider self-neglect as a potential differential diagnosis (Sect. 18.6.6).

18.6.3 Obtain Biopsychosocial History

(a) **General considerations**: It is preferable to obtain information directly from the patient whenever possible. When addressing sensitive issues and especially psychosocial history, the patient should be interviewed in private, separately from family, caregiver and/or suspected abuser [30]. Health providers should always address confidentiality, explaining health professionals' legal limitations as well as obligations, such as the duty to report according to local laws.

Questions, as well as responses, should be respectful and nonjudgemental, whether addressed to the patient, caretaker or suspected abuser.

Trying to understand the context, including the social and financial resources, is an important part of the evaluation [31]. It is important that providers understand and address barriers which may prevent elders from disclosing abuse even when asked directly (Sect. 18.6.7d).

Giving different answers/versions, especially if these do not seem to explain clinical findings (e.g. visible wounds), should be noted and documented [31].

Questions should explore risk factors for EAN; any symptom, sign or condition that may be considered as a "red flag" for EAN, conditions that may mimic EAN.

(b) **Asking the older patient about abuse or neglect**: Asking about abuse is not easy, but necessary at least when "red flags" or significant risk factors are observed. The Elder Abuse Suspicion Index—EASI©, shown in Table 18.8, is a simple tool developed for family physicians to assess for abuse in patients with a MMSE of 24 or greater in ambulatory settings [32]. It was used in a multi-country pilot study by the WHO working group on elder abuse and found to be a valid and simple tool covering all important categories, suitable for various geographical and cultural contexts [31].

(c) **Collecting information from a third party**: Collateral history may help obtain a full picture; however, some important aspects should be considered: (a) a possible breach of patient's confidentiality; (b) possible escalation of the violence, caused by pressuring the caretaker/family member who may be the perpetrator endangering the patient; and (c) possible legal consequences, including possible harm to the official investigation. Thus, whenever the patient is competent, HCPs should receive consent before any discussion with a third party. Whenever the patient is incompetent, the collateral history may be the only one available. In this case questions should be asked as far as necessary for immediate treatment and to establish a reasonable suspicion of EAN, with further actions directed according to local laws, e.g. formal report to APS.

Table 18.8 Elder Abuse Suspicion Index (EASI©) [32]

EASI© questions 1 to 5 asked to the patient; question 6 answered by doctor.			
Within the last 12 months:			
1 Have you relied on people for any of the following: bathing, dressing, shopping, banking or meals?	Yes	No	Did not answer
2 Has anyone prevented you from getting food, clothes, medication, glasses, hearing aides or medical care, or from being with people you wanted to be with?	Yes	No	Did not answer
3 Have you been upset because someone talked to you in a way that made you feel shamed or threatened?	Ye	No	Did not answer
4 Has anyone tried to force you to sign papers or to use your money against your will?	Ye	No	Did not answer
5 Has anyone made you afraid, touched you in ways that you did not want or hurt you physically?	Yes	No	Did not answer
6 *Doctor:* Elder abuse *may* be associated with findings such as poor eye contact, withdrawn nature, malnourishment, hygiene issues, cuts, bruises, inappropriate clothing, or medication compliance issues. Did you notice any of these today or in the last 12 months?	Yes	No	Not sure

The EASI© was validated for family physicians to administer to older persons with a Mini-Mental State Examination score of 24 or greater who are seen in ambulatory settings. A response of "yes" on one or more of questions 2 through 6 may establish concern

The Elder Abuse Suspicion Index (EASI©) by Yaffe MJ, Wolfson C, Lithwick M, Weiss D used with permission from Mark Yaffe, October 3, 2020 (mark.yaffe@mcgill.ca). For more information, see Yaffe MJ, Wolfson C, Lithwick M, Weiss D. *Development and validation of a tool to assist physicians' identification of elder abuse: The Elder Abuse Suspicion Index (EASI ©). Journal of Elder Abuse and Neglect,* 2008; 20 [3]: 276–300. https://www.mcgill.ca/familymed/research/projects/elder

18.6.4 Physical Examination

(a) **General considerations**: Whenever possible the examination should be carried out in private and should be proceeded by an explanation to and consent from the patient. Physical signs may reflect either injuries, including the use of restraints (such as ropes, belts, etc. which may leave ligature marks and are in many countries considered unacceptable), neglect or their consequences. The patient should be assessed for any abnormalities in vital signs, appearance, nutritional and hydration status. Signs of neglect or abuse may include lack of appropriate clothing, lack of hygiene (e.g. bad odour, dirty clothes, soiling), weight loss or malnutrition as presented in Table 18.7.

A complete physical exam should be performed to assess for general health and control of chronic conditions. A full mental status and neurological exam—including fundus examination—is necessary, especially whenever there is an abnormality or a possibility of a head injury.

(b) **Examination of injuries**: The patient should be carefully inspected from head to toe, looking for visible injuries, e.g. hematomas, bruises, burns, cuts/lacerations, abrasions, scars, deformations and object impressions (e.g. evidence of restriction or ligature marks, injuries caused by specific objects as belts, cigarette burns, etc.) [30]. Careful palpation should follow, to identify possible deeper injuries after the disappearance of the superficial signs.

Severity of injuries may vary widely, and different patterns may be found in different medical settings. A review of injuries associated with elder abuse found that two-thirds of injuries were to the upper extremity and maxillofacial region, followed by the skull and brain (12%), lower extremities (10%) and torso (10%). Though no injuries can be considered specific/pathognomonic some may be highly suggestive, considering possible mechanisms of injury, e.g. contusions and abrasions to axillae and inner aspects of arms as a result of grasping by the abuser, use of restraints or attempted self-defence by the victim [30, 33]. The majority of the injuries were of a mild nature, highlighting the opportunity and importance of identification and early intervention in primary care, possibly preventing significant morbidity or mortality [33].

(c) **Additional examinations by other specialists**: Whenever history or findings are suspicious of possible sexual abuse, the genitalia, rectal and oral regions should be examined by especially trained professionals [28]. Arranging for an examination by other specialists may also be necessary when abnormalities in other organs or systems are found such as ENT in cases of hemotympanum, nose bleeding, etc. Examination by a forensic specialist may also be indicated or required. Some of these experts may be available only in the hospital setting. The HCP in the community should take an active role in arranging for necessary examinations and if necessary hospitalising the patient, especially if there is a risk of noncompliance or loss of follow-up.

18.6.5 Laboratory and Imaging

When suspecting EAN, laboratory exams and imaging can offer useful information about general health, nutritional and hydration state, well or poorly controlled chronic conditions and potential differential diagnoses [30]. Some tests can be performed in primary care settings while others will require hospital settings depending on medical urgency, available facilities and patient and caretaker cooperation, among other factors. Consent to testing is essential, and in the case of an incapacitated older person, one must act according to the local laws (e.g. consent from the guardian, APS, court order, etc.).

(a) **Laboratory tests**: Various diseases and conditions can mimic abuse in older patients. For example, fractures may be caused by osteoporosis; hematomas or other skin marks could be caused by thrombocytopenia, senile purpura, steroid purpura, bleeding disorders or drugs [28]. Medical reasons for excessive bruising should be ruled out by performing blood coagulation studies and platelet counts [28, 30]. Specific exams should be considered according to abuse type: If sexual abuse is suspected, consider testing for STDs. Toxicological screening can be used to rule out poisoning or drug abuse. Medication blood levels should be tested when relevant, e.g. when intentional or unintentional misuse of medications is suspected. Low or undetectable levels of prescribed drugs may indicate neglect in a dependent older person; the presence of toxins or medications that were not prescribed to the patient may indicate intentional poisoning [28].

(b) **Radiology and imaging**: Radiographs and other imaging tests should be ordered to assess recent injuries as well as to rule out older ones. Despite the lack of pathognomonic lesions and signs of EAN, in a recent report of two emergency room cases, Wong et al. suggest that some of the findings in child abuse could also be found in elder abuse cases. Such shared characteristics may include (a) injuries which are not consistent with the reported mechanism, (b) injuries in multiple stages of healing which may include deformations as a result of old injuries and (c) patterns uncommon in accidental injury [34]. Several authors, mainly in emergency room settings, emphasise the importance of providing radiologists with detailed history when ordering radiographs, as well as the radiologist matching injury patterns with mechanisms of injury in the elderly. Improved bilateral cooperation between treating physicians and radiologists is critical for increasing the detection of elderly abuse cases [34, 35]. This is probably true in primary care settings as well.

It is of paramount importance to remember that in elders even minor head trauma can cause significant morbidity and mortality, as well as functional decline. Whenever there is a suspicion of such an injury, the evaluation should include a head CT [36].

18.6.6 Primary Management

(a) **Summarising information**: Possible differential diagnoses could be established after integration of data collected from history, physical examination, laboratory tests and imaging. Since there are no pathognomonic findings that distinguish accidental injuries from those caused by physical elder abuse, it is important to evaluate risk factors and circumstances as well [33]. One important possible differential diagnosis that should be considered is self-neglect. Creating a bio-psycho-social problem list which includes medical conditions, injuries, functional impairment, mental health issues as well as other consequences of abuse or neglect are useful for planning treatment, intervention and follow-up.

(b) **Treatment**: A comprehensive treatment plan should be based on the problem list, addressing each of the problems, and is beyond the scope of this chapter.

When suspecting self-neglect physicians should look for and address underlying conditions: cognitive impairment, depression, mental retardation, physical disability, psychological distress, lack of social support, etc. [4].

In cases of sexual abuse, WHO guidelines recommend that women should be given antibiotics to prevent and treat STDs without prior testing (chlamydia, gonorrhoea, trichomonas and syphilis if common in the area) as well as HIV preventive medications and offered hepatitis B vaccination [37]. When treating an older adult who was sexually abused, the HCP should consider these same principles, while weighing pros and cons according to the specific clinical case.

(c) **Documentation**: In cases of suspected EAN accurate documentation has medical, legal and forensic implications [30]. Documentation should use objective descriptive language, without interpretations or accusations. It is important to remember that the HCPs' main concern is the safety of the patient. Due to legal issues (e.g. guardianship of an incompetent older adult), the information might be available to the perpetrator. This is of major concern with the increasing use of electronic medical records and increasing access to the records by patients and caretakers. HCPs should document history as well as direct quotations and describe observations of patient behaviour, interaction between patient and caregiver, reactions to questions and physical examination findings. Injuries should be described and also drawn on body charts. Photographing injuries is also recommended, and consent should be obtained from patients with mental capacity. If a crime is suspected, photographs should be taken by the police. In the absence of a professional medical photographer, use a digital camera, and include the patient's name and date as well as a ruler in the photograph. Both close ups and distant pictures should be taken to provide perspective and location of lesions and at least two different angles for three-dimensional lesions [16, 28, 30].

(d) **Home visit**: A home visit by one of the HCPs or by social services may add valuable information, but the frequency of such visits differs significantly between countries. Discussing the possibility of EAN in the home setting can be tricky, as the perpetrator may be present [31]. Nevertheless, identification of neglect and self-neglect can be enhanced significantly by home visits. In an Irish study, 91 out of 120 GPs (76%) responded that they identified cases of EAN during a home visit. In this study self-neglect and neglect were more common than physical abuse [38]. A home visit may reveal numerous "red flags" which may be related to direct observation of relationships and living arrangements, neglect (e.g. unsuitable or unsafe living conditions including poor hygiene, lack of food, inadequate equipment) and signs of possible physical violence (e.g. marks on furniture; internal locks; objects used for restraining). The safety of the healthcare professionals should be taken into consideration when planning such visits. A joint visit by professionals from different disciplines may enhance the team's safety as well as effectivity.

(e) **Difficulties with a treatment plan**: Health providers should consider and address any possible factors, including those related to EAN, that may affect clinical findings or outcomes. For example, when a patient with an uncontrolled chronic illness is deprived of medications, the HCP should address the issue to make sure that medications will be available. Transfer to another medical provider should be considered in cases of resistance to or sabotage of medical interventions [39].

18.6.7 Consulting and Reporting

(a) **Action guided by the status of the patient**: As specified above the legal status of the patient is influenced by the decision-making capacity (DMC) and in some instances by functional dependence (Sect. 18.6.2). The older patient may not be able to take actions against an abuser due to either impaired DMC or significantly compromised physical functional ability. Thus, when abuse or neglect is suspected, the options on how to proceed depend on these parameters. All HCPs should know and follow local laws and criteria for mandatory reporting:

- **Competent and independent patient**: Whenever the patient's DMC is preserved, abuse or neglect should be discussed with the patient directly in private. We propose that the *LIVES* model's principles presented in WHO's clinical handbook for cases of intimate partner or sexual assault of women can be adapted for EAN cases. The LIVES model guides the health provider's response after disclosure of abuse, providing first-line support, and useful job aids can be found in the handbook [37].

    Listen and inquire about patient's needs and concerns: Listen to the patient closely with empathy, without judging. Ask open inviting questions such as "How can we help you?" "Is there anything that you need or are concerned about?" Notice the body language.

    Validate: Show that you understand and believe the patient and that she/he is not to blame. Respond to feelings, e.g. acknowledge that anger with perpetrator is a valid feeling.

    Enhance safety: Discuss the immediate risk of violence and a plan for protection if a violent event happens or if there is a threat of such an event. Examples of safety planning for elders include planning a place to go to and having essential phone numbers and a checklist of essential items to keep together in a safe place [16, 28]. When there is immediate danger, urgent measures to increase safety may include moving out temporarily (e.g. hospital admission, placement in a shelter or other type of facility) or a court protection order [31].

    Support: Provide information and help connect to services and social support. Resources may differ between countries and regions and may include both governmental and non-governmental organisations/services such as adult protective services (APS); helplines (telephone/internet) [5]; community services; legal services; day centre, etc. A patient-centred approach, discussing with patient various possibilities and asking for consent before sharing information are recommended.

- **Incompetent patient**: In most countries when an older person is not legally competent, there is a duty to report abuse or neglect to adult protective services, to the police or other specific agencies. Usually, in such cases the assessment and intervention regarding the abuse/neglect will be formally guided by them.

- **Unclear competence of the patient or physical dependence**: Further evaluation by an interdisciplinary team is necessary to determine the status of the patient and whether there is a duty to report and act according to formal guidance.

(b) **Addressing context, perpetrator, caretaker and caretaker burden**: PHC teams are in a unique position that enables them to meet and confer with various members of the family and address caretaker burden as well as relationship issues. Their ongoing relationship, which frequently involves multiple members of the same family, may enable them to perceive even subtle changes.

Addressing caretaker burden is a cornerstone in the management and prevention of EAN [5]. HCPs can help promote the connection and relationship between elderly people, their family and caregivers. Alleviating stressors that cause abuse may be necessary so that the family can provide care for the elderly at home [16]. In one study, for example, Korean social workers shared that they may decide not to carry out a mandatory report because they feel that the family member(s) can be helped to care for the elder in the home environment while improving in the areas that create abusive behaviours [40].

The perpetrator may be a family member or an external person, including a hired caretaker. Interventions with perpetrators of EAN will mostly be provided by other stakeholders, though there is not enough research on their long term effects [16]. Yet, we believe that whenever possible initial evaluation should include a health assessment of the perpetrator and treatment of any conditions which may contribute to the abusive behaviour. This may be possible specifically in the context of EAN occurring in family settings where the family physician cares for several members of the family but should be done discretely. When the perpetrator is also an older adult, he/she may have physical as well as mental health problems, occurring previously or arising at an older age, such as frontal lobe infarcts/injury, depression, dementia and substance abuse. These health issues may directly cause the abuse/neglect or indirectly contribute by decreasing the ability to function well enough as a caretaker for the older person (Table 18.7).

Relocation to nursing homes or to specialised shelter programs for elders, if available, should be considered whenever there is a need for providing security [5]. Nonetheless, it is important to note that EAN can occur also in such facilities [31, 41].

Important principles when managing EAN cases include a patient-centred approach, cultural sensitivity and adequate interventions for ethnic minorities—despite the lack of sufficient research on these topics [16].

(c) **Ethical and legal considerations**: It is believed that involving multidisciplinary teams is necessary both for evaluation and intervention in cases of elder abuse [5, 16, 28]. This may be limited by ethical and legal considerations. Specifically, every health professional should know whether the duty to report concerns only patients who are not legally competent or all cases of elder abuse; whether a suspicion of abuse is enough or there is a need for convincing evidence; whom to report to; and whether the reporter can remain anonymous or not. In the United States, for example, in most states there is a duty to report elder abuse to adult protective services whenever there is a reasonable suspicion, and most reports made by healthcare professionals cannot be anonymous [16].

Society should strive to protect the elderly while helping them maintain their autonomy, independence, culture and beliefs as well as their relationship with family whenever possible [6, 42]. Professionals should assume the ethical responsibility to protect elder abuse victims. Abuse, in principle, violates some ethical principles including autonomy, justice, beneficence and non-maleficence. Reporting violates the right to autonomy and confidentiality. In many EAN cases, beneficence and non-maleficence should be prioritised, and reporting is ethically acceptable when potentially will lead to activation of protective systems to help the victim and enhance safety. One should always remember that when such a system does not exist, reporting may cause more harm than good, putting the patient at risk of exacerbation of abuse or neglect [42]. HCPs must also understand that they may face penalties, including jail time and fines, for not reporting suspected abuse. Failure to report is considered by some as negligence or malpractice [27].

(d) **Addressing barriers**: HCPs under-diagnose and under-report cases of elder abuse. For example, in one study of primary care physicians in Ohio, more than half of the respondents reported that they had never identified a case of elder mistreatment [43]. Physicians' barriers include lack of knowledge and confidence, personal and professional beliefs, time constraints, concern with effects on the patient-doctor relationship, etc. [43, 44]. The HCPs' dilemmas are even more complex in specific situations, e.g. when the victim does not want measures to be taken and when there are complex family contextual factors [45]. An encouraging finding, on the other hand, comes from a more recent study from Ireland. The GP responders in this study were willing to confront the issue of elder abuse and neglect, sometimes at the risk of personal harm, and 73% of them perceived that the GP's role is not simply to provide medical treatment but also to be a part of the intervention and solution in abuse cases [38].

All professionals involved, including HCPs should be aware and address possible patients' barriers to disclosure as well as to taking action once EAN was disclosed or established. These may include various forms of dependence (emotional, physical, instrumental, financial, etc.); lack of accessibility to and lack of trust in services; self-blame; ambivalence or wanting to avoid possible harm to the perpetrator; various cultural and religious issues; shame and stigma; etc. [46, 47]. Any discussion should be patient-centred, adapted to the patient's capabilities and culture.

18.6.8 Follow-Up

(a) **General follow-up**: The importance of follow-up in cases of suspected or established EAN should not be underestimated. It should address among other issues medical conditions, injuries, functional impairment and mental health. A practical way is using the problem list. The HCP should examine injuries' healing process and functional consequences, to ensure maximal recovery and functionality. It is pertinent to examine for possible new injuries as well. Pain should be assessed and addressed to ensure the patient's well-being. Further follow-up planning is indicated whenever physical, emotional or functional consequences persist [16].

In cases of sexual assault, patients should be followed up 2 weeks, 1 month, 3 and 6 months following the assault, including mental health and psychosocial support assessment. When clinical findings included STDs, compliance to preventive measures that were recommended and test results should be followed [37].

(b) **Follow-up on EAN**: Follow-up is necessary to monitor ongoing abuse or neglect [16]. HCPs can discuss it directly with the competent patient. If the patient is incompetent, it is necessary to maintain ongoing contact with the relevant local services (e.g. APS, multidisciplinary team) as well as the legal guardian.

Close follow-up and a vigilant attitude may be considered when EAN was suspected but not proven or when there are relevant risk factors or "red flags".

When there are difficulties with follow-up, such as patients not showing up—the possibility of continued or worsening EAN should be considered, and actions should be taken accordingly. Follow-up by APS may sometimes be necessary to ensure medical treatment and follow-up [39].

18.7 Prevention of EAN

The MIPAA (Madrid International Plan of Action on Ageing) strongly recommended emphasising prevention and management through multi-sectoral, interdisciplinary community-based approaches to eliminate all forms of neglect, abuse and violence [31]. This is a complex task that requires the intervention of different professionals and agencies as well as a broad range of approaches. The WHO has recognised the need to establish a global strategy for the prevention of EAN improving cooperation between existing public health, social, medical and legal systems [31]. In this sense, it is important to point out the unique position of PHC professionals to detect EAN, raise awareness and promote effective interventions for this problem.

18.7.1 Types of Prevention and Their Aim

Based on the Cochrane reviewers' classification of levels of intervention [14], there are three fundamental types of preventive interventions, primary, secondary and tertiary prevention, as presented in Table 18.9. PHC teams and professionals could be involved at any of these levels.

Ayalon et al., in their systematic review and meta-analysis of interventions designed to prevent or stop elder abuse, identified three main categories of interventions:

1. Interventions designed to improve the ability of professionals
2. Interventions to detect or stop elder maltreatment that target older adults who experience elder maltreatment
3. Interventions that target caregivers who maltreat older adults

They concluded that currently, the most effective intervention was directly targeting physical restraint by long-term care facilities' paid carers (category 3 intervention) [48].

Another review indicates that community interventions focused on caretakers may have a protective effect against EAN. Such interventions include educational sessions provided by health professionals, trainings on coping skills for caretakers

Table 18.9 Type of preventive interventions

Type of prevention	Definition	Examples

Primary prevention	Interventions that prevent the abuse or neglect from occurring	• Health policies
		• Raising public awareness
		• Community interventions
		• General interventions for identification, reduction and treatment of risk factors, including:
		  – Addressing possible caretaker burden
		  – Advanced planning of care for an older person with a chronic condition that may worsen over time
		• Specific patient-/family-centred interventions: targeting the elderly, family members or caregivers
		• Encouraging research
		• Addressing ageism and advocacy for elders
		• Improving coordination of care
		• Training and education:
		  – For caretakers
		  – For HCPs
		  – For various community services (social services, police, judicial system, etc.)

Secondary prevention	Actions aimed at preventing further abuse: • Stopping abuse and escalating incidents • Improving patient's well-being	• Close monitoring of vulnerable older adults • Early EAN detection through screening or other tools • Mandatory reporting • Protective service interventions • Helplines • Support groups • Temporary placement, housing, emergency shelters • Training and education: programmes targeted at health and social care professionals • Dealing with the perpetrator: medically, socially and legally as required
Tertiary prevention	Actions to manage the consequences after the abuse has occurred	• Treatment of medical and mental health conditions resulting from EAN • Social services, police, legal support • Rehabilitation • Long term multidisciplinary support and counselling • Training and education: programmes targeted at health and social care professionals

(e.g. problem-focused strategies) as well as classes on the impact and of caring for people with dementia [49]. Some of these interventions fit well within the scope of the PHC teams' work.

It is uncertain whether specific educational interventions improve the knowledge of health care professionals and caregivers about EAN. Furthermore, it remains to be proved if such newly acquired knowledge actually leads to modification of professionals' and caretakers' behaviour resulting in a decrease of EAN [14].

Similarly, interventions such as supporting and educating EAN victims (category 2 interventions) appear to lead to more reporting. But it is unclear whether this indicates an actual increase in EAN cases or reflects only an increased awareness and inclination to report [14]. Nevertheless, there is evidence of moderate quality that shows teaching coping skills to family members caring for the elderly with dementia may possibly improve outcomes [50].

18.7.2 Screening as a Prevention Tool

The increased awareness of EAN has contributed to the development of screening protocols [51]; however, few of them have been accepted for extensive application in clinical settings. The variety of available tools reveals the urgent need to develop a reliable, practical and simple tool, easy and quick to use, with clear and appropriate wording, suitable for different contexts, with a high sensitivity rate [31].

The US Preventive Services Task Force (USPSTF) defines screening as the process of eliciting information about abusive experiences in a caring or family relationship from older or vulnerable adults who do not have complaints or obvious signs of abuse. Within such definition screening presents multiple goals as shown in Table 18.10 [52].

18.7.2.1 Screening Effectiveness and Employment

The effectiveness of EAN screening and its use in everyday practice are controversial. It is important to stress that screening refers to asymptomatic patients and in the context of EAN may be seen as older adults without obvious risk factors or "red flags" presented in Tables 18.7 and 18.9. The Canadian Task Force on Preventive Health Care, the United Kingdom National Screening Committee and the United States Preventive Services Task Force (USPSTF) do not recommend routine screening for EAN [53]. This is based on the lack of evidence that screening or early EAN detection reduces the exposure to abuse or its harmful consequences [54]. On the other hand, several associations such as the American College of Emergency Physicians, the American Medical Association and the National Gerontological Nursing Association do recommend routine EAN screening as there is a broad

Table 18.10 EAN screening

Screening definition	Screening goal
Process of eliciting information about abusive experiences in a caring or family relationship from older or vulnerable adults who do not have complaints or obvious signs of abuse (the US Preventive Services Task Force—USPSTF) [54]	• Identification of unrecognised EAN cases • Prevention of further and future abuse • Reduction of negative EAN health consequences [52]

agreement on encouraging and enhancing EAN prevention and early detection in order to reduce its potential negative impacts [52, 53].

18.7.2.2 Screening Tools

Among the existing validated screening tools, some can be suitable for clinical settings [53, 55]. They vary in length, type of abuse and psychometric appraisal, and they all represent useful tools to provide early identification and prevention.

The majority of screening tools include the direct questioning method used by clinicians to screen for abuse among the elderly in primary care or hospital settings [52]. Besides the EASI© tool (shown in Table 18.8), some other examples of open-ended questions that can reveal fear or any other potential indicators of abuse include [55]:

- "Is there anything going on at home that you would like to talk about?"
- "Has anyone touched you without your permission?"
- "Has anyone hurt, hit roughly or threatened you?"
- "Has anyone taken your personal possessions such as your money, car or valuables without your permission?"
- "Has anyone yelled or sworn at you?"
- "Has anyone made fun of you or hurt your feelings?"

It is important to emphasise that a positive screen for EAN does not indicate that abuse is taking place but that further information should be gathered [55]. In summary, HCPs should be aware of the high prevalence of EAN, educate themselves about elder abuse and consider actively searching and screening for EAN risk factors and "red flags", especially in high-risk populations [16].

18.7.3 Prevention: The State of the Art

The global elderly population is increasing dramatically worldwide [56], from 900 million in 2015 to nearly 2 billion in 2050. A higher ratio of elders in the population probably will mean a heavier burden of care for the younger population. As a result of these processes, the incidence and prevalence of EAN are expected to increase significantly as well.

Such concerning figures urge an action on prevention. But unfortunately the most recent scientific reviews on the topic concluded that there is not enough evidence demonstrating the effectiveness of existing interventions to reduce the occurrence or recurrence of EAN [48, 50]. High-quality trials regarding EAN prevention are urgently needed, including those from low- and middle-income countries. These should address cost-effectiveness, implementation assessment and equity considerations [14, 50]. At the same time, urgent steps should be taken by policymakers around the globe targeting the population changes and risk factors for EAN comprehensively, from every possible aspect. Societal issues as poverty, equity, adequate housing and health care as well as provision of adequate care for the elders and significant law enforcement for offenders are equally essential for a society striving to adequately control or abolish the sad phenomenon of EAN.

18.8 What's the Role of Family Physicians in Elder Abuse and Neglect?

Elder abuse and neglect are highly prevalent and significantly influence quality of life, morbidity and mortality of older adults. Family doctors should remain alert to major risk factors or "red flags". When suspicion arises, a proper evaluation should be done. This includes obtaining the bio-psycho-social history from the patient and/ or caretakers and family; evaluating cognition, competence and functional ability; performing a comprehensive physical examination; and considering possible differential diagnoses. A home visit or additional studies may be necessary. The family doctor, who usually knows well the patient, family and community, is in a unique position to recommend whether the evaluation could be done in the ambulatory setting or whether prompt hospitalisation for further workup or protection is necessary. This decision should be guided by the perceived risks, as well as the patient's wish when competent. Whenever the patient is incompetent or dependent, the physician should act according to the local reporting laws. Family physicians can identify EAN early and activate multidisciplinary teams to prevent further abuse as well as its consequences. They have an invaluable role in an ongoing management, support and follow-up. Furthermore, by actively addressing caretaker burden, physicians and their teams can sometimes prevent abuse before it happens. To do so family doctors and primary healthcare teams should be properly trained on this topic. Training should address necessary knowledge and skills as well as possible barriers to EAN identification. Last but not least, physicians should not treat these cases alone! They should keep the updated contact information of relevant consultants and community services; they should actively consult multidisciplinary teams; they should make sure to care for themselves and seek support services to prevent secondary trauma.

Acknowledgement A special thanks and sincere gratitude to Professor Tan Maw Pin (University of Malaya, Department of Geriatric Medicine, Faculty of Medicine) for the scientific review and precious suggestions.

References

1. Burston GR. Letter: Granny-battering. Br Med J. 1975;3(5983):592.
2. De Donder L, Luoma M-L, Penhale B, Lang G, Santos AJ, Tamutiene I, et al. European map of prevalence rates of elder abuse and its impact for future research. Eur J Ageing. 2011;8(2):129.
3. Yon Y, Mikton CR, Gassoumis ZD, Wilber KH. Elder abuse prevalence in community settings: a systematic review and meta-analysis. Lancet Glob Health. 2017;5(2):e147–56.
4. Dong X, Simon M, de Leon CM, Fulmer T, Beck T, Hebert L, et al. Elder self-neglect and abuse and mortality risk in a community-dwelling population. JAMA. 2009;302(5):517.

5. Pillemer K, Burnes D, Riffin C, Lachs MS. Elder abuse: global situation, risk factors, and prevention strategies. Gerontologist. 2016;56(Suppl 2):S194–205.
6. World Health Organization. WHO I Missing voices: views of older persons on elder abuse. WHO. 2015 [cited 2019 May 19].
7. Randel J, German T, Ewing D. United Nations principles for older persons. Ageing Dev Rep. 2018:197–8.
8. Official Journal of the European Communities. Charter of Fundamental Rights (EU) (2000/C 364/01). Encycl Big Data. 2018;1–3.
9. World Health Organization. European report on preventing elder maltreatment. 2011 [cited 2019 May 19].
10. van Bavel M, Janssens K, Schakenraad W, Thurlings N. Elder abuse in Europe. Eur Ref Framew Online Prev Elder Abus Negl. 2010.
11. Yon Y, Ramiro-Gonzalez M, Mikton CR, Huber M, Sethi D. The prevalence of elder abuse in institutional settings: a systematic review and meta-analysis. Eur J Public Health. 2019;29(1):58–67.
12. New definition of abuse. Action Elder Abus Bull. 1995;(11).
13. National Research Council (U.S.). Panel to Review Risk and Prevalence of Elder Abuse and Neglect, Bonnie RJ, Wallace RB. Elder mistreatment: abuse, neglect, and exploitation in an aging America. Washington, DC: National Academies Press; 2003. p. 552.
14. Baker PRA, Francis DP, Hairi NN, Othman S, Choo WY. Interventions for preventing abuse in the elderly. Cochrane Database Syst Rev. 2016;(8):CD010321.
15. Lachs MS, Pillemer KA. Elder abuse. N Engl J Med. 2015;373(20):1947–56.
16. Dong XQ. Elder abuse: systematic review and implications for practice. J Am Geriatr Soc. 2015;63(6):1214–38.
17. Castle N, Ferguson-Rome JC, Teresi JA. Elder abuse in residential long-term care. J Appl Gerontol. 2015;34(4):407–43.
18. Drennan J, Lafferty A, Treacy MP. Older people in residential care settings: results of a national survey of staff-resident interactions and conflicts. Dublin: NCPOP; 2012.
19. Levine JM. Elder neglect and abuse. A primer for primary care physicians. Geriatrics. 2003;58(10):37–40, 42–4.
20. Melchiorre MG, Di Rosa M, Lamura G, Torres-Gonzales F, Lindert J, Stankunas M, et al. Abuse of older men in seven European countries: a multilevel approach in the framework of an ecological model. PLoS One. 2016;11(1):e0146425.
21. Band-Winterstein T, Smeloy Y, Avieli H. Shared reality of the abusive and the vulnerable: the experience of aging for parents living with abusive adult children coping with mental disorder. Int Psychogeriatr. 2014;26(11):1917–27.
22. Band-Winterstein T, Avieli H, Smeloy Y. Harmed? Harmful? Experiencing abusive adult children with mental disorder over the life course. J Interpers Violence. 2016;31(15):2598–621.
23. Band-Winterstein T. Aging in the shadow of violence: a phenomenological conceptual framework for understanding elderly women who experienced lifelong IPV. [cited 2019 Nov 23].
24. Winterstein T-B, Band-Winterstein T. The impact of lifelong exposure to IPV on adult children and their aging parents. J Fam Issues. 2014;35(4):439–61.
25. Du Mont J, Macdonald S, Kosa D, Elliot S, Spencer C, Yaffe M. Development of a comprehensive hospital-based elder abuse intervention: an initial systematic scoping review network of sexual assault/domestic violence treatments centres. 2015.
26. Du Mont J, Kosa D, Macdonald S, Elliot S, Yaffe M. Determining possible professionals and respective roles and responsibilities for a model comprehensive elder abuse intervention: a Delphi consensus survey. PLoS One. 2015;10(12):e0140760.
27. Gibbs, Lisa M, Mosqueda L. The importance of reporting mistreatment of the elderly - American Family Physician. American Academy of Family Physicians. 2007 [cited 2019 Nov 23].
28. Hoover RM. Detecting elder abuse and neglect: assessment and intervention. 2014 [cited 2017 Aug 16];89(6).

29. Janofsky JS, McCarthy RJ, Foistein MF. The Hopkins Competency Assessment Test: a brief method for evaluating patients' capacity to give informed consent. 1992.
30. Pham E, Liao S. Clinician's role in the documentation of elder mistreatment interview and history-taking physical examination assessment Figure 1A and B: bruise with central clearing and linear demarcations. 2009.
31. WHO. A global response to elder abuse and neglect. Geneva: WHO; 2008.
32. Yaffe MJ, Wolfson C, Lithwick M, Weiss D. Development and validation of a tool to improve physician identification of elder abuse: The Elder Abuse Suspicion Index (EASI)©. J Elder Abus Negl. 2008;20(3):276–300.
33. Murphy K, Waa S, Jaffer H, Sauter A, Chan A. A literature review of findings in physical elder abuse. Can Assoc Radiol J. 2013;64(1):10–4.
34. Wong NZ, Rosen T, Sanchez AM, Bloemen EM, Mennitt KW, Hentel K, et al. Imaging findings in elder abuse: a role for radiologists in detection. Can Assoc Radiol J. 2017;68(1):16–20.
35. Russo A, Reginelli A, Pignatiello M, Cioce F, Mazzei G, Fabozzi O, et al. Imaging of violence against the elderly and the women. Semin Ultrasound CT MRI. 2019;40(1):18–24.
36. Walls R, Hockberger R, Gausche-Hill M, et al. Rosen's emergency medicine. 9th ed. Amsterdam: Elsevier; 2018. p. 328–9.
37. World Health Organization. Health care for women subjected to intimate partner violence or sexual violence: a clinical handbook. 2014 [cited 2017 Oct 20].
38. O'Brien JG, Riain AN, Collins C, Long V, O'Neill D. Elder abuse and neglect: a survey of Irish General Practitioners. J Elder Abuse Negl. 2014;26(3):291–9.
39. Halphen JM, Dyer CB. Elder mistreatment: abuse, neglect, and financial exploitation. UpToDate. 2019.
40. Doe SS, Han HK, Mccaslin R, Acsw P. Cultural and ethical issues in Korea's recent elder abuse reporting system. J Elder Abuse Negl. 2009;21(2):170–85.
41. Ben NM, Lowenstein A, Eisikovits Z. Psycho-social factors affecting elders' maltreatment in long-term care facilities. Int Nurs Rev. 2010;57(1):113–20.
42. Saghafi A, Bahramnezhad F, Poormollamirza A, Dadgari A, Navab E. Examining the ethical challenges in managing elder abuse: a systematic review. J Med Ethics Hist Med. 2019;12:7.
43. Kennedy RD. Elder abuse and neglect: the experience, knowledge, and attitudes of primary care physicians. Fam Med. 2005;37(7):481–5.
44. Mohd Mydin FH, Othman S. Elder abuse and neglect intervention in the clinical setting: perceptions and barriers faced by primary care physicians in Malaysia. J Interpers Violence. 2017;2017:886260517726411.
45. Killick C, Taylor BJ. Professional decision making on elder abuse: systematic narrative review. J Elder Abuse Neglect. 2009;21:211–38.
46. Chokkanathan S, Natarajan A, Mohanty J. Elder abuse and barriers to help seeking in Chennai, India: a qualitative study. J Elder Abuse Negl. 2014;26(1):60–79.
47. Dow B, Gahan L, Gaffy E, Joosten M, Vrantsidis F, Jarred M. Barriers to disclosing elder abuse and taking action in Australia. J Fam Violence. 2019;35:853–61.
48. Ayalon L, Lev S, Green O, Nevo U. A systematic review and meta-analysis of interventions designed to prevent or stop elder maltreatment. Age Ageing. 2016;45(2):216–27.
49. Fearing G, Sheppard CL, McDonald L, Beaulieu M, Hitzig SL. A systematic review on community-based interventions for elder abuse and neglect. J Elder Abuse Negl. 2017;29(2–3):102–33.
50. Baker PR, Francis DP, Mohd Hairi NN, Othman S, Choo WY. Interventions for preventing elder abuse: applying findings of a new Cochrane review. Age Ageing. 2017;46(3):346–8.
51. Van Den Bruele AB, Dimachk M, Crandall M. Elder abuse. Clin Geriatr Med. 2019;35:103–13.
52. Schofield MJ. Screening for elder abuse: tools and effectiveness. In: Elder abuse: research, practice and policy. Cham: Springer International Publishing; 2017. p. 161–99.
53. Perel-Levin S. Discussing screening for elder abuse at primary health care level. 2008.
54. Nelson HD, Bougatsos C, Blazina I. Screening women for intimate partner violence and elderly and vulnerable adults for abuse. Screening women for intimate partner violence and

elderly and vulnerable adults for abuse: systematic review to update the 2004 U.S. Preventive Services Task Force Recommendation. Agency for Healthcare Research and Quality (US); 2012 [cited 2019 Nov 17].

55. Burnett J, Achenbaum WA, Murphy KP. Prevention and early identification of elder abuse. Clin Geriatr Med. 2014;30:743–59.

56. World Health Organization. Aging and health. 5 Februray 2008. 2008 [cited 2019 Sep 5].

Part V

Quaternary Prevention

Polypharmacy, Overdiagnosis and Overtreatment

19

Ferdinando Petrazzuoli, Lucas Morin, Daniele Angioni, Nicola Pecora, and Antonio Cherubini

Abstract

In geriatric medicine, tools developed for identifying potentially inappropriate medications (PIMs) include the Beers criteria, the Swedish quality indicators developed by the Swedish National Board of Health and Welfare, the *STOPP/ START* criteria, the *EU(7)-PIM list*, and the *medication appropriateness index (MAI)*.

Two important factors which are very often related to polypharmacy are over-diagnosis and overtreatment.

Overdiagnosis is an unrecognised and growing worldwide problem in health-care. Disease definitions have been widened, and thresholds for treating risk

F. Petrazzuoli (✉)
Center for Primary Health Care Research, Clinical Research Center, Lund University, Malmö, Sweden
e-mail: ferdinando.petrazzuoli@med.lu.se

L. Morin
Inserm CIC 1431, Clinical Investigation Unit, University Hospital of Besançon, Besançon, France

D. Angioni
Eastern Piedmont, Primary Care Clinic in Novara South-District, Novara, Italy

Diagnostic Medical Sonographer in Vercelli, Vercelli, Italy

N. Pecora
AUSL Toscana Centro, Firenze, Italy

A. Cherubini
Geriatrics, Geriatric Emergency and Research Center on Aging, IRCCS INRCA, Ancona, Italy

© Springer Nature Switzerland AG 2022
J. Demurtas, N. Veronese (eds.), *The Role of Family Physicians in Older People Care*, Practical Issues in Geriatrics, https://doi.org/10.1007/978-3-030-78923-7_19

factors have been lowered. Finally, disease mongering is also continuously growing. Overdiagnosis is simply 'too much healthcare', too much screening of asymptomatic individuals, too much investigation of those with symptoms, too much reliance on biomarkers, too many quasi-diseases, too much diagnosis often leading to too much treatment, sometimes cost-ineffective medicines that are too costly and too rapidly approved for marketing, too many adverse reactions, and too much inappropriate monitoring. Too much healthcare leads almost inevitably to too little effective healthcare.

Overtreatment occurs when the best scientific evidence demonstrates that a treatment provides no benefit for the diagnosed condition. Patients are exposed to treatment harms, and waste of resources is inevitable on a grand scale.

General practitioners (GPs) have a crucial role in fighting overmedicalisation. Their role as passive enactors of specialist and public health ideas needs to be updated. GPs need to stand up and shape the clinical agenda from their unique perspective. To do this they need a stronger part in the creative process of evidence synthesis and policymaking.

Keywords

Polypharmacy · Overdiagnosis · Overtreatment · Overtesting · Adverse drug event · Inappropriate medication · Defensive medicine

19.1 Polypharmacy

19.1.1 Definition of Polypharmacy

Polypharmacy is defined as taking five or more long-term prescribed drugs [1–8], but definitions may vary widely, and appropriateness appears in only a minority of definitions. Indeed, numerical definitions of polypharmacy do not account for specific comorbidities and make it difficult to assess the safety and appropriateness of therapy in the clinical setting [9]. Older patients are often affected by multiple chronic diseases [10] and are consequently on polypharmacy. The risk of suffering from drug-related problems [11–14] is very high, since studies show that a substantial proportion of hospital admissions among older are due to adverse drug events (ADEs) [13, 15–18]. Most of these hospital admissions are avoidable [13, 19].

19.1.2 Prevalence of Polypharmacy

The prevalence of polypharmacy in adults and older adults has increased substantially in the last decades. In Scotland, for instance, the proportion of older adults exposed to five or more drugs rose from 11% in 1995 to 21% by 2010 [2, 20]. The prevalence of polypharmacy increases dramatically with age. In a study conducted in Scotland, the prevalence increased from 30% in those aged 60–69 years to almost

70% in those >80 years [7]. In the Netherlands, prevalence increased to 60% in a nursing home setting in older patients with an average age of 80 years [12]. In the United States, prevalence is also increasing [21]: 40% of adults aged ≥65 years take 5–9 medications and 18% take ≥10 medications [22].

19.1.3 List of Potentially Inappropriate Medications

Potentially inappropriate medications (PIMs) [23] can be defined as medications for which the risks outweigh the benefits for older patients [24]. Identification of PIMs can be performed using two different approaches. Implicit criteria are indicators that evaluate in depth the appropriateness of each drug, considering the patient who takes it, e.g. the medication appropriateness index. They are sensitive but also very time-consuming and heavily influenced by the expertise of the reviewer.

On the other hand, explicit criteria are lists of drugs whose use is inappropriate in general or in older individuals with specific conditions. Among them the *STOPP/START* criteria and the *Beers criteria* are the most commonly used.

The Swedish National Board of Health and Welfare has made a list of potentially inappropriate medications in the older [24]. This list includes 'anticholinergic drugs', 'long-acting benzodiazepines', 'tramadol', 'propiomazine', 'antipsychotic drugs', and 'non-steroidal anti-inflammatory drug (NSAID)'. The use of these drugs should be as low as possible, regardless of indication, for older patients.

19.1.4 Tools for Identifying Potentially Inappropriate Medications (PIMs)

Potentially inappropriate medications (PIMs) are one cause of DRPs. In many countries, guidelines concerning potentially inappropriate medication have been developed with *Beers criteria* being the best-known [25].

The *updated Beers criteria (2019)* [26] include five types of criteria:

1. Medications that are potentially inappropriate in older Adults
2. Medications that should typically be avoided in older adults with certain conditions
3. Drugs to use with caution
4. Drug-drug interactions
5. Drug dose adjustment based on kidney function

The problem with the *Beers* criteria is that it is based mainly on drugs present on the North American market. In Europe, it seems preferable using the Swedish quality indicators developed by the Swedish National Board of Health and Welfare [24], the *STOPP/START* criteria [27], and the *EU(7)-PIM list* [28].

STOPP/START: Screening Tool of Older Persons' Potentially Inappropriate Prescriptions (*STOPP*) and Screening Tool to Alert Doctors to Right Treatment (*START*).

STOPP is a list of potentially inappropriate prescriptions for common conditions in older people, considering drug effects as well as drug-drug and drug-disease interactions. *START* is a list of commonly omitted medications that are beneficial in older people developed by a research team and verified by consensus of experts via the Delphi method [29], as well as instances of prescribing omission, a list of medications that require specific consideration to avoid harmful drug-related adverse effects or which may be inappropriately omitted.

An implicit tool for identifying inappropriate medications is the *medication appropriateness index (MAI)* [30]: This an instrument that determines a drug's suitability to an individual and has been validated for evaluating drug use in the older [31]. The MAI is a 10-question index assessing prescription appropriateness in terms of drug choice and medication instruction accuracy associated with the detection of prescribing errors. The health outcome prediction, though, may require more time than typical visit makes feasible [32]. MAI, therefore, appears to be more time-consuming than explicit criteria and therefore more difficult to use in everyday care.

In the hospital setting the *lund integrated medicine management* (LIMM) [33] is an in-hospital intervention model with multi-professional teams, including clinical pharmacists. It has proved to reduce potentially inappropriate medications and unscheduled drug-related hospital revisits [33].

Recently another interesting tool has been tested in a multinational trial. This tool is called *SENATOR* and consists of a sophisticated software aimed at improving pharmacological therapy in older patients who are managed by specialists who are not geriatricians. The main aim was to reduce incident, adverse drug reactions. The *SENATOR* software produces a report designed to optimise older patients' current prescriptions by applying the published *STOPP/START* criteria, highlighting drug-drug and drug-disease interactions and providing non-pharmacological recommendations [34].

Even more relevant for the setting of primary care is the ongoing *OPERAM* trial [35]. The optimising therapy to prevent avoidable hospital admissions in multimorbid older people (*OPERAM*) trial will examine the effect of a structured medication review (*STRIP*) supported by the *STRIP* Assistant (*STRIPA*) clinical decision support software on drug-related hospital admissions (main endpoint) compared with usual care in older patients assisted in primary care.

19.1.5 Consequences of Polypharmacy

A study conducted in primary care has shown that about 93% of the older patients involved in the study had at least 1 drug-related problem (DRP) and that the average number of DRPs was 2.5 per patient [36]. Other studies in primary care found an average of 3.5–5.5 DRPs per patient [11, 12, 37], while studies performed in hospitals report 2.6–6.4 DRPs per patient [38–40].

The most important negative consequence related to polypharmacy, particularly inappropriate polypharmacy, is the higher risk of adverse drug events (ADE). Due to the fact that each drug has potential side effects, there is a higher probability of drug-drug, drug-nutrient, and drug-disease interactions, as well as a higher risk of error in the prescription, administration, and assumption of drugs. It should be also considered that older adults have a higher susceptibility to experience worsening health and functional status due to an ADE.

The negative consequences of polypharmacy also include poor medication adherence, reduced physical and social function, worse health outcomes, higher healthcare costs, and lower quality of life (QoL) [7, 41–43].

The consequences of polypharmacy by itself should not be overestimated [44]; for example, the use of drugs with anticholinergic properties in older patients has been proven to be independently associated with cognitive and functional decline [45], but dementia is not related to the number of drugs [46]. Sarcopenia seems to be not associated to polypharmacy in hospitalised older patients as well [47].

One of the most obvious examples of waste of resources is the questionable use of certain drugs [48] throughout the final year of life of older adults who died with dementia [48] and in general in older patients who reached the final part of their lives [20].

In this Swedish study 'Choosing Wisely? Measuring the Burden of Medications in Older Adults near the End of Life: Nationwide, Longitudinal Cohort Study [49]', polypharmacy increased throughout the last year of life of older adults. These drugs consisted of not only symptomatic medications but also long-term preventive treatments of questionable benefit [49]. The same study showed that in the final year before death, the proportion of individuals exposed to more than ten different drugs rose from 30.3% to 47.2% ($P < 0.001$ for trend). Angiotensin-converting enzyme inhibitors and statins were used by, respectively, 21.4% and 15.8% of all individuals during their final month of life [49].

The situation is particularly serious in nursing homes: A systematic review showed that almost one-half of nursing home residents are exposed to potentially inappropriate medications and suggests an increased prevalence over time [50].

19.1.6 Determinants of Polypharmacy

Polypharmacy has many causes [51]. The main one is the tendency to address chronic conditions with disease-specific guidelines that do not take into account that a patient is multimorbid [2]. These single-disease guidelines very often suggest treatment with medication without considering drug-drug and drug-disease interactions [52]. GPs/family doctors of course have to rely on these guidelines to treat chronic conditions, but when patients have multimorbidity, it is important to bear in mind that single-disease guidelines can increase the prevalence of polypharmacy and potentially inappropriate polypharmacy (PIP).

Figure 19.1 illustrates other possible drivers of polypharmacy. In real life what often happens is that patients who see multiple specialists may be prescribed a variety of drugs, but unfortunately GPs do not feel confident to reduce the dose or stop it. Preventive medications for cerebrovascular disease are the ones which contribute more to polypharmacy, since guidelines advise that patients at increased cardiovascular risk combine blood pressure-lowering medication, cholesterol-lowering medication, and platelet aggregation inhibitors.

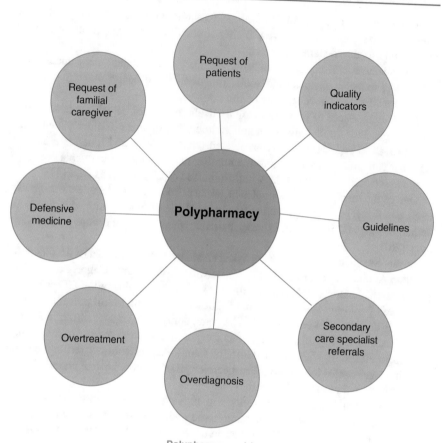

Polypharmacy: drivers

Fig. 19.1 Drivers of polypharmacy

Patient-related risk factors for polypharmacy may include:

- Incomplete knowledge of medications.
- Lack of ability to communicate medication history.
- Dishonesty about medication usage.
- ≥2 chronic medical conditions (increases the number of prescriptions per patient but increases the number of *medical practitioners* per patient as well) [53].

19.1.7 How to Address the Problem?

19.1.7.1 Medication Review

One way of preventing and reducing DRPs among older patients is to carry out medication reviews [10]. A medication review is a method to analyse, follow up, and review an individual's drug therapy, in a structured and systematic way, according to local guidelines and routines [54].

19.1.7.2 Benefits of Medication Reviews

In a hospital setting, medication reviews have been reported to improve drug use [55, 56] and to reduce repeat hospital visits [38]. Medication reviews in primary care can reduce the total number of drugs, reduce falls, and maintain self-rated health [57, 58].

However, highlighting the complexity of improving the appropriateness of polypharmacy, two systematic reviews could not demonstrate that interventions aimed at improving the appropriate polypharmacy neither substantial improvement in drug appropriateness nor in clinical outcomes of patients [59–63].

19.1.8 Role of Primary Care in Addressing Polypharmacy

Management of polypharmacy is a complex and time-consuming yet essential role of primary care clinicians, for which we could provide some recommendations. Knowing the list of inappropriate medications and deprescribing unnecessary medications are two key points.

Moreover, before adding new medications, specifically in patients with >5 medications, reviewing the patient's existing medications is essential. Lastly, avoid adding medications to treat symptoms caused by other drugs, or avoid adding duplicate medications to treat the same symptoms; it would be extremely significant [64, 65].

The role of primary care in facing this issue is crucial. There are values of primary care which are often underestimated: one of these values consist of 'integrating, prioritizing, contextualizing, and personalizing health care across acute and chronic illness, psychosocial issues and mental health, disease prevention, and optimization of health and meaning' [66]. This added value is difficult to see in the assessments at the level of diseases where wisdom, and caution is very often mistaken for clinical Inertia. This value is apparent, however, at the level of whole people and populations.

19.2 Overdiagnosis and Overtreatment

Two important factors which are very often related to polypharmacy are overdiagnosis and overtreatment.

19.3 Overdiagnosis

19.3.1 Definition of Overdiagnosis

Overdiagnosis is an unrecognised and growing worldwide problem in healthcare [67].

This is especially the case in high-income countries, where more sensitive tests, more testing, more screening, and earlier diagnosis are in focus, and more of the same will be implemented in the future [67]. Moreover, disease definitions have been, and are still being, widened; plus thresholds for treating, for example, risk factors, have been, and are still being, lowered. Finally, disease mongering is growing, because it is cheaper and faster to invent new 'diseases' than new pharmaceutical drugs [67].

Overdiagnosis has been defined simply as '… when people without symptoms are diagnosed with a disease that ultimately will not cause them symptoms or early death' and is also used as an umbrella term to include 'the related problems of overmedicalisation and subsequent overtreatment, diagnosis creep, shifting thresholds and disease mongering' [68]. Some commentators use 'too much medicine' to embrace such wider issues [69].

Broadly speaking overdiagnosis can be described as 'too much healthcare'. 'This includes too much screening of asymptomatic individuals, too much investigation of those with symptoms, too much reliance on biomarkers, too many quasi-diseases, too much diagnosis, often leading to too much treatment, sometimes cost-ineffective, medicines that are too costly and too rapidly approved for marketing, too many adverse reactions, and too much inappropriate monitoring' [70]. Too much healthcare leads almost inevitably to too little effective healthcare [70].

Overdiagnosis means transforming normal people into patients unnecessarily, by identifying problems that were never going to cause harm or by medicalising ordinary life experiences through expanded definitions of diseases [70].

The 'prostate cancer screening' case is a good example of that. The effectiveness of screening in reducing mortality rate and quality of life improvement represent a heated debate. Concerns regarding implementation of PSA screening and different guideline standards have led to a fear of mismanagement of prostate cancer [71].

19.3.2 Causes of Overdiagnosis

Overdiagnosis has two major causes: overdetection and overdefinition of disease. While the forms of overdiagnosis differ, the consequences are the same: diagnoses that ultimately cause more harm than benefit [70]. Confusion about what constitutes overdiagnosis undermines progress to a solution. Here we aim to draw boundaries around what overdiagnosis is and to exclude what it is not [70].

19.3.2.1 Drivers of Overdiagnosis

Drivers of overdiagnosis are well described. Advancing technology allows detection of disease at earlier stages or 'pre-disease' states. Well-intentioned enthusiasm and vested interests combine to lower treatment and intervention thresholds so that larger sections of the asymptomatic population acquire diagnoses, risk factors, or disease labels [72].

This process is supported by medicolegal fear and by payment and performance indicators that reward overactivity. It has led to a guideline culture that has unintentionally evolved to squeeze out nuanced, person-centred decision-making.

Underlying all this, there are little challenged, deeply intuitive narratives around the supposed benefits of early detection and intervention that are difficult to unpick for professionals and the public alike [68, 73].

19.3.2.2 Defensive Medicine

As Iona Heath states in her essay 'Role of fear in overdiagnosis and overtreatment', 'with the rise of neoliberal economics, health became a commodity like any other. The exploitation of sickness, and fears of sickness, for the pursuit of profit increased hugely over the subsequent decades, underpinned by the rapid commercialisation of healthcare' [74].

Popular scientific magazines terrify the population about this *epidemic of chronic diseases*, although many of those affected have no symptoms whatsoever. There is a toxic combination of good intentions, wishful thinking, and vested interest. One of the worst effects is detaching notions of disease from the experience of suffering, broadening the definitions of diseases, and turning risk factors into diseases and, most potent of all, fear [74].

19.3.2.3 Fears of Patients

Patients are afraid that their doctors will not understand what they try to describe and that an important diagnosis will be missed or made too late—through laziness, incompetence, or just bad luck. And of course, this is fuelled on a daily basis by newspapers, other news media, and, in those countries where it is allowed, direct to consumer advertising [74].

Doctors work every day in fear of missing a serious diagnosis and precipitating an avoidable tragedy for one of their patients. In our increasingly punitive societies, with all the easy talk of naming and shaming, doctors are also afraid of being publicly pilloried [74].

We should all remember that clinical work is hedged in by uncertainty on all sides because the application of the generalised truths of biomedical science to the unique context of an individual patient's life and circumstances will always be uncertain [74]. So doctors, and especially young doctors, are learning to be afraid of uncertainty [74]. Moreover, there is a growing fear of legal sues by patients.

19.3.2.4 What It Isn't

Overdiagnosis is not a false-positive result. False positives are abnormalities that turn out not to be diseases after further investigation. In overdiagnosis, the abnormality meets the currently agreed criteria for pathological disease (e.g. microscopic criteria for cancer), but the disease detected is not destined to cause symptoms or death [70].

19.3.2.5 Overtesting

Overtesting (sometimes referred to as overuse or overutilisation) can, but not always, increase the risk of overdiagnosis, but the risk increases proportionately with the degree of overuse [70].

For example, just to mention the same case as above, there is a relationship between how many prostate-specific antigen (PSA) tests are ordered in general practice and the incidence of prostate cancer [75] and between the number of male patients on a GP's list with a diagnosis of cancer and the number of PSA tests ordered [76]. GPs who undertake many PSA tests have many more male patients with overdiagnoses of prostate cancer, because the mortality rate is the same across clinics irrespective of the number of tests ordered [76].

19.3.2.6 Consequences of Overdiagnosis

Overdiagnosis is one of the most harmful and costly problems in modern healthcare [70]. It often triggers a cascade of overtreatment, although the two are not synonymous. To prevent and minimise overdiagnosis, we need more studies on the natural history of diseases, watchful waiting trials of very early/small or ambiguous abnormalities, studies of the effects of diagnostic language, intervention studies on known drivers of overdiagnosis, and studies of how to involve patients in decisions about diagnostic strategies [70]. Above all we need to ensure that new disease definitions are based on evidence [77], not financial interests [78].

19.3.2.7 Example of Not Effectiveness

Public health problems without easy solutions are fertile ground for large-scale overactivity in primary care [79]. NHS Health Checks were introduced nationally with a financial incentive as an apparent solution to metabolic disease, despite four decades of evidence showing such programmes do not affect population morbidity or mortality [80–82].

19.4 Overtreatment

19.4.1 Definition of Overtreatment

Overtreatment occurs when the best scientific evidence demonstrates that a treatment provides no benefit for the diagnosed condition, but it still is prescribed [70]. For example, middle ear infections in children and bronchitis in adults are often correctly diagnosed but overtreated with ineffective antibiotics [70].

19.4.1.1 Consequences of Overtreatment

Patients are exposed to treatment harms, from the mild to the fatal, and waste of resources is inevitable on a grand scale. The critical issue of opportunity cost may be raised but disregarded in cost-effectiveness decisions. This activity may feel sensible but lacks evidence and distracts from the need for more challenging solutions such as addressing the obesogenic environment or improving social care for people with dementia.

Lower treatment thresholds always create an increase in the number of patients taking medication for no benefit in order that a few might.

19.4.1.2 Overdiagnosis, Overtreatment, and Therapeutic Nihilism

Wishing to reduce overdiagnosis and overtreatment does not imply therapeutic nihilism or a desire to abandon preventive medicine [83]. Rather, it forces us to aim for an understanding of the evidence base that assists patients to make choices in a useful way, cognizant of benefits and harms [79, 84–86].

19.4.1.3 Research on Overdiagnosis and Overtreatment

Overdiagnosis is often misinterpreted as overutilisation or overtreatment. Overutilisation, overtreatment, and overdiagnosis are interrelated but represent three distinct topics [87]. Overdiagnosis can be caused by overutilisation and is nearly always followed by overtreatment [88]. Treating an overdiagnosed condition cannot improve the patient's prognosis and therefore can only be harmful. At the individual level, we can never be sure if the person is overdiagnosed. However, experiences and thoughts of individuals who are most likely overdiagnosed can be explored in qualitative interviews, e.g. men with a small screening-detected abdominal aortic aneurism [88].

19.4.1.4 Research Opportunities on Overdiagnosis: Role of the Qualitative Studies

If we want to know more about 'lived life' (e.g. the experiences and thoughts of individuals that have been overdiagnosed), we will most likely raise research questions that can be addressed in qualitative designs, such as interviews and observational fieldwork [88]. However, because we can never be certain that the individual has been overdiagnosed, we can interview those informants, who are most likely to be overdiagnosed, or informants that for a short period have had the experience of being overdiagnosed [88].

19.4.2 Awareness of the Problem in Primary Care

Modern concern has been articulated through worldwide movements such as the Preventing Overdiagnosis conferences, campaigns such as the BMJ's *Too Much Medicine*, JAMA's *Less is More*, Italy's *Slow Medicine* movement, the US (now international) *Choosing Wisely* project [79], and the WONCA Special Interest Group, *Quaternary Prevention & Overmedicalization* [84, 85].

In 2014 the Royal College of General Practitioners (RCGP) established its *Standing Group on Overdiagnosis* (Supporting Shared Decisions in Health Care).

19.4.2.1 What's the Role of Family Physicians in Polypharmacy?

Among the consequences of overmedicalisation, family physicians also carry the extra workload caused by it [79]. Iatrogenic multimorbidity creates a burden of complex and harmful polypharmacy for patients and their carers. Doctors with responsibility for one condition may not have the generalist, holistic overview needed to help the patient sort valuable interventions from low value [79].

Defending patients from the harms of *Too Much Medicine* needs to happen in the consulting room with a solid and longitudinal patient-doctor relationship, as well as at local and national policymaking level [79].

Every new innovation or intervention that is suggested for family physicians should be accompanied by opportunity costing, and, unless there is a new resource, current tasks should be identified to be stopped in order to fit new work in. Family physicians need to stand up and shape the clinical agenda from their unique perspective, drawing on the work and resources of academic primary care and the evidence-based medicine world [79].

Their role as passive enactors of specialist and public health ideas needs to be updated [79]. In order to do this, family physicians need a stronger part in the creative process of evidence synthesis and policymaking. They need to make sure that the 'common voice' is represented.

They call on the makers of guidelines to ensure that grassroots family physicians, with such a valuable, broad perspective, are enabled to have a greater influence in their production [79].

'Ordinary' family physicians are valuable family physicians, and they call on those who might think that their voice is not important to get involved in shaping the future of clinical practice for their patients and for themselves [79].

References

1. Anthierens S, Tansens A, Petrovic M, Christiaens T. Qualitative insights into general practitioners views on polypharmacy. BMC Fam Pract. 2010;11(1):65.
2. Guthrie B, Makubate B, Hernandez-Santiago V, Dreischulte T. The rising tide of polypharmacy and drug-drug interactions: population database analysis 1995–2010. BMC Med. 2015;13(1):74.
3. Haider S, Johnell K, Thorslund M, Fastbom J. Trends in polypharmacy and potential drug-drug interactions across educational groups in elderly patients in Sweden for the period 1992–2002. Int J Clin Pharmacol Ther. 2007;45(12):643–53.
4. Nishtala PS, Salahudeen MS. Temporal trends in polypharmacy and hyperpolypharmacy in older New Zealanders over a 9-year period: 2005–2013. Gerontology. 2015;61(3): 195–202.
5. Silwer L, Lundborg CS. Patterns of drug use during a 15 year period: data from a Swedish county, 1988–2002. Pharmacoepidemiol Drug Saf. 2005;14(11):813–20.
6. Gnjidic D, Hilmer SN, Blyth FM, Naganathan V, Waite L, Seibel MJ, et al. Polypharmacy cutoff and outcomes: five or more medicines were used to identify community-dwelling older men at risk of different adverse outcomes. J Clin Epidemiol. 2012;65(9):989–95.
7. Payne R, Avery A, Duerden M, Saunders C, Simpson C, Abel G. Prevalence of polypharmacy in a Scottish primary care population. Eur J Clin Pharmacol. 2014;70(5):575–81.
8. Qato DM, Alexander GC, Conti RM, Johnson M, Schumm P, Lindau ST. Use of prescription and over-the-counter medications and dietary supplements among older adults in the United States. JAMA. 2008;300(24):2867–78.
9. Masnoon N, Shakib S, Kalisch-Ellett L, Caughey GE. What is polypharmacy? A systematic review of definitions. BMC Geriatr. 2017;17(1):230.
10. Lenander C, Bondesson A, Viberg N, Beckman A, Midlov P. Effects of medication reviews on use of potentially inappropriate medications in elderly patients; a cross-sectional study in Swedish primary care. BMC Health Serv Res. 2018;18(1):616.

11. Brulhart MI, Wermeille JP. Multidisciplinary medication review: evaluation of a pharmaceutical care model for nursing homes. Int J Clin Pharm. 2011;33(3):549–57.
12. Finkers F, Maring J, Boersma F, Taxis K. A study of medication reviews to identify drug-related problems of polypharmacy patients in the Dutch nursing home setting. J Clin Pharm Ther. 2007;32(5):469–76.
13. Beijer H, De Blaey C. Hospitalisations caused by adverse drug reactions (ADR): a meta-analysis of observational studies. Pharm World Sci. 2002;24(2):46–54.
14. Morgan DJ, Dhruva SS, Coon ER, Wright SM, Korenstein D. 2019 Update on medical overuse: a review. JAMA Intern Med. 2019.
15. Davies EC, Green CF, Mottram DR, Rowe PH, Pirmohamed M. Emergency re-admissions to hospital due to adverse drug reactions within 1 year of the index admission. Br J Clin Pharmacol. 2010;70(5):749–55.
16. Conforti A, Costantini D, Zanetti F, Moretti U, Grezzana M, Leone R. Adverse drug reactions in older patients: an Italian observational prospective hospital study. Drug Healthc Patient Saf. 2012;4:75.
17. Salvi F, Marchetti A, D'Angelo F, Boemi M, Lattanzio F, Cherubini A. Adverse drug events as a cause of hospitalization in older adults. Drug Saf. 2012;35(1):29–45.
18. Sirois C, Domingues NS, Laroche M-L, Zongo A, Lunghi C, Guénette L, et al. Polypharmacy definitions for multimorbid older adults need stronger foundations to guide research. Clin Pract Public Health Pharm. 2019;7(3):126.
19. Pirmohamed M, James S, Meakin S, Green C, Scott AK, Walley TJ, et al. Adverse drug reactions as cause of admission to hospital: prospective analysis of 18 820 patients. BMJ (Clinical research ed). 2004;329(7456):15–9.
20. Wastesson JW, Morin L, Tan EC, Johnell K. An update on the clinical consequences of polypharmacy in older adults: a narrative review. Expert Opin Drug Saf. 2018;17(12):1185–96.
21. Steinman MA. Polypharmacy—time to get beyond numbers. JAMA Intern Med. 2016;176(4):482–3.
22. Budnitz DS, Lovegrove MC, Shehab N, Richards CL. Emergency hospitalizations for adverse drug events in older Americans. N Engl J Med. 2011;365(21):2002–12.
23. Lenander C, Bondesson A, Viberg N, Jakobsson U, Beckman A, Midlov P. Effects of an intervention (SAKLAK) on prescription of potentially inappropriate medication in elderly patients. Fam Pract. 2017;34(2):213–8.
24. Fastbom J, Johnell K. National indicators for quality of drug therapy in older persons: the Swedish experience from the first 10 years. Drugs Aging. 2015;32(3):189–99.
25. Fick D, Semla T, Beizer J, Brandt N, Dombrowski R, DuBeau C, et al. American Geriatrics Society 2015 Beers Criteria Update Expert Panel. American Geriatrics Society 2015 updated Beers criteria for potentially inappropriate medication use in older adults. J Am Geriatr Soc. 2015;63(11):2227–46.
26. Panel AGSBCUE, Fick DM, Semla TP, Steinman M, Beizer J, Brandt N, et al. American Geriatrics Society 2019 updated AGS Beers Criteria® for potentially inappropriate medication use in older adults. J Am Geriatr Soc. 2019;67(4):674–94.
27. O'Mahony D, O'Sullivan D, Byrne S, O'Connor MN, Ryan C, Gallagher P. STOPP/START criteria for potentially inappropriate prescribing in older people: version 2. Age Ageing. 2015;44(2):213–8.
28. Renom-Guiteras A, Meyer G, Thürmann PA. The EU (7)-PIM list: a list of potentially inappropriate medications for older people consented by experts from seven European countries. Eur J Clin Pharmacol. 2015;71(7):861–75.
29. Gallagher P, Ryan C, Byrne S, Kennedy J, O'Mahony D. STOPP (Screening Tool of Older Person's Prescriptions) and START (Screening Tool to Alert doctors to Right Treatment). Consensus validation. Int J Clin Pharmacol Ther. 2008;46(2):72–83.
30. Hanlon JT, Schmader KE, Samsa GP, Weinberger M, Uttech KM, Lewis IK, et al. A method for assessing drug therapy appropriateness. J Clin Epidemiol. 1992;45(10):1045–51.

31. Samsa GP, Hanlon JT, Schmader KE, Weinberger M, Clipp EC, Uttech KM, et al. A summated score for the medication appropriateness index: development and assessment of clinimetric properties including content validity. J Clin Epidemiol. 1994;47(8):891–6.

32. Hanlon JT, Schmader KE. The medication appropriateness index at 20: where it started, where it has been, and where it may be going. Drugs Aging. 2013;30(11):893–900.

33. Hellström LM, Bondesson Å, Höglund P, Midlöv P, Holmdahl L, Rickhag E, et al. Impact of the Lund Integrated Medicines Management (LIMM) model on medication appropriateness and drug-related hospital revisits. Eur J Clin Pharmacol. 2011;67(7):741–52.

34. Lavan AH, O'Mahony D, Gallagher P, Fordham R, Flanagan E, Dahly D, et al. The effect of SENATOR (Software ENgine for the Assessment and optimisation of drug and non-drug Therapy in Older peRsons) on incident adverse drug reactions (ADRs) in an older hospital cohort - trial protocol. BMC Geriatr. 2019;19(1):40.

35. Adam L, Moutzouri E, Baumgartner C, Loewe AL, Feller M, M'Rabet-Bensalah K, et al. Rationale and design of OPtimising thERapy to prevent Avoidable hospital admissions in Multimorbid older people (OPERAM): a cluster randomised controlled trial. BMJ Open. 2019;9(6):e026769.

36. Milos V, Rekman E, Bondesson Å, Eriksson T, Jakobsson U, Westerlund T, et al. Improving the quality of pharmacotherapy in elderly primary care patients through medication reviews: a randomised controlled study. Drugs Aging. 2013;30(4):235–46.

37. Sorensen L, Stokes JA, Purdie DM, Woodward M, Elliott R, Roberts MS. Medication reviews in the community: results of a randomized, controlled effectiveness trial. Br J Clin Pharmacol. 2004;58(6):648–64.

38. Gillespie U, Alassaad A, Henrohn D, Garmo H, Hammarlund-Udenaes M, Toss H, et al. A comprehensive pharmacist intervention to reduce morbidity in patients 80 years or older: a randomized controlled trial. Arch Intern Med. 2009;169(9):894–900.

39. Christensen AB, Holmbjer L, Midlöv P, Höglund P, Larsson L, Bondesson Å, et al. The process of identifying, solving and preventing drug related problems in the LIMM-study. Int J Clin Pharm. 2011;33(6):1010–8.

40. Blix HS, Viktil KK, Moger TA, Reikvam Å. Characteristics of drug-related problems discussed by hospital pharmacists in multidisciplinary teams. Pharm World Sci. 2006;28(3):152.

41. Payne RA, Abel GA, Avery AJ, Mercer SW, Roland MO. Is polypharmacy always hazardous? A retrospective cohort analysis using linked electronic health records from primary and secondary care. Br J Clin Pharmacol. 2014;77(6):1073–82.

42. Ahmed B, Nanji K, Mujeeb R, Patel MJ. Effects of polypharmacy on adverse drug reactions among geriatric outpatients at a tertiary care hospital in Karachi: a prospective cohort study. PLoS One. 2014;9(11):e112133.

43. Montero-Odasso M, Sarquis-Adamson Y, Song HY, Bray NW, Pieruccini-Faria F, Speechley M. Polypharmacy, gait performance, and falls in community-dwelling older adults. Results from the gait and brain study. J Am Geriatr Soc. 2019;67(6):1182–8.

44. Morin L, Larrañaga AC, Welmer A-K, Rizzuto D, Wastesson JW, Johnell K. Polypharmacy and injurious falls in older adults: a nationwide nested case-control study. Clin Epidemiol. 2019;11:483.

45. Brombo G, Bianchi L, Maietti E, Malacarne F, Corsonello A, Cherubini A, et al. Association of anticholinergic drug burden with cognitive and functional decline over time in older inpatients: results from the CRIME project. Drugs Aging. 2018;35(10):917–24.

46. Soysal P, Perera G, Isik AT, Onder G, Petrovic M, Cherubini A, et al. The relationship between polypharmacy and trajectories of cognitive decline in people with dementia: a large representative cohort study. Exp Gerontol. 2019;120:62–7.

47. Agosta L, Bo M, Bianchi L, Abete P, Belelli G, Cherubini A, et al. Polypharmacy and sarcopenia in hospitalized older patients: results of the GLISTEN study. Aging Clin Exp Res. 2019;31(4):557–9.

48. Morin L, Vetrano DL, Grande G, Fratiglioni L, Fastbom J, Johnell K. Use of medications of questionable benefit during the last year of life of older adults with dementia. J Am Med Dir Assoc. 2017;18(6):551e1–7.

49. Morin L, Vetrano DL, Rizzuto D, Calderon-Larranaga A, Fastbom J, Johnell K. Choosing wisely? Measuring the burden of medications in older adults near the end of life: nationwide, longitudinal cohort study. Am J Med. 2017;130(8):927–36.e9.

50. Morin L, Laroche ML, Texier G, Johnell K. Prevalence of potentially inappropriate medication use in older adults living in nursing homes: a systematic review. J Am Med Dir Assoc. 2016;17(9):862e1–9.

51. Aubert CE, Streit S, Da Costa BR, Collet T-H, Cornuz J, Gaspoz J-M, et al. Polypharmacy and specific comorbidities in university primary care settings. Eur J Intern Med. 2016;35:35–42.

52. Boyd CM, Darer J, Boult C, Fried LP, Boult L, Wu AW. Clinical practice guidelines and quality of care for older patients with multiple comorbid diseases: implications for pay for performance. JAMA. 2005;294(6):716–24.

53. Salive ME. Multimorbidity in older adults. Epidemiol Rev. 2013;35(1):75–83.

54. Cipolle RJ, Strand LM, Morley PC. Pharmaceutical care practice. New York: McGraw-Hill; 1998.

55. Bergkvist A, Midlöv P, Höglund P, Larsson L, Eriksson T. A multi-intervention approach on drug therapy can lead to a more appropriate drug use in the elderly. LIMM-Landskrona Integrated Medicines Management. J Eval Clin Pract. 2009;15(4):660–7.

56. Spinewine A, Swine C, Dhillon S, Lambert P, Nachega JB, Wilmotte L, et al. Effect of a collaborative approach on the quality of prescribing for geriatric inpatients: a randomized, controlled trial. J Am Geriatr Soc. 2007;55(5):658–65.

57. Lenander C, Elfsson B, Danielsson B, Midlöv P, Hasselström J. Effects of a pharmacist-led structured medication review in primary care on drug-related problems and hospital admission rates: a randomized controlled trial. Scand J Prim Health Care. 2014;32(4):180–6.

58. Zermansky AG, Alldred DP, Petty DR, Raynor DK, Freemantle N, Eastaugh J, et al. Clinical medication review by a pharmacist of elderly people living in care homes—randomised controlled trial. Age Ageing. 2006;35(6):586–91.

59. Johansson T, Abuzahra ME, Keller S, Mann E, Faller B, Sommerauer C, et al. Impact of strategies to reduce polypharmacy on clinically relevant endpoints: a systematic review and meta-analysis. Br J Clin Pharmacol. 2016;82(2):532–48.

60. Rankin A, Cadogan CA, Patterson SM, Kerse N, Cardwell CR, Bradley MC, et al. Interventions to improve the appropriate use of polypharmacy for older people. Cochrane Database Syst Rev. 2018;9:Cd008165.

61. Martin P, Tamblyn R, Benedetti A, Ahmed S, Tannenbaum C. Effect of a pharmacist-led educational intervention on inappropriate medication prescriptions in older adults: the D-PRESCRIBE randomized clinical trial. JAMA. 2018;320(18):1889–98.

62. Tannenbaum C, Martin P, Tamblyn R, Benedetti A, Ahmed S. Reduction of inappropriate benzodiazepine prescriptions among older adults through direct patient education: the EMPOWER cluster randomized trial. JAMA Intern Med. 2014;174(6):890–8.

63. Thio SL, Nam J, van Driel ML, Dirven T, Blom JW. Effects of discontinuation of chronic medication in primary care: a systematic review of deprescribing trials. Br J Gen Pract. 2018;68(675):e663–e72.

64. Morin L, Todd A, Barclay S, Wastesson JW, Fastbom J, Johnell K. Preventive drugs in the last year of life of older adults with cancer: is there room for deprescribing? Cancer. 2019.

65. Morin L, Wastesson JW, Laroche ML, Fastbom J, Johnell K. How many older adults receive drugs of questionable clinical benefit near the end of life? A cohort study. Palliat Med. 2019;33(8):1080–90.

66. Stange KC, Ferrer RL. The paradox of primary care. Ann Fam Med. 2009;7(4):293–9.

67. Brodersen J. Overdiagnosis: an unrecognised and growing worldwide problem in healthcare. Slovenian J Public Health. 2017;56(3):147–9.

68. Moynihan R, Glasziou P, Woloshin S, Schwartz L, Santa J, Godlee F. Winding back the harms of too much medicine. BMJ (Clinical research ed). 2013;346:f1271.

69. Carter SM, Rogers W, Heath I, Degeling C, Doust J, Barratt A. The challenge of overdiagnosis begins with its definition. BMJ (Clinical research ed). 2015;350:h869.

70. Brodersen J, Schwartz LM, Heneghan C, O'Sullivan JW, Aronson JK, Woloshin S. Overdiagnosis: what it is and what it isn't. BMJ Evid Based Med. 2018;23(1):1–3.

71. Kale MS, Korenstein D. Overdiagnosis in primary care: framing the problem and finding solutions. BMJ (Clinical research ed). 2018;362:k2820.

72. Starfield B. Is patient-centered care the same as person-focused care? Perm J. 2011;15(2):63.

73. Heath I. Overdiagnosis: when good intentions meet vested interests—an essay by Iona Heath. BMJ (Clinical research ed). 2013;347:f6361.

74. Heath I. Role of fear in overdiagnosis and overtreatment—an essay by Iona Heath. BMJ (Clinical research ed). 2014;349:g6123.

75. Mukai TO, Bro F, Pedersen KV, Vedsted P. [Use of prostate-specific antigen testing]. Ugeskr Laeger. 2010;172(9):696–700.

76. Hjertholm P, Fenger-Gron M, Vestergaard M, Christensen MB, Borre M, Moller H, et al. Variation in general practice prostate-specific antigen testing and prostate cancer outcomes: an ecological study. Int J Cancer. 2015;136(2):435–42.

77. Doust J, Vandvik PO, Qaseem A, Mustafa RA, Horvath AR, Frances A, et al. Guidance for modifying the definition of diseases: a checklist. JAMA Intern Med. 2017;177(7):1020–5.

78. Moynihan RN, Cooke GP, Doust JA, Bero L, Hill S, Glasziou PP. Expanding disease definitions in guidelines and expert panel ties to industry: a cross-sectional study of common conditions in the United States. PLoS Med. 2013;10(8):e1001500.

79. Treadwell J, McCartney M. Overdiagnosis and overtreatment: generalists—it's time for a grassroots revolution. Br J Gen Pract. 2016;66(644):116–7.

80. Krogsbøll LT, Jørgensen KJ, Larsen CG, Gøtzsche PC. General health checks in adults for reducing morbidity and mortality from disease: Cochrane systematic review and meta-analysis. BMJ (Clinical research ed). 2012;345:e7191.

81. Jørgensen T, Jacobsen RK, Toft U, Aadahl M, Glümer C, Pisinger C. Effect of screening and lifestyle counselling on incidence of ischaemic heart disease in general population: Inter99 randomised trial. BMJ (Clinical research ed). 2014;348:g3617.

82. Capewell S, McCartney M, Holland W. Invited debate: NHS Health Checks—a naked emperor? J Public Health. 2015;37(2):187–92.

83. Stegenga J. Medical nihilism. Oxford: Oxford University Press; 2018.

84. Jamoulle M. Quaternary prevention: first, do not harm. Revista Brasileira de Medicina de Família e Comunidade. 2015;10(35):1–3.

85. Martins C, Godycki-Cwirko M, Heleno B, Brodersen J. Quaternary prevention: reviewing the concept. Eur J Gen Pract. 2018;24(1):106–11.

86. Morin L, Barclay S, Wastesson JW, Johnell K, Todd A. Reply to Deprescription during last year of life in patients with pancreatic cancer: optimization or nihilism? Cancer. 2019;125(19):3471–2.

87. Korenstein D, Chimonas S, Barrow B, Keyhani S, Troy A, Lipitz-Snyderman A. Development of a conceptual map of negative consequences for patients of overuse of medical tests and treatments. JAMA Intern Med. 2018;178(10):1401–7.

88. Brodersen J. How to conduct research on overdiagnosis. A keynote paper from the EGPRN May 2016, Tel Aviv. Eur J Gen Pract. 2017;23(1):78–82.

Part VI

Palliative and Supportive Care for Older Patients

Supportive and Palliative Approach to the Older Persons

20

Simone Cernesi, Jacopo Demurtas, Carlos Centeno, Katherine Pettus, Scott A. Murray, and Eduardo Bruera

Abstract

In the majority of high-income settings, palliative care (PC) still relies on hospital care and palliative care specialists, while the involvement of other healthcare professionals, notably general practitioners (GPs), is undefined and incomplete. Moreover, to develop the full potential of palliative care, the participation of the public is needed, from patients' associations and caregivers to health advocacy associations and to national health systems.

S. Cernesi (✉)
AUSL, Modena, Italy
e-mail: dott.cernesi@gmail.com

J. Demurtas
Primary Care Department, USL Toscana Sud Est, Grosseto, Italy

C. Centeno
Unidad de Medicina Paliativa y Control de Síntomas, University of Navarra, Pamplona, Spain

K. Pettus
International Association for Hospice and Palliative Care, Houston, TX, USA

S. A. Murray
Primary Palliative Care Research Group, Usher Institute of Population Health Sciences and Informatics, University of Edinburgh, Edinburgh, UK

E. Bruera
Department of Palliative, Rehabilitation and Integrative Medicine, The University of Texas MD Anderson Cancer Center, Houston, TX, USA

© Springer Nature Switzerland AG 2022
J. Demurtas, N. Veronese (eds.), *The Role of Family Physicians in Older People Care*, Practical Issues in Geriatrics, https://doi.org/10.1007/978-3-030-78923-7_20

For this to occur, the silent palliative care revolution must spread a palliative care culture among all stakeholders and participants in the care process.

Fear of death, stigmatization of patients and their relatives when facing a complex disease like cancer or organ failure, or dementia, leads to palliative care being similarly stigmatized, neglected, or unacceptable.

Early identification of patients for discussions of goals of care based on their needs and wishes is fundamental, keeping in mind that dying is a multidimensional process. GPs can play a pivotal role here, leading to improved quality of care and quality of life and in due course dying for both patients and caregivers.

Keywords

Palliative care · Advocacy · Early palliative care · Simultaneous palliative care Death · Quality of care

20.1 Introduction

Palliative care has been defined by the World Health Organization (WHO) as an approach that "improves the quality of life of patients and their families facing the problem associated with life-threatening illness" [1]. The International Association for Hospice and Palliative Care (IAHPC) published a consensus definition in 2019 that emphasized the serious health-related suffering as opposed to "life-threatening illness." Palliative care is the active holistic care of individuals across all ages with serious health-related suffering [2][1] due to severe illness [2] and especially of those near the end of life. It aims to improve the quality of life of patients, their families, and their caregivers.

Over the past few decades, palliative care has evolved from a philosophy of care to an accredited professional discipline, with a growing number of clinical programs and accumulation of expertise related to symptom control, psychosocial, and spiritual care, communication, decision making, and end-of-life care [3].

It is well-known that the demographic pyramid is fundamentally changing and increasing the palliative care needs among fragile patients and chronically ill patients [4].

To face these new challenges, palliative care must be *universally* recognized as an essential element of the human right to health that is accessible to all who need it, in all settings [1].

Cultural and linguistic barriers often assimilate palliative care to futile treatment, in some cases confining it to terminality. Palliative care can include *active treatments* that embrace the patient and family in four dimensions [5].

---

[1] https://hospicecare.com/what-we-do/projects/consensus-based-definition-of-palliative-care/ definition

In addition to palliative care specialist and hospice care, it is essential, in order to be able to take care of the whole eligible population, to promote a widespread model of palliative care that includes a fundamental role for primary care and among the profession of family doctors [6–8].

For each dimension, the GP should identify the needs and formulate possible realistic solutions adapting them to the local resources and organization [1, 6].

The identification and analysis of needs should result in an advance care planning ACP, this both at home, in nursing homes, and in hospices, involving the patient, family, and all the professionals [9].

Fulfilling this fundamental right by making it accessible and sustainable, primary care has a unique potential to deliver palliative care to patients with all illnesses, at all times during the illness trajectories, to reach all dimensions of need, in all settings and in all countries [1].

In addition to this first level, specialist palliative care and hospices must be available when more expertise is needed.

20.2 Factors Related to the Medical and Health World

One of the main obstacles to the spread of palliative care in primary care is the limited number of cases directly managed by GPs.

The stereotype that palliative care and end-of-life care are synonymous remains widespread in the primary care setting and needs to be debunked.

This stereotype moreover contributes to late recognition of eligible palliative patients, especially non-oncological patients, which leads to the failure of many palliative care projects [10].

The belief that palliative care is aimed primarily at cancer patients is still deep-rooted, while the management of non-oncologic patients and patients with end-stage organ failure or disease remains nebulous.

It is not yet clear that palliative care is a step-by-step process (see Box 20.1) and cannot be assimilated into pain treatment [11].

There is no consensus on essential tools and models to detect patients who could potentially benefit from supportive and palliative care [12].

It is necessary to define which tool is more viable and accessible in family practice and primary care, especially in dealing with older persons [12, 13].

Patients should be identified in an *early stage* [14], if possible during the period when curative treatment is ongoing but when the patient could benefit from supportive treatment (*simultaneous palliative care*) [15, 16] and family physicians should pay special attention to early introduction of these supportive treatments (*early palliative care*) [17–20].

A clear schedule of the steps to follow after early identification is described in Box 20.1

Box 20.1 The Several Steps from Patients' Identification (Courtesy of Doctor Simone Cernesi)

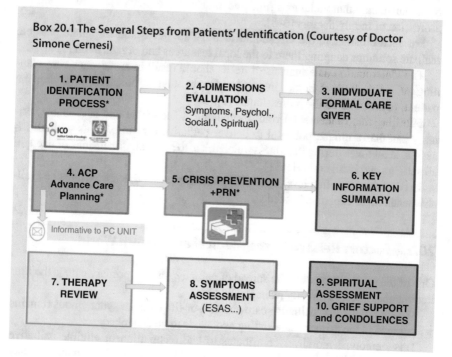

20.3 Early Identification

Early identification is critical. If this basic (and complex) step is lacking, the "palliative care cascade" doesn't begin.

Most models (GSF, SPICT, NecPal) are based on the *surprise* or *surprising question*:

Would I be surprised if this patient died in the next 12 months?

Depending on the answer, general and specific indicators of deterioration should be assessed and evaluated.

The first intervention with the surprise question in the community setting was published in 2001. Primary care physicians were challenged to identify those patients most likely to die in the next 6–12 months among those they have seen recently with diagnoses such as Alzheimer's, cancer, and chronic lung or heart disease.

Based on their perception of the likelihood of death of the patient, identify referrals to the palliative care clinic [21].

The importance of this assessment is evident from the fact that approximately 1% of the population of a single GP practice could benefit from a palliative care intervention [22].

This step should be followed by a 4D assessment (as following), and if the patient lacks capacity, it is important to identify one or more caregivers or legal representatives depending on national regulations.

Also, a thorough discussion of the potential trajectory of deteriorating patients is necessary and can guide goals of care and interventions. These are discussed with the patient and/or caregiver.

This decision should be clear and recorded in an ACP.

20.4 Trajectories of Illness and the Dynamic "Four-Dimensional" Pattern of Needs

Typical trajectories of physical decline have been described for people with end-stage disease. It is possible that social, psychological, and spiritual levels of distress may also follow characteristic patterns.

The dynamic "four-dimensional" pattern of needs is different on the three typical trajectories of functional decline towards the end of life (rapid, intermittent, and gradual), and in this chapter we suggest how it can be incorporated into disease-specific care (https://www.youtube.com/watch?v=vS7ueV0ui5U).

20.4.1 Rapid Functional Decline (Fig. 20.1)

In people with advanced cancer, social functioning typically declines in parallel with physical decline, whereas psychological and spiritual well-being often fall together at four key times: around diagnosis, at discharge after initial treatment, as the illness progresses, and in the terminal phase.

Patients and family members report that the time around diagnosis is one of the most traumatic, psychologically and existentially, with further emotional turmoil as the patient gets more ill. All people whose cancer may be life-limiting, but not necessarily untreatable, should be considered for palliative care from diagnosis. They

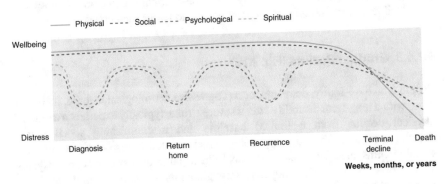

Fig. 20.1 Well-being trajectories in patients with conditions such as cancer causing rapid functional decline [14]. (Courtesy of Scott A. Murray)

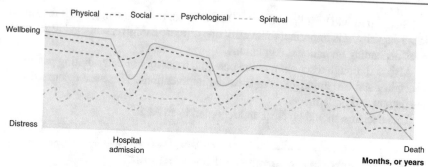

Fig. 20.2 Well-being trajectories in patients with an intermittent decline (typically organ failure or multimorbidity) [14]. (Courtesy of Scott A. Murray)

can benefit from holistic care and support as well as planning care even when they may be relatively well physically.

20.4.2 Intermittent Decline (Fig. 20.2)

In people with life-limiting, long-term conditions or multiple illnesses, the dynamic "four-dimensional" pattern of needs is different from that for most progressive cancers. Social and psychological decline both tend to track the physical decline, while spiritual distress fluctuates more and is modulated by other influences, including the person's capacity to remain resilient.

During the increasingly frequent exacerbations of conditions such as heart failure, liver failure, or chronic obstructive pulmonary disease, patients and their carers are anxious, need information, and often have social problems. Support for these needs might be more effective and likely to reduce hospital admissions than interventions focusing on disease management or physical well-being, especially as multimorbidity is the norm in these conditions. Planning for exacerbations should include dealing with multidimensional needs and communicating current plans and patient wishes regularly and routinely to out-of-hour care providers and hospitals. This facilitates appropriate management during and after such crises.

20.4.3 Gradual Decline (Fig. 20.3)

People who have frailty, dementia, or a progressive neurological disease, including those with a long-term disability after a severe stroke, typically experience a gradual physical decline from a limited baseline and a diminishing social world. Psychological and existential well-being sometimes fall in response to changes in social circumstances or an acute physical illness but a decrease in social, psychological, or existential well-being can herald global physical decline or death.

Some older people reach a tipping point when they feel unable to live usefully or with dignity and experience increasing psychological and existential distress before dying.

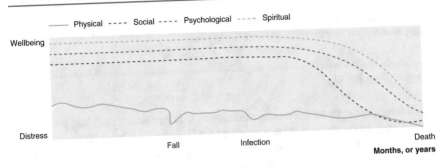

Fig. 20.3 Well-being trajectories in patients with a gradual decline (typically frailty or cognitive decline). (Courtesy of Scott A. Murray [14])

Actions to promote optimum physical health should be combined with help to engage with social support and care that let frail older people maintain a *sense of self and purpose* even in the face of increasing dependence. Allowing older people to raise and discuss their greatest fears—of losing independence, dementia, or being a burden to others—is person-centered early palliative care. Anticipating and planning for deteriorating health in older age can reduce distress while promoting a realistic understanding of normal aging and how death occurs at the end of a long life. People with early dementia or progressive neurological conditions need holistic palliative care and support to plan ahead from the time of diagnosis.

The trajectories of social, psychological, and spiritual needs elsewhere described for organ failure [23] and notably for oncologic patients [23] may apply also to older people with frailty.

In advanced heart failure, social and psychological decline ran in parallel with physical deterioration. Spiritual distress fluctuated more and was modulated by various other influences, including a perceived lack of understanding of these issues by health professionals.

People may react in different ways to illness, and many external factors can impinge on any typical patterns.

Separating spiritual needs from psychological/emotional needs is especially challenging.

Individual patients will die at different stages along each trajectory, and rates of progression vary. Comorbidity and social circumstances may intervene, and priorities and needs change, but there is usually a dominant trajectory of physical decline.

The clinical implications of these concepts imply that care planning must be (at least) four-dimensional. Optimizing quality of life with a view to achieving a timely, dignified, and peaceful death is the primary endeavor of palliative care. Understanding and considering typical trajectories of need may help professionals anticipate when, and in which dimension, an individual patient is likely to be distressed so that they are in a better position to plan care proactively.

Advance care planning is known as "anticipatory care planning" in Scotland, which is less stigmatizing to patients and even doctors, and this has promoted uptake to 70% of people who die.

Such plans should be communicated to all settings electronically, if possible using a common information system [24].

20.5 Pro Re Nata

Once these initial tasks have been completed, it is necessary to define pro re nata (*PRN*) medication for symptom control and relief (e.g., dyspnea, vomit, delirium, pain) [25, 26]. PRN medication is essential in home care and nursing home settings, with PRN patients may avoidable futile suffering (symptom controls) and hospital admissions are less likely.

Deprescribing, avoiding overtreatment and medication reconciliation are also advised. It is important to have clear goals, in palliative care the aims are to maintain good quality of life and symptoms management.

It is important that all information regarding the palliative care patient is summarized and available to other healthcare professionals.

Please circle the number that best describes:

	0	1	2	3	4	5	6	7	8	9	10	
No pain	0	1	2	3	4	5	6	7	8	9	10	Worst possible pain
Not tired	0	1	2	3	4	5	6	7	8	9	10	Worst possible tiredness
Not nauseated	0	1	2	3	4	5	6	7	8	9	10	Worst possible nausea
Not depressed	0	1	2	3	4	5	6	7	8	9	10	Worst possible depression
Not anxious	0	1	2	3	4	5	6	7	8	9	10	Worst possible anxiety
Not drowsy	0	1	2	3	4	5	6	7	8	9	10	Worst possible drowsiness
Best appetite	0	1	2	3	4	5	6	7	8	9	10	Worst possible appetite
Best feeling of wellbeing	0	1	2	3	4	5	6	7	8	9	10	Worst possible feeling of wellbeing
No shortness of breath	0	1	2	3	4	5	6	7	8	9	10	Worst possible shortness of breath
Other problem	0	1	2	3	4	5	6	7	8	9	10	

Patient's Name _____

Date _____ Time _____

Complete by (*check one*)
☐ Patient
☐ Caregiver
☐ Caregiver assisted

Fig. 20.4 ESAS scale for palliative care

Symptoms and pain should be regularly reassessed with the ESAS, as shown in Fig. 20.4 (Edmonton Symptoms Assessment Scale) [27].

20.6 Potential Issues and Barriers to Palliative Care

The GP who delivers palliative care can expect to face several challenges
Those can be categorized into five subgroups:

- Language
- Culture
- Sociodemographic
- Organizational
- Advocacy

20.6.1 Language (Denial, Palliphobia, Pallilalia, Palliactive) [28]

The term palliative care was coined by Dr. Balfour Mount in 1975. It was used to describe his hospice program and later gained widespread acceptance.

Confusion still permeates discussions about palliative care, and the variety of terms used to describe this process cause even more confusion in the process of establishing a viable program.

In recent years a vast amount of definitions such as "care of the dying," "terminal care," "end-of-life care," "continuing care," "total care," "holistic care," "comprehensive care," "comfort care," "pain and symptom management," and "quality-of-life care" have been used synonymously, while the more recent "supportive care" and "best supportive care" seem more popular [15, 29].

The discussion about the need for standardized definitions continues as there is still confusion about the terms and their significance. In some countries—notably Italy—palliative care is still commonly considered an irrelevant intervention, which further blocks its dissemination.

The first stage in the process of acknowledging the need for a palliative care program is "denial": At this stage, individuals and organizations are unaware of the need for palliative care programs.

The second is "palliphobia": In this phase some individuals or organizations recognize that there is a problem, but this usually meets with consistent fear about the consequences of the problem and the possible solutions. This step is followed by "pallilalia": It takes place between 2 and 4 years after the establishment of a palliative care initiative and consists of repetitive nonsense spoken about palliative care without anything being done to advance its development. Individuals and teams have overcome the first two stages but are unable or unwilling to commit the necessary resources for the establishment of a team. This stage results in a significant amount of burnout among palliative care professionals.

Stage IV is the *palliactive* stage. This is the final stage in the cultural development of individuals and institutions. It is recognized by the appointment and funding of healthcare professionals, the designation of an administrative structure such as a department or a division, and the allocation of formal curriculum space and training program rotations and, very importantly, by a budget. This stage is reached when colleagues actively refer patients to the palliative care team and encourage other colleagues to do the same.

20.6.2 Cultural

This is a sociological problem. The global north discusses global aging as an economic problem rarely addressing the health challenges or discussing end-of-life care [30, 31].

Another aspect of the problem concerns training relating to health workers, although this is improving thanks to national regulations in many European countries. There are still too few professors in palliative care and too few hours dedicated to university education.

We are still too accustomed to reasoning about the existing problem (acute) and less to reasoning in terms of possible foreseeable complications. This also challenges organizations when appropriate medical and nursing care is lacking.

Older persons are less likely to receive adequate palliative care than cancer patients [32].

Although palliative care has begun to appear in medical and nursing study plans, there remains a lack of standardization between different countries and sometimes also within individual countries [33].

The European multicountry PACE project was launched to improve training in care homes [32].

The project reveals the challenges of defining and evaluating the effectiveness of training interventions in care homes, highlighting the extent to which this area needs further study. It also anticipates the increase in palliative care needs for these settings, which could also represent a prototype for future home care.

Increasing skills related to the geriatric field and palliative care in a multidisciplinary and multi-professional collaboration within an integrative framework could represent a realistic answer in a sea of still unanswered questions.

20.7 Advocacy

Palliative care policy advocacy consists of structured communication between national, regional, and global palliative care associations (nongovernmental organizations) and government representatives, at the local, national, regional, and international levels.

Advocacy encourages governments to improve access to internationally controlled essential medicines such as morphine by collaborating, upon request, to review and revise unduly restrictive laws and regulations, educate prescribers, and raise public awareness on the likely benefits of rational access to controlled medicines. Promote Palliative Care under UNIVERSAL HEALTH COVERAGE [3, 34], considerating the mission: palliative care for everyone and everywhere [35] including vulnerable population (Older persons, prisoners, people with psychiatric problems, people who live in poverty, etc.).

Everyone, including patients and caregivers, ideally participates in advocacy activities.

Both individuals and institutions engage in advocacy.

Some examples of advocacy:

1. Join your national, regional, and international palliative care organizations.
2. Get to know your lawmakers and regulators. Invite them to visit your program and see your work firsthand.
3. Participate in social media.
4. Ensure your association designates an advocacy focal point to engage in direct communication: letters, emails, etc. with lawmakers and with regional and international palliative care organizations.
5. Get to know journalists and representatives of traditional media: Learn to write press releases, editorials, and co-author journal articles.
6. Participate in a delegation with your national, regional, or international association in meetings where public health issues are debated and policy goals are set out in resolutions and consensus documents.

By recognizing and specifying palliative care as an essential service under UHC, the draft 2018 Astana Declaration reflects the incremental progress since Alma Ata 1978, in the global development of palliative care [36].

20.8 Burnout Risk in GP Palliative Care

One condition that often impairs GP activity is represented by burnout. While providing palliative care, healthcare professionals (HCPs) and among those GPs daily work directly with dying patients and their families and caregivers, with a high risk of distress and burnout.

Recent evidence suggests that, at least in the US, clinician burnout exceeds the national average in the palliative care workforce.

HCPs working in palliative care may be at risk of experiencing feelings of helplessness, meaninglessness, and fear of death. These psychological states may lead to disengagement from patients and compassion fatigue and facilitate the development of burnout symptoms.

To help HCPs professionally cope with palliative care and recover from the psychological burden, measures to reduce stress and burnout and support engagement and health were developed, including a 13-item, evidence-based palliative clinician self-care checklist made by MD Anderson's palliative care service [37] (see Box 20.2).

Box 20.2 Adapted from a Survey of Palliative Care Clinicians' Weekly Self-Care Practices [36]

Palliative care clinician burnout checklist [37]

1. Exercise most days
2. Healthy food most days
3. Practice meditation, yoga, mindfulness most days
4. Literature reading (no junk reading)
5. Art movie/theater (no junk movies)
6. Watch visual art
7. Meet with family members in person
8. Meet with friends in person
9. Participate in spiritual/religious activities
10. One pall care professional education activity
11. Avoid noise most days (TV, sponsored web, BB after work)
12. Achieve at least one personalized self-care goal

Complete success: >8/12 items; partial success 4–7/12 items; <4/12 there is always next week.

20.9 Conclusions

As in many other scenarios, family physicians have a "privileged" position, and this can be meaningful for patients' treatment, even in palliative care. Family doctors should detect as early as possible those patients which may need palliative care and start as soon as possible a palliative care management, bearing in mind patients' needs and preferences. Moreover, the role of family doctors in these cases is extended to the management of symptoms and symptom control, so the family doctor should be aware and taught about the use of pro re nata medications. Family doctors should also participate and advocate for palliative care. Finally, it has to be considered that caring for people and, notably, end-of-life care may affect doctors with the burden of burnout. Therefore, it is necessary for family physicians to team up with other professionals, keep the network of services, and save some time for themselves and their families.

References

1. World Health Organization. Why palliative care is an essential function of primary health care. Geneva: World Health Organization; 2018.
2. Radbruch L, De Lima L, Knaul F, Wenk R, Ali Z, Bhatnaghar S, et al. Redefining palliative care–a new consensus-based definition. J Pain Symptom Manage. 2020;60(4):754–64.

3. Munday D, Boyd K, Jeba J, Kimani K, Moine S, Grant L, et al. Defining primary palliative care for universal health coverage. Lancet (London, England). 2019;394(10199):621.
4. Scholten N, Günther AL, Pfaff H, Karbach U. The size of the population potentially in need of palliative care in Germany—an estimation based on death registration data. BMC Palliat Care. 2016;15(1):29.
5. Ferrell BR, Coyle N, Paice J. Oxford textbook of palliative nursing. Oxford: Oxford University Press; 2014.
6. Thomas K, Noble B. Improving the delivery of palliative care in general practice: an evaluation of the first phase of the Gold Standards Framework. Palliat Med. 2007;21(1):49–53.
7. Mahmood-Yousuf K, Munday D, King N, Dale J. Interprofessional relationships and communication in primary palliative care: impact of the Gold Standards Framework. Br J Gen Pract. 2008;58(549):256–63.
8. Banks I, Weller D, Ungan M, Selby P, Aapro M, Beishon M, et al. ECCO essential requirements for quality cancer care: primary care. Crit Rev Oncol Hematol. 2019;142:187–99.
9. Ranganathan A, Gunnarsson O, Casarett D. Palliative care and advance care planning for patients with advanced malignancies. Ann Palliat Med. 2014;3(3):144–9.
10. Mitchell S, Tan A, Moine S, Dale J, Murray SA. Primary palliative care needs urgent attention. BMJ. 2019;365:l1827.
11. Murray SA, Mitchell S, Boyd K, Moine S. Palliative care: training the primary care workforce is more important than rebranding. BMJ. 2019;365:l4119.
12. Gómez-Batiste X, Martínez-Muñoz M, Blay C, Amblàs J, Vila L, Costa X, et al. Utility of the NECPAL CCOMS-ICO© tool and the Surprise Question as screening tools for early palliative care and to predict mortality in patients with advanced chronic conditions: a cohort study. Palliat Med. 2017;31(8):754–63.
13. Maas EAT, Murray SA, Engels Y, Campbell C. What tools are available to identify patients with palliative care needs in primary care: a systematic literature review and survey of European practice. BMJ Support Palliat Care. 2013;3(4):444–51.
14. Murray SA, Kendall M, Mitchell G, Moine S, Amblàs-Novellas J, Boyd K. Palliative care from diagnosis to death. BMJ. 2017;356:j878.
15. Fadul N, Elsayem A, Palmer JL, Del Fabbro E, Swint K, Li Z, et al. Supportive versus palliative care: what's in a name? A survey of medical oncologists and midlevel providers at a comprehensive cancer center. Cancer. 2009;115(9):2013–21.
16. Meyers FJ, Linder J, Beckett L, Christensen S, Blais J, Gandara DR. Simultaneous care: a model approach to the perceived conflict between investigational therapy and palliative care. J Pain Symptom Manag. 2004;28(6):548–56.
17. Greer JA, Pirl WF, Jackson VA, Muzikansky A, Lennes IT, Heist RS, et al. Effect of early palliative care on chemotherapy use and end-of-life care in patients with metastatic non–small-cell lung cancer. J Clin Oncol. 2012;30(4):394–400.
18. Temel JS, Greer JA, Muzikansky A, Gallagher ER, Admane S, Jackson VA, et al. Early palliative care for patients with metastatic non–small-cell lung cancer. N Engl J Med. 2010;363(8):733–42.
19. Zimmermann C, Swami N, Krzyzanowska M, Hannon B, Leighl N, Oza A, et al. Early palliative care for patients with advanced cancer: a cluster-randomised controlled trial. Lancet. 2014;383(9930):1721–30.
20. Finucane AM, Bone AE, Evans CJ, Gomes B, Meade R, Higginson IJ, et al. The impact of population ageing on end-of-life care in Scotland: projections of place of death and recommendations for future service provision. BMC Palliat Care. 2019;18(1):1–11.
21. Pattison M, Romer AL. Improving care through the end of life: launching a primary care clinic-based program. J Palliat Med. 2001;4(2):249–54.
22. Elliott M, Nicholson C. A qualitative study exploring use of the surprise question in the care of older people: perceptions of general practitioners and challenges for practice. BMJ Support Palliat Care. 2017;7(1):32–8.

23. Murray SA, Kendall M, Grant E, Boyd K, Barclay S, Sheikh A. Patterns of social, psycho-logical, and spiritual decline toward the end of life in lung cancer and heart failure. J Pain Symptom Manag. 2007;34(4):393–402.

24. Finucane AM, Davydaitis D, Horseman Z, Carduff E, Baughan P, Tapsfield J, et al. Electronic care coordination systems for people with advanced progressive illness: a mixed-methods evaluation in Scottish primary care. Br J Gen Pract. 2020;70(690):e20–e8.

25. Care WIP. Symptom relief into primary health Care: a WHO guide for planners, implementers and managers. Geneva: World Health Organization; 2018.

26. Russell BJ, Rowett D, Currow DC. Pro re nata prescribing in a population receiving palliative care: a prospective consecutive case note review. J Am Geriatr Soc. 2014;62(9):1736–40.

27. Bruera E, Kuehn N, Miller MJ, Selmser P, Macmillan K. The Edmonton Symptom Assessment System (ESAS): a simple method for the assessment of palliative care patients. J Palliat Care. 1991;7(2):6–9.

28. Bruera E. The development of a palliative care culture. J Palliat Care. 2004;20(4):316–9.

29. Hui D, De La Cruz M, Mori M, Parsons HA, Kwon JH, Torres-Vigil I, et al. Concepts and defi-nitions for "supportive care," "best supportive care," "palliative care," and "hospice care" in the published literature, dictionaries, and textbooks. Support Care Cancer. 2013;21(3):659–85.

30. Kluge H, Kelley E, Swaminathan S, Yamamoto N, Fisseha S, Theodorakis PN, et al. After Astana: building the economic case for increased investment in primary health care. Lancet. 2018;392(10160):2147–52.

31. Barishansky RM. The silver tsunami: are you ready? America's elderly population is explod-ing, and EMS services will have to reflect that. EMS World. 2016;45(8):53–6.

32. Moore DC, Payne S, Van den Block L, ten Koppel M, Szczerbińska K, Froggatt K. Research, recruitment and observational data collection in care homes: lessons from the PACE study. BMC Res Notes. 2019;12(1):1–6.

33. Arias N, Garralda E, Rhee JY, Lima L, Pons-Izquierdo JJ, Clark D, et al. EAPC Atlas of pal-liative care in Europe 2019. Vilvoorde: EAPC; 2019.

34. WHO, editor. Declaration of Astana. Global Conference on Primary Health Care; 2018.

35. Centeno C, Sitte T, De Lima L, Alsirafy S, Bruera E, Callaway M, et al. White paper for global palliative care advocacy: recommendations from a PAL-LIFE Expert Advisory Group of the Pontifical Academy for Life, Vatican City. J Palliat Med. 2018;21(10):1389–97.

36. Pettus K, Moine S, Kunirova G, De Lima L, Radbruch L. Palliative care comes of age in the 2018 declaration of Astana. J Palliat Med. 2019;22(3):242.

37. Bruera E, Anderson AE, Williams JL, Liu DD. A survey of palliative care clinicians' weekly self-care practices. J Clin Oncol. 2019;37(31_suppl):59.

Dying at Home

21

Ana Nunes Barata, Andrea Salvetti, Alessandro Bussotti, and Jacopo Demurtas

Abstract

When faced with the prospect of dying with an advanced illness, the majority of people, notably older patients, prefer to die at home, surrounded by their beloved ones and relatives. Nevertheless, in many countries around the world, those patients are still most likely to die in a hospital.

Home palliative care increases the chance of dying at home and reduces symptom burden in particular for patients with cancer, without impacting on caregiver grief or burden.

When home palliative cares are available, the chances of these patients dying at home more than double. Home palliative care services also help in relieving symptoms' burden and seem to have a positive impact on caregiver burden, not influencing bereavement.

Family doctors have a role of utmost importance in home palliative care, thanks to their knowledge of patient's context, preferences, beliefs, and families, and several experiences in Europe and the United States have proven the important role of family physicians in this complex situation.

A. Nunes Barata (✉)
USF Águas Livres, Amadora, Portugal
e-mail: anunesbarata@gmail.com

A. Salvetti · J. Demurtas
Primary Care Department, USL SudEst Toscana, Grosseto, Italy

A. Bussotti
Florence, Italy

© Springer Nature Switzerland AG 2022
J. Demurtas, N. Veronese (eds.), *The Role of Family Physicians in Older People Care*, Practical Issues in Geriatrics, https://doi.org/10.1007/978-3-030-78923-7_21

Doctors to achieve the best results in this setting have to be supported by a team and need the possibility to refer these patients to hospice or second-level palliative care.

The role of family physicians does not end with the patient's death but goes on, encompassing the aspects of caring of bereavement of caregivers and families.

Keywords

Palliative care · Home care · Team · Caregivers · Bereavement

21.1 Introduction

The topic of death is still a taboo in today's day and age, making it difficult to cover and specially for healthcare professionals to talk about it [1], in case they did not have the required training to do so. When dealing with the elderly population, there is a greater sense of the end, which, in some cases may even make this topic even more controversial [2].

The aging population, associated with a high prevalence of chronic conditions, will condition a greater need for palliative care. Palliative care is provided by a multidisciplinary team with the purpose to alleviate the suffering, independently of the disease, status, or other therapeutic requirements [3].

Palliative care need is expected to increase by 42% by 2040 [4], increasing out of proportion to deaths.

Palliative care delivered by specialists has been shown to improve outcomes for patients and family carers. However, only a minority of older people receive specialist palliative care at the end of life [4].

It's frequent for older patients to live and die with chronic conditions, which are preceded by long periods of physical decline and functional incapacity. So, it is important to assess all symptoms when providing palliative care to older individuals [5].

Establishing a diagnosis and treating and sharing the prognosis are tasks that are attributed to a physician. In the last century, technological advancements have made it possible that some diseases are identified in an earlier stage and cure has been offered to conditions that were previously fatal. Therefore, "prognosis" has been slowly forgotten as years went by [6].

Many physicians feel intimidated when they are asked questions like "Doctor, how long do I still have?" as they consider it a difficult process and emotionally disturbing. Generally, physicians try not to do predictions, and they look for means to keep them for themselves (they do not share them with the patient unless they are requested to do so). When sharing information, they try not to be very specific and even offer positive expectations [6].

Even if the notion of prognosis is multidimensional, and much larger than only living or dying as it also includes all the aspects that are related to the progression of the disease (e.g., future symptoms, incapacity, limitations, suffering, etc.), it is usually the life expectancy that is asked when someone asks about a prognosis [7].

21.2 Better at Home?

Three decades of research on the effectiveness of home palliative care have resulted in clear evidence of the benefit of home palliative care in helping patients to die at home and reducing symptom burden without impacting on caregiver grief [8]. Studies show that if people are given the opportunity, the greater majority would choose to die at home and not in a different environment or even at a hospital. With well-organized services, especially high-quality home care, this is in many times possible.

A patient's place of care may become her place of death. For some patients this is a strong preference and a significant reason for wanting to be cared for at home [9].

Despite the expectations of patients, relatives, and professionals, offering a choice about the place of care can be problematic. In circumstances where others would experience significant burdens or risk by caring for a patient at home, it can be argued that offering a choice of home care is inappropriate. The same may be true where limited resources in community care cannot stretch to home care for highly dependent individuals without being stripped from other people in need [10].

Recent meta-analyses (including seven trials with 1222 patients, with three high-quality RCTs) showed that having access to home palliative care services more than double the odds for patients with illnesses such as cancer, CHF, and COPD to die at home [8].

The authors of that review showed also the evidence of small but statistically significant positive effects on the symptom burden of people having severe illnesses [8].

Studies show that if people are given the opportunity, the greater majority would choose to die at home and not in a different environment or even at a hospital. With well-organized services, especially high-quality home care, this is many times possible. Also cost-effectiveness of home palliative care has been investigated, with some evidences reporting lower costs [11].

In Brumley's trial [11] in-home palliative care delivered by a multidisciplinary team significantly increased patient satisfaction, decreasing at the same time the use of medical services and global care expenses at the end of life.

Nevertheless, even if many people would prefer to be cared for and to die at home, in practice death in hospitals remains common in many countries, especially in those where the hospice movement and palliative cares are still "young."

In the white book of palliative care, advocacy policymakers are invited to acknowledge the societal and ethical value of palliative care, therefore modifying existing healthcare structures, policies, and outcome measures, in order to ensure universal access to palliative care for all patients in need [12].

They are also strongly invited to ensure an integrated health system, to allow a smooth flow of patients between the different levels of care, in a way that patients with complex problems may be referred to secondary and tertiary levels, as needed, and referred back to home care, eventually [12].

The variation in place of death suggests that the organization of services plays an important role in determining the options that people can consider.

This possibility is further suggested by detailed studies in the United States [13]. Those studies found that the proportion of people dying at home ranges from 18% to 32% and appears to vary primarily with the availability of hospital beds [13].

Patient preferences, physician training, and availability of community services were either irrelevant to the place of death or of minimal importance compared to the number of hospital beds per head of population [13].

Studies show that if people are given the opportunity, the greater majority would choose to die at home and not in a different environment or even at a hospital. With well-organized services, especially high-quality home care, this is many times possible [14].

One of these studies, carried along Europe and involving several countries (Belgium, Spain, the Netherlands, Italy), was the Sentinel GP Networks Monitoring End of Life Care (SENTIMELC) study [15].

In many European countries, GPs can provide a good health perspective on end-of-life care and people dying [15].

In this study GPs were the observational units. Considering the enhanced accessibility of GP across Europe, GPs were adopted to gather data and produce a population-based sample of deaths.

One important exception was represented by the extensive specialist nursing home network in the Netherlands, where nursing home residents were treated and managed by their own doctors, without any intervention from GPs [14, 15].

For this, there are some standards that need to be met (Box 21.1):

1. **A family member that has the capacity to adapt himself to a highly demanding condition**

   Recent analysis made in Europe showed how caregivers in European regions were emotionally overburdened [16]. In some cases these difficulties were reported also in covering the cost of palliative care. Patients' age, cause of death, place of death, and specialist palliative care provision were associated with physical or emotional and financial burden [16, 17].

2. **Nurses that are able to visit the patient at least once a day**

   Both in nursing homes and at homes, the intervention of nurses is crucial. This close follow-up of the patient and of his/her family allows a comprehensive and integrated care, aiding in patient education and the assessment of his/her well-being [18]. Nurses are used to the role of coordination which gives them the experience when it comes to handling a case and navigating the road of care. Nurses can act as a link between the different levels of care, considering healthcare professionals as well as the patient and the individual. When considering the fundamentals of care when it comes to nursing, nurses are tailored to provide individualized palliative care to patients with life-threatening illnesses and their relatives.

Circumstances that nurses face in palliative care challenge them in practical, relational, and moral dimensions of care which consequently causes that their role is provided in a comprehensive way [19].

3. **An attentive physician**
   GPs should take care of both patient and family member, with early detection of symptoms worsening regarding the patient and burnout/breakdown risk for the caregiver. Doctors should focus whereas possible on patient preferences, needs, and dignity. Family physicians should also provide basic teaching to the patient, caregivers, and relatives of what will happen, sharing trajectories of illness, answering questions, and providing a tailored individual plan of care for the patient [3].

4. **Ability for the team to quickly answer to new problems**
   Pro re nata medications, relief of symptoms, and guaranteeing the best care and comfort to the terminally ill patient are core activities in the team. The different professionals managing the case should adapt themselves to the scenario, also in terms of adaptive leadership, with the goal to address the individual needs of the patient [13].

5. **Having the guarantee of a quick admission to hospice or a second palliative care level, or palliative care team on place in case there is any complication** [10].

Box 21.1 The Core Players and Required Skills to Guarantee the Best End-of-Life Care at Home

Players	What is needed
Caregivers	He/she needs to have the capacity to cope with a highly demanding situation
Dedicated nurses	Close follow-up, both in nursing homes and at home
Attentive GP	Early detection of symptoms worsening and caregiver's risk of breakdown. Education of patient and caregiver
Team reactivity and capacity to deal with situations	The team should rapidly respond to the sudden demands of assistance, including pro re nata medications, relief of symptoms, and guaranteeing comfort
Palliative care team or services	An integrated network of services, within the community with the possibility for patients to receive second-level care or to be admitted to hospice

It is crucial for the healthcare professionals to collaborate with the patient and the family so that they understand what may happen, starting from the description of trajectories of illness, and in what ways they can receive the required support [3].

For this, patient and family education is of utmost importance, so that they are able to take the decisions firsthand according to what is happening at the moment. But for this, both patient and family need to feel supported. In order to guarantee their psychological and physical well-being, it is important for the physician to routinely do home visits and to show that he/she is available in case any emergency may happen. Therefore, it is counterproductive to tell the patient and the family that the physician will only visit in case "something happens" as this will make them much more anxious and raise expectations.

It is known that the majority of the circumstances at home may be managed by the patient and the family, as long as they are prepared beforehand and they feel supported, both during the day and at night.

The circumstances of a dying patient may change rapidly. In each home visit, the situation might change. So, common circumstances should be discussed with the family members, so that they are psychologically and practically prepared for the event. The healthcare professional needs to leave at the patient's home a supply of the required material in case of a causality. However, causalities need to be predicted as much as possible. The physician should leave a prepared prescription at the patient's home, so that they can be applied by a nurse, for example, as is the case of a bleeding or any other acute change.

Considering all what was explained above, a person who lives in the company of a family member who is notable to take on the care at home will need to be admitted to the hospital eventually. A long progressing terminal disease is also many times associated to an admission at the hospital.

Elderly patients require comprehensive, palliative care, especially when considering the circumstance of dying at home. Only by creating the required environment that meets the needs of the patient and the family will it be possible to provide care until the end of life, respecting the wishes of the patient when dying at home.

21.3 Patient's Choice

Why is patient choice desirable in these situations? The choice for patients is considered to be ethically desirable. Supporting the exercise of choices about healthcare provision is fundamental to respecting a patient's autonomy [10]. Promoting choices about how and where healthcare is received enhances patients' quality of life; this is also due to partly retaining an element of control over their lives which results often compromised by the severe illness [10].

Despite the benefits that follow from offering choice, there are times when patients have fewer choices than they have preferences. (Patients would prefer not to have a terminal illness, but do not have any choice about this.) If professionals are not clear in their thinking as to this distinction, then they may be left feeling uncomfortable when what are perceived to be choices (but are actually only preferences) about the place of care are not achieved. The role of healthcare professionals is to facilitate those choices that do exist and to help patients understand why other preferences are unachievable [9, 10].

21.4 Discharge Planning

When planning discharge for patients with life-limiting illnesses, whether in a palliative care setting or elsewhere, professionals must consider whether the patient in question has the mental capacity required to make a decision about the place of care. Further considerations include the risks a home discharge would pose to those providing care, the views of these individuals, and issues of resource allocation [10]. Evaluation of these factors can aid the team in their interactions with patients and carers and guide the process of discharge planning. This will ensure that patient choice is facilitated wherever possible, but that harm is prevented where it is not possible or not right to facilitate a patient's choice. In this way, teams will take account of patient autonomy and will also consider the best interests of the patient, those involved in providing care, and other patients. The process of planning a complex discharge can take several weeks; it is therefore imperative that this is initiated as early as possible following the patient's admission. Unnecessary delays may risk the patient missing any window of opportunity for care at home and will also limit the time available for decision-making [9].

21.5 Bereavement and Grief

Grief may be described in three main phases: shock/negation, chaos/despair, and reorganization. In the first phase, the reactions of anger may assume many different types and forms of expression (negative comments, sarcasm, passive-aggressive behaviors, or explicitly aggressive behaviors) [20]. When a patient is in his/her final days of life, this is mostly shown as:

- He/she is aware that he/she is deprived of his/her dreams for the future.
- Physical pain and suffering.
- Others who turn their back (as they know he/she is dying).

The patient who is terminally ill goes through a process of a "preparatory grief," where he/she prepares to go away from this world. The patient will think about the past and will try to avoid family/friends in times of greater sadness, pain, or anxiety [21].

In the final days of life, it is usual to find traces of a depressive suffering by the patient and the family which needs to be identified in order to better answer to their needs. In this view, there are four situations that may occur: demoralization, the desire to anticipate death, the intention of suicide, and the request for assisted suicide or euthanasia. It is important that the healthcare professionals are able to identify the specifics of each situation so that they may provide the required support and follow-up that ensure the dignity of the patient and of his/her family [20–22].

Diseases that have a long and irreversible outcome are associated with an inevitable loss for the patient, family members, and healthcare professionals, which leads to suffering and grief processes that are sometimes difficult.

A complicated grief process should be diagnosed in an early stage, so that a pertinent help process can be applied and done at an adequate timing.

The loss is a change that includes someone being deprived of something that is tangible (a home, car, job) or not tangible (a project of life, hope for an outcome, etc.) that activates reactions that are linked to affection, cognitive, and behavioral reactions or, in other words, a process of grief. When death is approaching, different types of loss may occur which may be important challenges for the dying patients and their families and, as such, need to be diagnosed and monitored by the healthcare professionals that are committed to helping in those stages.

It is important to assess objectively the most important dimensions of the loss. Without this careful assessment, it will be difficult to start a meaningful help project that will answer the true needs of the patient and the family at that precise moment.

One also needs to take into account that a loss, many times, brings other losses that need to be integrated into the person's context. So, healthcare professionals, notably general practitioners need to assess both main/primary losses and any types of secondary losses.

21.6   The Role of Primary Care Physicians

Physicians in primary care are in the first line of contact with the healthcare system. They provide holistic care, based on a patient-centered approach that answers the needs of the patients and their families in order to offer a fully comprehensive care [23]. This connection allows family physicians to uphold an important standard when it comes to trust, as they build a long-standing relationship of care with each individual and with his/her family.

It is known that in a list of 2000 patients that are followed up by a family physician, there is a mean of 20 patients entering a terminal phase every year. In this last year of life, five patients will die of cancer, five because of organ failure, seven to eight due to multiple pathologies (e.g., dementia), and two to three patients will die because of a sudden death [24].

The growing number of patients needing palliative care is rapidly increasing due to the aging nations and expanding populations. Aging nations and expanding populations mean annual numbers of deaths are predicted to rise by as much as 17% over the coming years [25]. Considering this scenario, it is crucial to have more healthcare professionals available in order to deliver high-quality palliative care.

As family physicians are in a privileged role with patients due to holistic care they provide, they have the possibility to deliver palliative care integrating this knowledge into their day-to-day practice. If palliative care is provided by family physicians, this will leave a room for the organization and establishment of more specialized palliative care services. With this collaboration in hand, it is possible to distribute tasks more effectively, allowing community palliative care teams to address and support the cases that have a more demanding management.

In order to facilitate implementing palliative care teams in primary care, the European Association for Palliative Care (EAPC) Taskforce in Primary Palliative Care developed a *Toolkit for The Development of Palliative Care in The Community* [26]. To this list, one also has to take into account the public health strategy of WHO that is upheld on four pillars: adequate policies, availability for education, access to medication, and implementation at all levels of society.

With these resources it is possible to build a strong, personalized palliative care network at the community level that guarantees the best quality of life possible.

21.7 Conclusion

Family doctors' role is crucial in understanding patients' preferences and detect whether patients and family would prefer "at home." Nevertheless, this is less effective or ineffective if home palliative care services and networks are not established and functioning. A possible solution would be the development and spread of palliative care in the community.

References

1. Bruera E. The development of a palliative care culture. J Palliat Care. 2004;20:316–9.
2. Barbosa A, Neto I. Manual de cuidados paliativos, vol. 200. Lisboa: Faculdade de Medicina de Lisboa; 2006.
3. Davies E, Higginson IJ, World Health Organization. Better palliative care for older people. Copenhagen: WHO Regional Office for Europe; 2004.
4. Bone AE, Gomes B, Etkind SN, Verne J, Murtagh FE, Evans CJ, Higginson IJ. What is the impact of population ageing on the future provision of end-of-life care? Population-based projections of place of death. Palliat Med. 2018;32:329–36.
5. Alliance WPC, World Health Organization. Global atlas of palliative care at the end of life. London: Worldwide Palliative Care Alliance; 2014.
6. Twycross R. Temas Gerais. In: Twycross R, editor. Cuidados Paliativos. 2nd ed. Lisboa, Portugal: Climepsi Editores; 2003. p. 15–28.
7. Bluethmann SM, Mariotto AB, Rowland JH. Anticipating the "silver tsunami": prevalence trajectories and comorbidity burden among older cancer survivors in the United States. Cancer Epidemiol Biomark Prev. 2016;25:1029–36.
8. Gomes B, Calanzani N, Curiale V, McCrone P, Higginson IJ. Effectiveness and cost-effectiveness of home palliative care services for adults with advanced illness and their caregivers. Cochrane Database Syst Rev. 2013;(6):CD007760.
9. Townsend J, Frank A, Fermont D, Dyer S, Karran O, Walgrove A, Piper M. Terminal cancer care and patients' preference for place of death: a prospective study. BMJ. 1990;301:415–7.
10. Wheatley VJ, Baker JI. "Please, I want to go home": ethical issues raised when considering choice of place of care in palliative care. Postgrad Med J. 2007;83:643–8.
11. Brumley R, Enguidanos S, Jamison P, Seitz R, Morgenstern N, Saito S, McIlwane J, Hillary K, Gonzalez J. Increased satisfaction with care and lower costs: results of a randomized trial of in-home palliative care. J Am Geriatr Soc. 2007;55:993–1000.

12. Centeno C, Sitte T, De Lima L, Alsirafy S, Bruera E, Callaway M, Foley K, Luyirika E, Mosoiu D, Pettus K. White paper for global palliative care advocacy: recommendations from a PAL-LIFE Expert Advisory Group of the Pontifical Academy for Life, Vatican City. J Palliat Med. 2018;21:1389–97.
13. Weitzen S, Teno JM, Fennell M, Mor V. Factors associated with site of death: a national study of where people die. Med Care. 2003;41:323–35.
14. Van den Block L, Deschepper R, Bossuyt N, Drieskens K, Bauwens S, Van Casteren V, Deliens L. Care for patients in the last months of life: the Belgian Sentinel Network Monitoring End-of-Life Care study. Arch Intern Med. 2008;168:1747–54.
15. Van den Block L, Onwuteaka-Philipsen B, Meeussen K, Donker G, Giusti F, Miccinesi G, Van Casteren V, Alonso TV, Zurriaga O, Deliens L. Nationwide continuous monitoring of end-of-life care via representative networks of general practitioners in Europe. BMC Fam Pract. 2013;14:73.
16. Pivodic L, Van den Block L, Pardon K, Miccinesi G, Vega Alonso T, Boffin N, Donker GA, Cancian M, López-Maside A, Onwuteaka-Philipsen BD. Burden on family carers and care-related financial strain at the end of life: a cross-national population-based study. Eur J Public Health. 2014;24:819–26.
17. Adelman RD, Tmanova LL, Delgado D, Dion S, Lachs MS. Caregiver burden: a clinical review. JAMA. 2014;311:1052–60.
18. Ferrell BR, Coyle N, Paice J. Oxford textbook of palliative nursing. Oxford: Oxford University Press; 2014.
19. Sekse RJT, Hunskar I, Ellingsen S. The nurse's role in palliative care: a qualitative meta-synthesis. J Clin Nurs. 2018;27:e21–38.
20. Kissane D. Family focused grief therapy: the role of the family in preventive and therapeutic bereavement care. Bereavement Care. 2003;22:6–8.
21. Kissane DW, McKenzie M, Bloch S, Moskowitz C, McKenzie DP, O'Neill I. Family focused grief therapy: a randomized, controlled trial in palliative care and bereavement. Am J Psychiatr. 2006;163:1208–18.
22. Rumbold B, Aoun S. Bereavement and palliative care: a public health perspective. Prog Palliat Care. 2014;22:131–5.
23. van Weel C, Roberts R, Kidd M, Loh A. Mental health and primary care: family medicine has a role. Ment Health Fam Med. 2008;5:3–4.
24. Watson M. Oxford handbook of palliative care. Oxford: Oxford University Press; 2019.
25. Gomes B, Higginson IJ. Where people die (1974–2030): past trends, future projections and implications for care. Palliat Med. 2008;22:33–41.
26. Brogaard T, Neergaard MA, Murray SA. Promoting palliative care in the community: a toolkit to improve and develop primary palliative care throughout Europe. Scand J Prim Health Care. 2016;34:3–4.

Integrating Spiritual Care in the Frame

Daniel Nuzum, Jacopo Demurtas, and Christina Puchalski

Abstract

The recognition of the place of spiritual care in healthcare has been growing in recent decades and complements a growing awareness of the importance of person-centred care. There has been increasing evidence of the place of spirituality in the overall wellbeing and health of patients. While for many historically spirituality and religious faith were synonymous, it is accepted that spirituality is a broader reality which for many does not include religious expression. For the older person, the recognition of and attention to their spiritual reality provide an important opportunity to acknowledge their values, perspective and approach to life and illness. To include spirituality in the overall care of the older person is to provide a comprehensive approach to medical care, caring for the person rather than simply treating the illness. This chapter provides an introduction to the

D. Nuzum (✉)
Cork University Hospital & Marymount University Hospital and Hospice, Cork, Ireland

Association of Clinical Pastoral Education (Ireland) Ltd., Dublin, Ireland

Department of Obstetrics & Gynaecology, College of Medicine and Health, University College Cork, Cork University Maternity Hospital, Cork, Ireland
e-mail: daniel.nuzum@ucc.ie

J. Demurtas
Primary Care Department, USL Toscana Sud Est, Grosseto, Italy

C. Puchalski
Medicine and Health Sciences, The George Washington University, Washington, DC, USA

© Springer Nature Switzerland AG 2022
J. Demurtas, N. Veronese (eds.), *The Role of Family Physicians in Older People Care*, Practical Issues in Geriatrics, https://doi.org/10.1007/978-3-030-78923-7_22

place of spirituality in the care of older persons and also provides an introduction to spiritual assessment for healthcare professionals working in general practice.

Keywords

Spiritual care · Wellbeing · Older · Values · Person-centred approach

22.1 Introduction

Spirituality can be described as the essence of 'who we are' as human beings. As a core dimension of identity and purpose, the acknowledgement and care of the human spirit should be an integral part of the overall care of all patients. Spirituality should, at its best, be integrated and woven through the tapestry of all interventions and care for older persons and their families by the whole healthcare team. Recognising the spiritual dimension of the person being cared for is to provide a truly person-centred approach to medical care. Much has been written in the literature in recent years concerning the role and influence of spirituality and belief on the lifestyle choices, medical decisions and wellbeing of patients. There has also been a greater understanding and appreciation of the global breadth of spirituality that includes both religious and nonreligious perspectives and influences and how these come to bear on health and wellbeing.

The aim of this chapter is to provide a rationale for the inclusion of spirituality in the medical care of older patients and to provide an introductory outline to spiritual assessment for healthcare professionals in their care of older patients and service users.

22.2 What Is Spirituality?

There has been much discourse concerning the nature of spirituality and seeking to define the concept of spirituality. At its broadest, spirituality encompasses an existential understanding of the nature of how we as human beings make sense of who we are. Spirituality contributes to how we find meaning in our life, relationships, values, purpose and for many the approach to the end of life and what happens after death. For some, spirituality and religion are synonymous; however, it is important to remember that while religious faith is important for many, spirituality is a broader concept which may include religious faith but is not confined to it. For others, spirituality is experienced and expressed in secular and humanistic ways without reference to the sacred. For all, spirituality characterises the 'essence' of who we are.

There has been a growing desire to arrive at a common understanding and definition of spirituality in healthcare. A 2009 national consensus conference in the USA defined spirituality as 'the aspect of humanity that refers to the way individuals seek and express meaning and purpose and the way they experience their connectedness to the moment, to self, to others, to nature and to the significant or sacred' [1]. This was further developed at a later meeting in Geneva in 2014 with international consensus to give a more global perspective and also to include the expression of spirituality and was defined as 'Spirituality is a dynamic and intrinsic aspect of humanity through which persons seek ultimate meaning, purpose and transcendence and experience relationship to self, family, others, community, society, nature and the significant or sacred. Spirituality is expressed through beliefs, values, traditions and practices' [2]. The European Association of Palliative Care has also focussed on the importance of spirituality with the establishment of a spirituality reference group. These consensus definitions have gained widespread global respect as working definitions of spirituality across the lifespan but in particular in palliative care and end-of-life care. In many ways the discipline of palliative care has led the way in naming and integrating spirituality in the formal definition of palliative care adopted by the World Health Organization (WHO) in 2004 and further expanded by resolution of the 67th WHO Assembly in 2014 to 'palliative care is an approach that improves the quality of life of patients (adults and children) and their families who are facing the problems associated with life-threatening illness, through the prevention and relief of suffering by means of early identification and correct assessment and treatment of pain and other problems, whether physical, psychosocial or spiritual' [3, 4]. This resolution also emphasised the ethical duty of healthcare professionals '…to alleviate pain and suffering, whether physical, psychosocial or spiritual, irrespective of whether the disease or condition can be cured…' [4].

While palliative care has included spirituality as an essential component of care, spirituality has also been recognised in the wider medical field not least in psychiatry. In an increasing secularisation of society, some see spirituality as a very personal or private matter that should not be the business of healthcare professionals. However, to see spirituality in this way is to misunderstand an essential nature of the human person for whom spirituality and meaning are core dimensions of who there are and how they view life and their vision of health which in turn can impact on the healthcare choices especially when it comes to care directives, intervention and end-of-life care discussions and planning. It may also have a bearing on compliance with healthcare treatment and overall quality of life. So, if spirituality is important to patients and families, then it should be important to healthcare professionals too.

A 2019 meta-synthesis of spiritual care understanding and needs in the final year of life highlighted the importance of spiritual care in the published literature for both patients and family members/caregivers [5]. This review highlighted the importance of relationships, managing remaining life, dealing with dying and after death and finding meaning in illness. However, the literature also points to challenges for healthcare professionals and their lack of comfort in addressing spiritual needs [6]. Not to include spiritual matters is to deny a whole dimension of our humanity which in turn may have negative implications for overall health and wellbeing. Spiritual wellbeing is also recognised as contributing to better overall health outcomes, quality of life and wellbeing [7–9].

22.3 Assessing Spiritual Need

At its most basic level, to assess spiritual need in general practice is to get to know the person of the patient: 'Who are you?'. In addition to providing good spiritual care, this approach also fosters a trusting therapeutic relationship between the physician and the patient. This therapeutic relationship when based on trust and respect provides a supportive environment where the patient feels valued, and this includes the spiritual dimension of who they are and what is important to them. Out of this relationship the physician—indeed the whole healthcare team—can and should integrate spiritual care alongside physical and emotional care to support the older person and their family/loved ones as they adjust to increasing frailty and old age. This approach is captured well in the narrative approach to medicine promoted by Charon as being essential for fostering empathy, reflection, professionalism and trust between physicians and patients [10].

Navigating the natural processes of growing older places many spiritual realities on the journey for older patients. These include the areas of loss, hope, identity, joy, faith, fulfilment, frailty, purpose, pride, meaning, purpose, transcendence, function, relationship and dependence to name but a few. These named spiritual concerns provide both burden and benefit to older persons as they deal with illness and loss of function. Indeed the loss of function can also increase isolation and the withdrawal from the usual supports of community. Where physical and mental function decreases, the capacity for challenging spiritual feelings to surface and remain present is increased with the associated impact on self, wellbeing and overall health. For a physician to be mindful of spiritual dynamics is to open up a further and important dimension of care as well as identifying potential burdens and resources associated with spirituality that can be drawn upon for overall care and wellbeing of the older person. This can be easily integrated into the medical consultation and review of and with the older person by the physician and the wider healthcare team and where indicated, by drawing on the expertise of spiritual care practitioners/pastoral carers. The increasing realities of periods of isolation associated with seasonal infection outbreaks and global pandemics also pose challenges requiring novel ways of remaining connected to older and more vulnerable populations to care for their spiritual health alongside their physical and emotional needs [11].

While for some, spiritual practice is closely linked with religious and cultural practice, it is important not to make assumptions about spiritual/religious practice and tradition but rather to invite patients or family members to share what the particular practices and preferences of the patient/service user are. For patients where religious or cultural practice is important, these can be important resources to be accessed in times of frailty or illness. For those with a secular/humanistic understanding of life and wellbeing, various practices such as mindfulness, reflection and yoga, to name but a few, take on a spiritual dimension and practice. As older persons with increasing frailty can become more isolated from their peers, religious, spiritual and secular practices can help them to remain connected in non-physical ways to communities of faith/practice and in this way to feel less isolated. It is also the case that older patients often experience a renewed perspective on life as physical capacity reduces and find new meaning and perspective in spiritual practices.

22.4 Know Your Patient: Know the Person

The key to good overall care is getting to know the life story of the person you are caring for. Taking time to get to know the story of the patient from their younger years helps to weave a rich spiritual tapestry which can then be continued into the older years of life. This approach to care helps to set the person in their broader life context that is not defined by the challenges of older age, increasing frailty or illness. It also honours the fullness of the life of the older patient and maintains their dignity and sense of self. In addition to the information shared by the patient, it is helpful to gain collateral information from close family members who can paint a rich picture of the patient as an individual. From a spiritual perspective, it is helpful to gain insights into the particular preferences, resources and traditions (if any) of the patient, a number of which may influence lifestyle, medical and ethical choices in healthcare. Some have argued in the past that enquiring about spiritual matters is too personal or intrusive in medical practice. However, the evidence highlights that spiritual needs are important to patients [5]. To help a patient to share their story requires a trusting relationship where a patient feels safe that their story will be heard without negative judgement. This requires a readiness for the professional to practice compassionate presence, to listen compassionately and to be sensitive to the subtleties of spiritual distress or concern that are shared in the story of the patient and then to interpret how to respond to these concerns appropriately or to refer to a spiritual care professional. As a general practice point, it is helpful to remember that enquiring about spiritual needs is just that: an inclusion of what is important to the patient. When framed in this way as part of overall care, the patient retains the autonomy to share as little or as much as they wish about what is important to them. For this author, the experience is that patients and their families appreciate the opportunity to share their story. So how does one do this?

22.5 Spiritual History Tools

As the physician listens attentively to the story of the patient, it is likely that spiritual issues will arise as part of the overall narrative conversation and rarely as a separate 'spiritual section' of a conversation or consultation. Alongside the professional intuitive assessment of the professional, generally speaking it is more helpful for the healthcare professional to ask open ended questions of a conversational nature such as 'How have you been coping with [...your situation, illness, etc.] recently?' 'Has anything been helping you?' 'What do you enjoy in life?' 'What gives you meaning, strength, etc.?' 'Are there any particular relationships that are supportive or that are a concern just now?' 'Is there anything that you feel it would be helpful for us to know in terms of your spiritual life/practices so that we can care better for you?' As the relationship with a general practitioner is likely to be over a period of time, the importance of non-verbal cues and changes in behaviours should also be noted as possible indicators of spiritual/existential distress. In addition to the above narrative questions, it is also helpful to use a spiritual history tool, to help to get a clearer overall picture of a patient's possible spiritual or existential concern(s).

There are a number of recognised spiritual history/screening tools available for general use by healthcare professionals use (healthcare chaplains are trained to use more in-depth spiritual assessment tools). One such tool is the *FICA Spiritual History Tool©* developed by Professor Christina Puchalski of the George Washington Institute for Spirituality and Health [12]. This tool provides a helpful conversational guide for the healthcare professional as part of a spiritual history and is included in Appendix [13].[1]

While tools are helpful, they should not be used rigidly and work best when applied sensitively to the needs of each individual patient/service user. It is recommended to receive some training in their use. In recent years the George Washington Institute for Spirituality and Health has also developed an innovative and respected Interprofessional Spiritual Care Education Curriculum (ISPEC) which has sought to provide robust spiritual care training for clinicians and other healthcare professionals [14]. (There are also other broad spiritual care programmes available for healthcare professionals and provided by clinical pastoral education supervisors/educators; the 'Introduction to Clinical Pastoral Education for Healthcare Professionals' run at University College Cork, Ireland, is one such example https://www.ucc.ie/en/cpd/options/medhealth/cpd1621/).

22.6   Responding to Spiritual Need

Using a spiritual screening tool such as FICA© as part of overall clinical assessment, issues of spiritual concern or distress as well as spiritual resources can be identified. The information that is received should be recorded in the medical record and care plan of the patient. When issues of spiritual concern are identified, a referral can be made to a spiritual care provider or chaplain who is trained to assess and respond to spiritual need or distress. In community settings, the provision of spiritual care may very much depend on local resources. However, the therapeutic and supportive impact of the recognition of spiritual concern through the interest, inquiry and conversation of the healthcare professional should not be underestimated. Simply asking the question as a physician conveys interest and person-centred care as well as giving the physician a richer understanding of the person they are caring for. Primary care spiritual care initiatives have identified some promising results concerning the value of spiritual care in promoting overall wellbeing in community practice settings [15–17].

---

[1]The *FICA Spiritual History Tool©* has been included with the kind permission of Professor Christina Puchalski and is included at Appendix.

22.7 Spirituality in End-of-Life Care

Naturally as we get older, we reflect on the reality of mortality and therefore end-of-life issues. Spirituality can have an influential role in how we approach the end of life, and in particular it is important that end-of-life preferences can be discussed and established in advance so that all care that is planned and provided can be in accordance with the expressed wishes and preferences of the patient. Regardless of religious expression or not, facing and experiencing the dying process and death is a profoundly spiritual and existential experience for most people and their families and caregivers. The importance of spiritual sensitivity in this area cannot be overestimated. Spiritual sensitivity provides a valuable level of human comfort as part of good medical care. A point of good practice is to provide an opportunity for end-of-life wishes and preferences to be recorded so that caregivers and healthcare staff know what a particular patient's wishes are for end-of-life care, rituals, practices and customs in advance so that they can be sensitively provided at end of life. This also prevents inappropriate interventions.

22.8 Spirituality in Dementia

Spirituality can have an important role to play in dementia. As cognitive function declines, the place of spirituality and previously known and familiar rituals can provide a comforting routine and can help to access habitual patterns of relating. It is often the case that older practices, both religious and spiritual, remain recognisable in dementia for the patient. This is particularly the case with music, prayer and ritual practices which can provide a familiar and comforting solace amidst the distress of uncertainty associated with dementia as cognitive function declines. Enabling a patient to access these spiritual practices also helps to maintain their dignity and value as well as providing valuable spiritual support and wellbeing.

22.9 What Is the Role of General Practitioner in Spiritual Needs of the Patients?

The general practitioner (GP)—which is taken in this context to include all healthcare professionals in the general practice team—has an important first point of contact with patients usually in a community setting. The nature of the therapeutic relationship between patients and their GP in a community setting provides a valuable opportunity for longer-term care as well as a broader appreciation of the patient and wellbeing in their community setting. The GP is particularly well placed to know her/his patient over a longer time frame and to know intimately the life story of their patient. This places the GP in a good position to have an appreciation of the spiritual dimensions and expression of a patient and how they might impact on their wellbeing and health. In addition the GP is well placed to observe more subtle changes in the overall wellbeing of a patient and to be able to appreciate in depth what the individual strengths and resources are for a patient to access for their recovery and treatment. This should naturally include the spiritual resources and concerns of the patient. In this way the GP perhaps is uniquely placed amongst healthcare professionals to recognise the integrated care of a patient physically, socially, spiritually and emotionally. As a GP relates to other professionals to support her/him in their role, this should also apply to spiritual matters and experience from other sectors can make a case for the development of these relationships as part of the overall suite of services and care that a GP can access for her/his patients. Where a GP identifies spiritual or existential distress or concern, in addition to the acknowledgement of this distress through compassionate listening and presence, a referral should be made to a spiritual care provider for more in-depth accompaniment, intervention and care. This is best done alongside the continuing care by the GP. In places where access to professional spiritual care is not available, it can help to refer the patient to their own spiritual/religious advisor.

22.10 Conclusion

The provision of good medical care to older persons includes good spiritual care. Building on a global awareness and recognition of the importance of spiritual care in overall healthcare and wellbeing, to recognise and include spiritual care is to offer a truly person-centred approach to comprehensive medical care that honours the needs, values and unique dimensions of each patient in a holistic way in both general practice and in residential care settings. Good spiritual care upholds the autonomy of the older person and recognises the unique gifts and strengths of her/his life story and spiritual/existential/humanistic beliefs as a resource for their ongoing care. Building on a trusting therapeutic relationship, the healthcare team by including spiritual care provides an opportunity for an older person to experience dignified, respectful and affirming person-centred care that is attentive to their overall needs and the promotion of their wellbeing.

Appendix: FICA Spiritual History Tool©™

The FICA Spiritual History Tool was developed by Dr. Puchalski and a group of primary care physicians to help physicians and other healthcare professionals address spiritual issues with patients. Spiritual histories are taken as part of the regular history during an annual exam or new patient visit but can also be taken as part of follow-up visits, as appropriate. The FICA tool serves as a guide for conversations in the clinical setting.

The acronym FICA can help structure questions in taking a spiritual history by healthcare professionals.

F: Faith and Belief

'Do you consider yourself spiritual or religious?' or 'Is spirituality something important to you' or 'Do you have spiritual beliefs that help you cope with stress/difficult times?' (Contextualize to reason for visit if it is not the routine history).

If the patient responds 'No', the healthcare provider might ask, 'What gives your life meaning?' Sometimes patients respond with answers such as family, career or nature.

(The question of meaning should also be asked even if people answer yes to spirituality.)

I: Importance

What importance does your spirituality have in your life? Has your spirituality influenced how you take care of yourself, your health? Does your spirituality influence you in your healthcare decision making? (e.g. advance directives, treatment, etc.)

C: Community

'Are you part of a spiritual community? Communities such as churches, temples, and mosques or a group of like-minded friends, family or yoga can serve as strong support systems for some patients. Can explore further: Is this of support to you and how? Is there a group of people you really love or who are important to you?'

A: Address in Care

'How would you like me, your healthcare provider, to address these issues in your healthcare?' (With the newer models including diagnosis of spiritual distress, A also refers to the 'assessment and plan' of patient spiritual distress or issues within a treatment or care plan).

© C. Puchalski, 1996.

Puchalski, C., & Romer, A. L. (2000). Taking a spiritual history allows clinicians to understand patients more fully. *Journal of palliative medicine, 3*(1), 129–137.

References

1. Puchalski C, Ferrell B, Virani R, Otis-Green S, Baird P, Bull J, et al. Improving the quality of spiritual care as a dimension of palliative care: the report of the Consensus Conference. J Palliat Med. 2009;12(10):885–904.

2. Puchalski CM, Vitillo R, Hull SK, Reller N. Improving the spiritual dimension of whole person care: reaching national and international consensus. J Palliat Med. 2014;17(6):642–56.
3. Vitillo R, Puchalski C. World Health Organization authorities promote greater attention and action on palliative care. J Palliat Med. 2014;17(9):988–9.
4. W.H.O. Strengthening of palliative care as a component of comprehensive care throughout the life course. WHA67.19. Geneva: World Health Organization; 2014.
5. Clyne B, O'Neill SM, Nuzum D, O'Neill M, Larkin J, Ryan M, et al. Patients' spirituality perspectives at the end of life: a qualitative evidence synthesis. BMJ Support Palliat Care. 2019.
6. Abarshi E, Echteld M, Donker G, Van den Block L, Onwuteaka-Philipsen B, Deliens L. Discussing end-of-life issues in the last months of life: a nationwide study among general practitioners. J Palliat Med. 2011;14(3):323–30.
7. Steinhauser KE, Fitchett G, Handzo GF, Johnson KS, Koenig HG, Pargament KI, et al. State of the science of spirituality and palliative care research Part I: Definitions, measurement, and outcomes. J Pain Symptom Manag. 2017;54(3):428–40.
8. Chen J, Lin Y, Yan J, Wu Y, Hu R. The effects of spiritual care on quality of life and spiritual well-being among patients with terminal illness: a systematic review. Palliat Med. 2018;32(7):1167–79.
9. Fitchett G. Recent progress in chaplaincy-related research. J Pastoral Care Counsel. 2017;71(3):163–75.
10. Charon R. The patient-physician relationship. Narrative medicine: a model for empathy, reflection, profession, and trust. JAMA. 2001;286(15):1897–902.
11. Byrne MJ, Nuzum DR. Pastoral closeness in physical distancing: the use of technology in Pastoral Ministry during COVID-19. Health Social Care Chaplaincy. 2020;8(2).
12. Puchalski C, Romer AL. Taking a spiritual history allows clinicians to understand patients more fully. J Palliat Med. 2000;3(1):129–37.
13. Puchalski C. FICA: The George Washington Institute for Spirituality and Health. 1996.
14. Puchalski C, Jafari N, Buller H, Haythorn T, Jacobs C, Ferrell B. Interprofessional spiritual care education curriculum: a milestone toward the provision of spiritual care. J Palliat Med. 2020;23(6):777–84.
15. Kevern P, Hill L. 'Chaplains for well-being' in primary care: analysis of the results of a retrospective study. Prim Health Care Res Dev. 2015;16(1):87–99.
16. Alan G, Debbie B. Community chaplaincy listening in a community mental health group. Health Social Care Chaplaincy. 2019;7(1):42.
17. Austyn S, Alan G, Rebecca G. What is the impact of chaplaincy in primary care? The GP perspective. Health Social Care Chaplaincy. 2018;6(2).

Part VII

Self-Determination, Dignity and Humanism

An Introduction to Dignity Therapy

23

Giovanna D'Iapico

Abstract

The life expectancy of people at birth has lengthened, and chronic diseases that require constant care by the team of professionals, family members, and friends of the person-patient have appeared on the threshold of the world. The dignity therapy approach, in this sense, offers the person that space to reflect on their life, its value, the meaning, and the significance of their existence. Dignity is a nebulous term, a very elusive and changing concept. The term dignity refers to everything that deserves honor, respect, and esteem. Harvey Chochinov attempted to define the term dignity for people in palliative care, leading to the construction of the model of dignity. The intervention that arises from this model embraces all areas of interest of the person and is the map to guide the interventions in support of the sense of dignity of the person.

Keywords

Chronic diseases · Chochinov · Dignity therapy · Self-perception · Dignity · Palliative care

23.1 Introduction

The promotion of well-being and the best possible quality of life, the protection of dignity, and respect for the person must be the primary objectives of those who work for the care of people who are frail due to the aging process or an incurable disease.

G. D'Iapico (✉)
Primary Care Department, AUSL, Modena, Italy

Nurse Palliative Care, AUSL, Modena, Italy
e-mail: diapo70@hotmail.it

© Springer Nature Switzerland AG 2022
J. Demurtas, N. Veronese (eds.), *The Role of Family Physicians in Older People Care*, Practical Issues in Geriatrics, https://doi.org/10.1007/978-3-030-78923-7_23

Person-centered care has the potential to increase the perception of dignity of the person requesting care. The logic means that the person can choose to value his last days, despite the illness and/or terminality. This is the goal of a holistic approach centered on the person who also deals with the psychological and spiritual aspects and needs to characterize the path of the disease and the approach to death [1]. Thanks to the improvement in the quality of life and with scientific and technological progress, the life expectancy of people at birth has lengthened, and chronic diseases that, by their nature, cannot be eradicated from the person's body have appeared on the threshold of the world, but they require constant care by the team of professionals, the family, and friends of the person-patient [2]. Palliative care refers precisely to the reception and care of the person as a whole, and usually the main target is the frail elderly person [3]. Therapeutic interventions in favor of these fragile people must be imbued with dignity, so that they are effectively dignity-conserving cures [4]. The approach of dignity therapy (DT), in this sense, offers the person that space to reflect on their life, its value, the meaning, and the significance of their existence.

23.2 The Concept of Dignity

Dignity is a nebulous term, a very elusive and iridescent concept. It is a fluid construct, closely related to the culture in which it is used. The term dignity relates to everything that deserves honor, respect, and esteem, and healthcare personnel who work with fragile people must imbue their therapeutic actions with dignity to transmit consideration, respect, and kindness to patients [4]. It is not possible to speak of dignity without trying to define it. This is what Harvey Chochinov did when he arrived at the construction of a model of dignity that had a good empirical basis. This model investigates what dignity represents for people whose lives are threatened or limited by an incurable disease. Many patients, interviewed by Chochinov et al. [5], when asked "What is dignity for you?", replied that this concept is closely linked to the quality of the care offered and the support provided by the network in which these treatments are provided (social dignity). Others have replied that dignity is linked to the severity of the disease (illness-related issues), while still others believe that the sense of dignity is linked to personal characteristics and to one's philosophical and existential beliefs [4]. Dignity, therefore, is strictly connected with the deepest sense of oneself and of one's own nature as a person. The good management of symptoms and pain, feeling accepted and supported, and seeing personal needs recognized and satisfied reduce the likelihood that the person feels their dignity is threatened. Dignity is respect for oneself, for one's values, and for what makes us ourselves: dignity is the freedom of choice. The person who at that moment is the patient of palliative care does not stop being a subject and therefore cannot be reduced to an object: he is the source of the information that guides the path of palliative care and cannot be ignored in any way. It is the reference point for every decision made by the team of professionals and must be listened to. This indicates that there are no sociodemographic factors (gender, marital status, education, ethnicity, origins, religion) that a priori influence the perception of the sense of dignity [5]. The only significant difference between those who had an intact sense of dignity and those who felt they had lost it was where they were interviewed: people with a low sense of dignity were more likely to be hospitalized than those who still had one good perception of one's dignity. This suggests that hospitalization or, on the contrary, the possibility of staying at home assisted by professionals greatly influences the sense of dignity and, in turn, also psychophysiological indicators. This study also showed that people with lower levels of perception of dignity were those at greatest risk of experiencing distress and the desire to die [5]. This research also demonstrates that the concept of dignity is closely linked to personal history and cannot be subjected to standardization, as it is an extremely complex concept. Finally, dignity is a flexible and resilient concept even in the face of the most important and difficult challenges such as a terminal illness (ibidem). Dignity is a concept that transcends time: it depends on how the person sees himself in the past, in the present, and in the future. Knowing that something of us can go beyond death and that it can remain with the people we love increases the sick person's sense of dignity [6]. Furthermore, dignity is a concept that is expressed in the relationship with the other and derives from how I perceive that the other sees me [7]. In fact, it is embodied in the person's experience and is influenced by the experiences of decay and decay of one's own body [8]. The profound transformations caused by the disease or by the therapies change the physical appearance of the person who can no longer recognize his own image reflected in the mirror [4]. This experience risks arousing in the person a sense of loss of their own self, the true target of the disease, which can be further diminished by the looks of the people around the patient who are unable to go beyond the present image and remember the intrinsic value of the person despite the disease (ibidem). If the professional can only see a sick patient, the person will also feel only a sick person, and the part of his identity linked to the disease will take over, canceling all the other facets of his identity. However, if the professional works within a perspective of global personal care and is interested with genuine curiosity in the personal history of the person in front of him, he will also be able to see emerging identities linked to other roles of spouse, parent, and child, and this will allow to expand the possibilities of the person and the perception that he has of himself. This will give the person the certainty that his identity, in all its facets, has been heard, accepted, and affirmed [9].

23.3   The Therapy of Dignity

The basis of dignity therapy (DT) is the model of dignity, Chochinov started from reality, from people's needs to understand the factors that affect the sense of dignity. The intervention that arises from this model embraces all areas of personal interest and is the map for guiding interventions in support of the person's sense of dignity [9]. According to the empirical model developed by Chochinov et al. [5], there are three sources of primary influence on dignity: physical factors linked to illness, psychological and spiritual factors, defined by the authors as a "catalog of indicators of the conservation of dignity," and external factors dependent on the "social environment" defined as an "inventory of social dignity" [4]; these themes are composed of further subcategories that add complexity to the model, mirroring the complexity of human reality [9].

Dignity therapy (DT) focuses on the generative tasks of dignity: concluding unfinished business, sharing words of love, and leaving a final document for loved ones [1]. Dignity therapy, in fact, is a brief and personalized psychotherapy that aims to reduce existential, psychological and spiritual stress, and to promote the quality of life of the last days of people whose life is limited or threatened by incurable diseases. This therapy investigates the personal concept of dignity of those facing terminal illness, wondering what determines the quality of the person's remaining days, offering them the opportunity to reflect on their own lives and tell it to a person genuinely interested and ready to listen. The resulting story will become the legacy that the person will be able to give to their loved ones, as a reminder of a life worth remembering and words of encouragement, warning, or love for those who remain [4].

Originally, Chochinov carried out this intervention in 2002 as a short psychotherapy to increase the sense of dignity in patients with low levels of distress; later the application was also extended to other areas.

The person who is approaching the end of his life often experiences existential fears and faces spiritual and psychological difficulties that may not be recognized by health personnel and consequently are not subject to intervention [4]. The person, or at least a part of him, is thus abandoned to the anxieties related to the unknown, and an important part of him, especially the spiritual and emotional one, is not embraced and welcomed in the treatment path. In this sense, DT is an approach that reinforces the perception of value of the person in a supportive context and offers the possibility of sharing the moments of one's life that are considered most significant and talking about topics that you want to be remembered by friends and family members [10]. DT aims to promote self-affirmation, supporting the person in recognizing himself within his story [4], thus also changing the way in which family members look at the sick person, remembering that it is above all the person who is part of their family and their lives, worthy of respect and value. In randomized controlled trials (RCTs), participants who also received DT intervention in addition to standard palliative care (SPC) reported DT as the best tool for reducing suffering and depression [11], possibly because the generative document allows the person to give himself and give his words and experiences to the most important and significant people. Dignity therapy does not intervene on external reality: it is not an intervention for the healing of the person, it does not prevent death, but it offers a space for reflection on one's own existence, successes, and failures and promotes awareness and autobiographical awareness that it allows the person to return to be in control of his own actions in his own environment [4]. The reflections concern the person's past, rather than the future; in this dialogue on one's own history, the difficulties and failures are reread through new eyes and inserted into a new perspective, allowing one to look at one's life as a global and original unit as well as how she lived. The person feels important and appreciates that someone cares about them and their conditions in a genuine and disinterested way. DT fits into the vein of existential therapeutic interventions such as reminiscence therapy (RT), life storybooks, ethical testament, or narrative medicine. However, it differs from it since it has an experimental basis [4] and does not aim to collect all the memories and details of the person's life but to highlight and bring to light the most significant and important experiences and memories for the person [12]. A study conducted by Vuksanovic et al. [13] showed that DT is superior to life review (LR) interventions as it increases the generativity and integrity of the ego. LR's intervention favors the vision of death as part of the life cycle and as an antidote to depression and death anxiety that arise from the encounter with death [1]; however, it lacks the aspect of generativity represented from the generative document. From these studies it emerges that DT is perceived as more supportive and helpful not only to the people involved in the path but also to family members both when they receive the generative document and after the death of the loved one [13]. However, both DT and LR were considered helpful and supportive, and both were recommended by participants to other patients, as people perceived an improvement in their levels of well-being, sense of dignity, and worth. Both of these interventions have a high acceptability and satisfaction; they have helped people feel more active and important in their world of love. DT has the potential to reduce aspects of stagnation, apathy, low contribution, and participation in relationships, despair, guilt, and regret [13]. It is positively associated with psychological and emotional well-being and reduces levels of anxiety, depression, and distress, especially in the short term, for a period of 30 days [10, 13]: perhaps the levels of depression and anxiety decrease thanks to the creation of the generative document [10].

Where there is very great pain, DT can help the person recognize past pain and try to soothe it by sharing that experience. However, the therapist must never forget that DT is not psychotherapy; therefore, it is unthinkable to use it as a path that can lead to the origin of pain, traumatic event, or emotional block, since it is not suitable for this purpose: this could be one of the limits of DT, but in reality it simply defines its range of action. It must be understood that some stories can be too painful to be told and the therapist, but also family members, must have respect for the person's history and give them permission to keep the memories that they consider too intimate, which can make them feel too vulnerable [4]. The story can be composed of narratives and silences, and this makes the generative document that will be born unique (ibidem). Participants use therapy for more personal purposes: some express their love for family and friends while others describe regrets and remorse for some of their actions (ibid.). For most people, therapy is a way of remembering special and important events to be passed on as an inheritance (ibidem). DT is an opportunity available to the person; it serves to tell them what they need to be remembered: it may happen that the person does not want to reconstruct their story, but only remember the mistakes made, and ask for forgiveness from family members wishing them the good fortune to stay away from the same mistakes [4]. For this reason, the intervention, although it has a stable frame, cannot be standardized but must be tailored around the person and tailored for her.

Dignity therapy can be carried out at the person's home, in nursing homes, hospices, and in the palliative care departments of hospitals and mainly concerns the physical, psychosocial, existential, and spiritual issues that worry the person or are a source of stress [6]. Some subsequent research suggests that DT may be of greater benefit to patients with a high level of psychological distress at baseline [10], although Chochinov does not recommend DT to people with severe depression, as they may present with vision distorted of oneself and one's life and generate "horrible stories" [4]. In conclusion, DT is an intervention that starts from the needs, desires, and values of the person and recognizes and supports them, promoting better communication with loved ones.

23.4   The Therapist

The questions of the DT protocol provide the framework within which the capacities and abilities of the therapist who guides the interview are revealed and act, who is capable of welcoming people's confidences and organizing their intertwining into a coherent generative document and significant [4]. Guiding the person means helping him to structure the story and organize it through questions on the temporal sequence and the connections between events, asking to better contextualize the scene, and favoring the memory of details [6]. This is why training is important, because the therapist needs to be trained and at ease with existential questions and the issues related to them; must be able to be a good active listener and a worthy interlocutor aware of the range of emotions that can manifest themselves during the interview, from joy to gloom; and must be able to manage the silences and emotions that will emerge [4]. Another key skill of the therapist is the attention he places in making sure that the person has been given all possible opportunities to say what he wanted to be remembered: this is the therapist's greatest responsibility towards the person he relies on him [4].

The therapist's role is to facilitate the revelation of an important life worthy of being told even just because it was lived and to underline the profound meaning of sharing this unique story.

Having said that, which professional figure could include the DT in his daily practice and which figures could not effectively complete the task? According to the meta-analysis by Fitchell and colleagues [1], psychologists, nurses, and spiritual fathers could be the right figures to guide the person along the path of therapy, as, thanks to their profession, they welcome the person in toto, have a holistic approach, and are familiar figures in constant contact with the person. Despite these specific skills, all health and care personnel that gravitate around the sick person must be trained so that their behaviors and attitudes towards the person are supportive of their dignity, and every therapeutic action is impregnated with dignity [1, 4]. The training must have as a reference point the experience of the person who will conduct the interview in such a way as to arouse that sense of authenticity that will allow the interview to be truly generative of meaning and not a trivial checklist [14].

23.5   The Protocol

First of all it is important to understand which people to propose the therapy to.

Inclusion criteria. Careful evaluation is necessary because although the person may appear to be in a condition of physical and mental well-being; he is not necessarily at peace with himself [4]. An idiographic approach must be adopted, which allows knowledge of the person in such a way as to understand and recognize their needs. DT can be offered when you think you can give people comfort and serenity to face the final days of their life.

Exclusion criteria. DT is not a panacea, it cannot be offered to anyone, because not everyone benefits from it. This does not mean that a person will never be able to access DT but that being in that particular situation and with certain characteristics, it is better if you do not participate. How anyone who is too sick and can die before 2 weeks and shows a cognitive impairment that limits the ability to give sensible and reasoned answers.

Introduction meeting In the first meeting between the therapist and the patient, DT is presented and described. Chochinov [15] recommends that DT be presented as a positive opportunity for subjective reflection, offered to people to tell each other and tell their story. The therapist must ensure that the person decides freely and without pressure; furthermore, he must remind the participant that he is the protagonist of the therapy and therefore is free, if he deems it necessary, to withdraw from the path at any time because the consent must always be current and valid for the present moment. The therapist leaves a copy of the protocol of the questions to the person so that they can prepare for the next meeting. Knowing the questions that will be asked allows you to feel as calm and comfortable as possible with the approach of the interview meeting and evaluate if there are any thematic areas not investigated by the questions but that the person would like to address [4]. The person, in this first meeting, decides to whom to allocate the generative document. This will allow the DT to be directional and meaningful and not just an autobiographical tale. Personalizing the document, thinking of addressing someone in particular, helps to create a true and original document, without it appearing impersonal and vague [4]. In addition, the person can decide whether to do the therapy alone or together with a friend.

The interview Before the interview, it is important for the therapist to take care of preparing the setting, in order to make the DT similar to a chat in a welcoming, intimate, and safe environment that maximizes privacy and comfort. Of course, this goal is more likely to be achieved when DT takes place in the person's home rather than in a hospice or institutional setting. Before turning on the recorder, the therapist must make sure that the person no longer has questions for clarification to ask him [4]. At this point, the interview can begin; it is audio-recorded so that, on the one hand, the therapist can be genuinely and completely listening and, on the other hand, the words are really those spoken by the person (ibidem)/human experience and are closely linked to the sense of being a person, to the essence and deep self of the person [4]. The first questions refer to the person's biography and personal history:

- Tell me something about your history; in particular, the parts that have remained with her or which she considers most important.
- When did you feel most alive?
- Are there specific things you want your family members to know and specific things they would like them to remember?
- What were the most important roles in your life (e.g., family, professional, volunteer roles)? Why were they so important to you, and what results do you think you have achieved within these roles?
- What are your most important goals? What are you most pride of?

The following questions, on the other hand, investigate the most emotionally demanding part:

- Are there specific things that you feel the need to say to loved ones or things to repeat that you would like to take time for?
- What are your hopes and dreams for the people you love?
- What have you learned about life that you would like to pass on to others?
- What advice or address words would you like to convey to your/her/his/hers [son, daughter, husband, wife, parents, others]?
- Are there important words, or even instructions, that you would like to offer to family members?
- In creating this permanent legacy, are there other things you would like to see included?

During the interview, the "photo album technique" can be used to put the person at ease and promote memories. Choosing this visual approach creates a bubble of time around the person, in which she can immerse herself to recall the episodes and emotions of the memories of her life. This imaginary and mental photograph allows people to more easily describe the moments they remember and want to tell [4]. It is important that both the person and the therapist remain focused on the goal of DT, in order to create a cohesive and harmonious document. In addition, the therapist must make sure that the story is clear for those who will read it and, therefore, asking for some more details can favor contextualization and greater clarity of the events narrated. In conclusion to the interview, it is important to collect feedback from the person. We must always thank the person for the honor and privilege of having had the opportunity to hear those words: this is also a behavior in support of the dignity of the person. The exchange of memories with family members can take place before the interview meeting or after the interview but before the final (or almost) printing of the generative document. If the family member or friend is present during the interview, the therapist must be trained to manage the situation, so that the protagonist of the DT receives the necessary space to express himself and that the family member/friend only has the role as a facilitator [4].

Transcription and editing   It is the editor's task to organize the person's speech into a complete and cohesive text [1, 4]. The editing process is divided into four tasks or "primary phases" [4]:

1. Cleaning the transcript. It consists in eliminating the phrases that make the text more similar to conversation than to prose, for example. The unclear phrases typical of spoken language and the therapist's interventions are deleted.
2. The improvement of narrative clarity.
3. Correction of time sequences. Reading chronologically inconsistent text can threaten understanding.
4. The identification of an adequate conclusion.

Usually the generative document contains only the words spoken by the person, consequently the questions are also integrated into the text, in such a way as not to break the narrative and make it more like a story told than an interview. The editor must never forget that the last word belongs to the person, the protagonist of the path of DT and of the generative document; in this way the empowerment of the autonomy and self-determination of the person is supported, and nothing of the content of the document generative will be against his will [1].

Delivery meeting and corrections. In the third meeting, the edited text is presented to the person. The therapist reads the text aloud and then leaves room for the person to make any changes, corrections, clarifications, or additions, always listening to their wishes. Once the document is completed, the person can request as many copies as they wish. It may also happen that the person has no desire to leave it to someone in particular and therefore the document is added to the person's papers, together with documents, diaries, letters, etc.

Final meeting   In the fourth meeting, the completed and refined generative document is delivered to the person. The person delivers it to the recipient, and the feedback, impressions, and thoughts about the path just concluded are collected.

23.6   The Generative Document

The generative document preserves the most precious memories of the person. The generative document is something that remains and allows the person to leave a part of himself to his loved ones, the part they consider most important. Through this tool, the story of the person, as told by the person himself, remains alive in the memories of family members, and over time the words that he himself spoke echo.

The generative document is an opportunity to tell someone what you cannot express in person; it is a dialogue in which the person talks about what is most important to them, an opportunity for communication to introduce loved ones to new parts and different perspectives in the life of the author of the document. The generative document is usually created thinking about the person it is intended for. It happens, therefore, that the author may be worried about the reaction that the recipient might have. It is the therapist's job to help the person reread the document, perfecting and refining it, so that it adheres to the author's wishes and does not threaten the relationship he has with the loved one [4]. It is important that the therapist is trained and skilled in guiding people to avoid the possible negative consequences of DT, who is always vigilant about the contents that could cause suffering to those who remain (ibidem). The fact that the generative document is a written legacy offers the advantage of separating the person's words from the his image, which can be deteriorated by the course of the disease [4]. The DT and its final product give special words to the loved ones of the protagonist. The generative document is a tangible sign of the person's value and gives him the certainty that his thoughts and words are still worth listening to [9].

23.7   Acceptability and Satisfaction of the DT

The person's perspective. DT has proved to be a simple and useful tool in reflecting on the sense and meaning of the existence of the person involved in the therapy. However, it is not clear how it acts on the various characters who participate in it: first of all the person and then the family members and health personnel [11]. Research shows that most of the participants feel satisfied (91%) and consider DT useful or very useful for themselves and their families. More than 50% say that DT's intervention has increased their perception of well-being, dignity, hope. and purpose in life. About 47% report that DT has increased their desire to live [11]. People are welcomed into a safe space where they remember their life, an existence that has not always been characterized by suffering and illness. They remember their journey, the challenges they faced, and the values that guided them. They reflect on their history, and the development of themselves and share it with loved ones. The existential reflection that emerges from the interview and from the story of one's own story increases the sense of direction and purpose in the life of the person who takes part in it. Although the feelings and fears of being a burden to loved ones do not diminish, the person feels worthy of value and has the opportunity to "close one's business" and prepare to leave the world peacefully. DT allows you to capture the crucial moments of life and share them with those you love.

The perspective of family members. Most of the family members whose loved one participates in DT affirm the usefulness of the intervention for the patient. Nearly 70% say that DT increases a person's sense of dignity, the perception of a purpose in life, and general well-being [11]. Family members find a source of satisfaction and help in the generative document. This object is a comfort both in the present moment in which it is given to the family and in the future to face the death of the person; it becomes an anchor and a symbol of the life of a loved one, a beacon that gives meaning to an unspeakable and incomprehensible event such as the death of a loved one.

The generative document transmits the love and value of a life that was worth living; this therapy legitimizes life and gives an opportunity to put on paper what the person hopes is his legacy [4]. Through the generative document, the deceased is able to give support for the elaboration of mourning, because the recipient receives words from him that he can keep for life as a special gift (ibidem).

The therapist's and healthcare professional's perspective. DT not only supports end-of-life individuals and their families but helps care professionals perceive their work as meaningful and valuable [14]. Therapists benefit from DT as the path brings them emotionally closer to the person followed and promotes better understanding, increasing satisfaction with the chosen profession. All this increases the awareness of their work and the quality of the care provided.

23.7.1 PDQ (Patient Dignity Question)

Dignity can be increased by respecting the person's values and preferences, i.e., when importance is given to the person's voice and decisions through the patient dignity question (PDQ). This is a simple and open question: "What do I need to know about you as a person to give you the best possible care?" Research has shown that this single question can identify problems and stressors that may be important to consider when planning care. The intent is to reveal "invisible" factors that may not otherwise come to light and identify the patient's concerns early in the care process. The question about the dignity of the patient is useful during every phase of care and treatment, and anyone who works in health care can consider the question as it helps to provide adequate care to people and their families. The intent is to involve everyone in the healthcare community by thinking of patients as unique human beings, rather than just focusing on a specific disease or set of symptoms. Dignity care does not just refer to interventions and actions that may involve interaction, but it also extends to the way the healthcare professional thinks about the patient and the attitude with which they carry out these support actions [8]. Care can never be standardized, because each person is unique, and it is important to value their personal path, but it is important to find guidelines that can help health professionals in their delicate accompanying work (ibidem). Interventions in support of the dignity of the person should be calibrated after a careful analysis of which stressors influence and weaken a person's sense of dignity, and each action must be tailored around the person to whom it is addressed. It is important that in the planning of the interventions, the person has a voice to express their ideas about the treatment path of which he is the protagonist. Relieving symptoms with drug and nondrug therapy (such as meditation, massage, and relaxation) and taking care of the person's general comfort, for example, through hygiene and bed position, are effective strategies to reduce the impact of symptoms on the suffering of the person (symptom distress) (ibidem). Clear communication on the type of intervention and the possible outcomes decreases the psychological distress resulting from medical uncertainty and fear of death, so that both the patient and family can anticipate and prepare to face illness and death without losing hope and serenity [8]. The balance between truthtelling and therapeutic hope is important and, therefore, understanding how much the person is willing to listen and accept (ibidem). Contrary to what one might think, open and sincere communication, without exceeding in frankness, helps people to reflect and express their experiences regarding diagnosis and prognosis (ibidem). Dialogue, the exchange of ideas and concerns and empathic listening promote a person's awareness of existential issues, reassuring and allowing them to calmly face the last phase of life. It is good to remember that familiarity is a strength for maintaining and enhancing the independence of the person (level of independence). Words, places, people, and family routines help the person not to feel stranger in his environment and offer a quiet, familiar, silent place, with the possibility of keeping a pet, improves the person's sense of privacy [8]. At the base of these interventions, there is a deep knowledge of the person and his history, possible only thanks to a genuine interest and curiosity that lead to communication and careful and person-centered dialogue (ibidem). To maintain and support the independence of the person, it is important to find the right balance between the active care of the person by the healthcare staff, and the space cut out within the daily routine so that the person himself actively takes care of himself, balancing the risk of taking the place of the person by making him feel passive experiences and the opposite risk of neglecting him, arousing in him feelings of abandonment. Living at home or in hospice has proved not to be a determining factor: familiarity and hospitality can also be achieved in healthcare facilities, as, moreover, the risk of passivity and the feeling of "being cast aside" can characterize even the home environment if family members are not first trained and adequately informed [8]. Helping the person to maintain their role (maintenance of pride) means allowing patients to participate in activities that are meaningful to them, and this is possible only if one undertakes to know the person's history, tastes, hobbies, and interests [8]. Whenever the health and care staff approaches the person-patient, it is important that they transmit respect for the person and for his age, fostering a sense of personal pride and dignity; these attentions make the person feel important and worthy [8]. In fact, in the life of people with a disease that threatens their lives, small things matter a lot: the name by which the person wishes to be called, the courtesy of the medical staff, and the possibility of chatting and laughing in company increase the sense of importance. of the person, the perception of control helping to maintain a routine of "normalcy" (ibidem). The person can exercise control (autonomy/control) as often as he has a "say in the matter," choosing to accept interventions and requesting the assistance of others and organizing his activities on the basis of new priorities [8]. As for the aspect of spirituality, physical contact and attention on the part of the health and care staff favor the person's reflection on their relationship with spirituality. This also means the ability to forgive and be forgiven, to settle meaningful relationships, family, and friends. In the field of spirituality, it is important to listen to the patient, to be curious and interested in his history and the most significant aspects of his life, and to be with him on his existential journey [8]. In order to address this, healthcare professionals must be trained and prepared to have conversations with patients about existential issues and the meaning and significance of life. Staff training, therefore, is of fundamental importance so that they are able to stay close to the patient even during the last months or days: in fact, lower levels of "vital exhaustion" and depression of staff derive from the awareness of their role, at the same time increasing the perception of self-efficacy (ibidem). To favor the proximity of friends and relatives, it is important to adopt an organization that facilitates contacts thanks to wide and flexible visiting hours and through technologies such as letters, telephone, and the Internet. The possibility of having photographs of people or significant moments for the person also increases the feeling of belonging to a community [8]. To increase social support, it is important to favor the presence of the family and support in care, to be available to provide information on the patient's health, and to work with the family to favor the elaboration of the situation and reflection on death, as well as communication of emotions and feelings regarding the situation and fear of death between family and patient (ibidem).

23.8 Dignity Therapy Outside Palliative Care

When dignity therapy is applied outside the context in which it was born, particular attention is needed to the inclusion criteria of the people to whom it is addressed to ensure that the therapy does not cause harm. Below are some researches that have led DT beyond the oncology field. There are usually no impediments of an emotional or mnemonic nature that hinder the completion of DT: people, whose disease is in the early stage of development, know how to remember the important things they want to talk about and give as a personal inheritance to loved ones [12]. However, the help of family members acquires importance in the event that there are communication difficulties, for example, the family members of people diagnosed with advanced dementia can help shape some answers [4].

DT with elderly people in a nursing home. Starting from the evidence that low levels of perception of one's dignity are associated with high levels of psychological and spiritual distress and the loss of the will to live, some studies have proposed DT to elderly people living in a care facility, with an objective of verifying the effectiveness of DT in improving the quality of life of institutionalized elderly people [7, 11]. The results show that the sense of dignity increases after a week after surgery, although it does not remain constant over time, while the levels of hope and quality of life remain high. In conclusion, the dignity therapy is a feasible, effective, and desirable intervention to improve the quality of life and well-being of both the elderly person and his family (ibidem).

DT with older people with mild cognitive impairment (MCI) or with an onset of dementia. Some studies affirm that it is desirable to propose palliative care starting from the diagnosis, that is, from the moment in which the person with a poor prognosis is taken care of. Dementia is a disease that limits the life of individuals and for this reason the person suffering from it can benefit from a path of palliative care. DT offers the possibility to the person to feel himself again, be understood, be accepted, and accept himself for who he is, increasing the perception of purpose and meaning of his life [12]. The well-being of the person with early-stage dementia can be threatened by changes in relationships with family and friends, the sense of loneliness, the inevitability of the course, and the loss of hope that lead to an ever-increasing and terrifying perception of detachment, both from the true self and from significant others (ibid.). Dignity therapy can offer these people the opportunity to enclose their values and important memories in a "time capsule," which escapes the inexorable deterioration brought about by the disease (ibidem). Johnston et al. [12] investigated the efficacy of DT in reducing the psychophysical and spiritual stress of people in the early stages of a diagnosis of dementia, improving their quality of life. Research demonstrated its feasibility, acceptability, and effectiveness. The World Health Organization (WHO) declares that people with dementia are extremely fragile and too often their rights are overruled [12]: the culture you want disseminating through the models of palliative care is a culture attentive to people in the most fragile and vulnerable phases of their lives, affirming the intrinsic value of the human being [4]. Some participants in the study [12] stated that if DT had been conducted while they were still at home and not in a facility suitable for welcoming people with their disease, they would probably have felt more at ease and more willing to do the introspection that DT requires. They would have found themselves in a familiar and protected environment, surrounded by objects that witness their history. For this reason, it could be important to propose DT in the very early stages of dementia disease, thus going against the common thought that DT is aimed at those who are about to die [4, 12]. Despite this, DT was welcomed positively by the people invited, by family members, and by health personnel as it improved communication and relationships between people. Participants spoke freely about themselves and the most intimate and precious details and were willing to be guided in the exploration of their history [12]. In these cases, as people diagnosed with dementia are not at the end of their life, it happens that the generative document is not the final document: the person has the opportunity to add photos, letters, additional material, and new thoughts to it [12]. In this way the generative document can be seen as an evolving document, available to the person to fix and bequeath the most important thoughts.

In conclusion, many family members, after experiencing DT, pointed out that if DT had been proposed in the early stages of the disease, when the care-recipient was able to better communicate their thoughts and emotions, perhaps the person would have benefited more [16].

References

1. Fitchett G, Emanuel L, Handzo G, Boyken L, Wilkie DJ. Care of the human spirit and the role of dignity therapy: a systematic review of dignity therapy research. BMC Palliat Care. 2015;14(1):8.
2. De Beni R, Borella E, editors. Psicologia dell'invecchiamento e della longevità. Italy: Il Mulino; 2015.
3. Venturiero V, Tarsitani P, Liperoti R, Ardito F, Carbonin P, Bernabei R, Cambassi C. Cure palliative nel paziente anziano terminale. G Gerontol. 2000;48(4):222–46.
4. Chochinov HM. Terapia della dignità. In: Moretto G, Grassi L, editors. Parole per il tempo che rimane. Roma: Il Pensiero Scientifico Editore; 2015.
5. Chochinov HM, Hack T, Hassard T, Kristjanson LJ, McClement S, Harlos M. Dignity in the terminally ill: a cross-sectional, cohort study. Lancet. 2002;360(9350):2026–30.
6. Hall S, Edmonds P, Harding R, Chochinov H, Higginson IJ. Assessing the feasibility, acceptability and potential effectiveness of dignity therapy for people with advanced cancer referred to a hospital-based palliative care team: study protocol. BMC Palliat Care. 2009b;8(1):5.
7. Hall S, Chochinov H, Harding R, Murray S, Richardson A, Higginson IJ. A phase II randomised controlled trial assessing the feasibility, acceptability and potential effectiveness of dignity therapy for older people in care homes: study protocol. BMC Geriatr. 2009a;9(1):9.
8. Östlund U, Brown H, Johnston B. Dignity conserving care at end-of-life: a narrative review. Eur J Oncol Nurs. 2012;16(4):353–67.
9. Chochinov HM. Dignity and the eye of the beholder. J Clin Oncol. 2004;22(7):1336–40.
10. Julião M, Barbosa A, Oliveira F, Nunes B, Carneiro AV. Efficacy of dignity therapy for depression and anxiety in terminally ill patients: early results of a randomized controlled trial. Palliat Support Care. 2013;11(6):481–9.
11. Martínez M, Arantzamendi M, Belar A, Carrasco JM, Carvajal A, Rullán M, Centeno C. 'Dignity therapy', a promising intervention in palliative care: a comprehensive systematic literature review. Palliat Med. 2017;31(6):492–509.
12. Johnston B, Lawton S, McCaw C, Law E, Murray J, Gibb J, et al. Living well with dementia: enhancing dignity and quality of life, using a novel intervention, dignity therapy. Int J Older People Nursing. 2016;11(2):107–20.
13. Vuksanovic D, Green HJ, Dyck M, Morrissey SA. Dignity therapy and life review for palliative care patients: a randomized controlled trial. J Pain Symptom Manag. 2017;53(2):162–70.
14. Puchalski CM, Jafari N. Acknowledging the person in the clinical encounter: whole person care for patients and clinicians alike. Commentary on Chochinov et al. J Pain Symptom Manage. 2015;49(6):973.
15. Chochinov HM, McClement S, Hack T, Thompson G, Dufault B, Harlos M. Eliciting personhood within clinical practice: effects on patients, families, and health care providers. J Pain Symptom Manag. 2015;49(6):974–80.
16. Aoun SM, Chochinov HM, Kristjanson LJ. Dignity therapy for people with motor neuron disease and their family caregivers: a feasibility study. J Palliat Med. 2015;18(1):31–7.

The Role of the General Practitioner in the Last Developmental Task of the Elder People About Death, Identity, Narratives and Dignity

Ines Testoni

Abstract

Contemporary Western society resists any form of existential reflection on the fact that we are mortal, whereas the media represent death as an exceptional event that takes place in situations that are very far from everyday realities. Some negative effects derive from this cultural removal. In the last decades, the debates surrounding death have taken on greater importance in both clinical and academic fields. Older people often die in retirement homes. The cultural denial of death means that tools and structured paths are rarely prepared to equip them with appropriate instruments. This chapter presents the concept of the last developmental task, which is a time when the elder people should reconstruct their sense of existence. In particular, it is considered how the dignity of the older persons can be enhanced by the general practitioner. In fact, the general practitioner is a central figure in the care of older people, because he knows their medical history and has often established a relationship of trust with them. Dignity therapy represents a valid instrument for helping terminally ill patients. The possibility for the general practitioner of utilising it with elder people has been hypothesised. In fact, the psychological literature has already shown how narrative methodologies facilitate talking about the past as a function of the future, even when one is facing death. Being able to narrate the trials that one has already overcome and remembering how the difficulties that have been overcome have affected the future may help one think beyond death.

I. Testoni (✉)
FISSPA Department, University of Padova, Padova, Italy
e-mail: ines.testoni@unipd.it

© Springer Nature Switzerland AG 2022
J. Demurtas, N. Veronese (eds.), *The Role of Family Physicians in Older People Care*, Practical Issues in Geriatrics, https://doi.org/10.1007/978-3-030-78923-7_24

Keywords

Dignity therapy · Denial of death · Terror management theory · Developmental
tasks · Narratives

24.1 Introduction

The general practitioner is often a crucial reference point in the lives of older people,
even when they are approaching death. However, the relationship with people
approaching death requires special attention and the ability to manage the relationship with competence and empathy. Psychology may offer important suggestions to
help general practitioners in this task, first of all explaining some aspects of individual transformation in the cycle of life. In fact, the problem is that in contemporary
culture, the last phase is always considered a mere decline, because of the general
resistance to any form of existential reflection on the fact that we are mortal [1]. All
this has been abundantly illustrated by the researchers who posited terror management theory (TMT) to explain why individuals and societies are so psychologically
focused on producing situations and artefacts that distract them from reflecting on
transience. TMT's explanation is based on the assumption that humans, like all forms
of life, are biologically predisposed toward self-preservation in the service of survival. However, they are equipped with two particularly important adaptive capacities: a high degree of self-awareness and the capacity to think in terms of past, present
and future. On the one hand, these characteristics give people a high degree of flexibility that helps them stay alive, but on the other hand, they also produce the extraordinarily unsettling realisation that death is inevitable and that it is generally
unpredictable and uncontrollable. The awareness that death is inevitable and makes
people psychologically vulnerable because of their consciousness that they are tran-
sitory creatures in a passing universe in turn produces potentially paralysing existential terror and despair. Therefore, humans banish death from their consciousness and
shield themselves from existential terror by embracing cultural worldviews that help
them keep death anxiety under control, removing it at an unconscious level [2].

Moreover, after the Second World War, thanks to peace and the increasingly
systematic respect for fundamental human rights, the levels of well-being in the
West have grown exponentially compared to previous centuries, and people's life
expectancy has proportionally expanded. The result is that our capacity to postpone
death grows in direct proportion to our inability to cope with it and then the conceal-
ment of death runs parallel with a notable increase in the preoccupation with physical perfection and in the scientific urge to explain, measure and control everything.
People want to live longer, but they also want to remain youthful, so death is increasingly considered a failure, and the weakening of the body, the natural consequence
of ageing, has been interpreted as an imperfection. In this milieu, the denial of death
is also distanced from social life through the displacement of cemeteries from inter-
urban areas to the outskirts of cities and the increased practices of ash dispersion
after the cremation of the body [3].

All this means that general practitioners work in a community that has lost the sense of solidarity with those who grow old and those who die. Indeed, when people become seriously ill or have to cope with the effects of old age, they are abandoned. As Norbert Elias ([4], p. 10) clearly pointed out, nowadays, one of the more general problems is our inability to give dying people the help and affection they need, because another's death is a reminder of our own. As TMT points out, people build a wall against the idea of their own deaths by distancing themselves from the dying. Behind an overwhelming need to believe in one's own health, beauty and success, there is the need to deny the foreknowledge of one's own death, which the vision of the sick and the elder persons calls into question, forcing people to remember that 'I was what you are and you will be what I am now'.

24.2 Harm Reduction of Ageing

The harm reduction model is a public health policy designed to reduce the negative consequences associated with various human conditions. Usually it is related to the management of social behaviours that can create negative effects in people who adopt risky behaviours such as recreational drug use and sexual activity. We use such an expression in this context rhetorically to evoke the generalised perception that ageing is the result of an unhealthy way of managing life. However, it is one paradoxical effect arising from the systematic denial of death. In the last few decades, the debates surrounding this problem have taken on greater importance in both clinical and academic fields. In fact, this phenomenon has produced generations of families who have abandoned the rituals of the memory of their ancestors and at the same time are unable to manage serious illnesses, the elder people and dying processes at home. This mentality has made it common to abolish old age, for either health or aesthetic reasons, as if eliminating this period would permit us to live forever, or at least to live within that illusion [5] (Box 24.1).

> **Box 24.1 Geropsychology**
> Geropsychology focuses on the study of ageing and the provision of clinical services for older adults, expanding knowledge of the normal ageing process and designing interventions to help older persons and their families overcome problems, enhance Well-being and achieve maximum potential during later life. Traditionally, this field has focused on solving late-life difficulties that can result in depression and anxiety arising from coping with physical health problems and caring for a disabled spouse or grieving the death of loved ones [6]. In fact, addressing these problems results in decreased emotional suffering and improved quality of life for older adults and their families. Geropsychologists usually provide services to older adults in a variety of settings, including healthcare facilities, community-based private or group practices and places where older adults reside. Geropsychologists collaborate with other professionals, including medical and mental healthcare service providers, to ensure their clients are given comprehensive care.

However, one of the most important and recent areas of research is inherent to the management of death-related thoughts in elder persons, especially when they are recovering in long-term care and assisted-living facilities or hospices. The general practitioners have to intervene with a particular ability in managing death-related topics, which have been widely shunned in everyday communication and relationships. Indeed, in the families they have to face the phenomenon called 'conspiracy of silence', which indicates an incapacity of relatives to raise the issue of death with people who are at the end of their lives [7]. The main concern that causes this effect is the fear of activating death anxiety and dynamics that cause depression in elder and dying people. This is the consequence of the removal of the memento mori, which means 'do not forget that you have to die'. It has been practised throughout the history of humanity, thanks to which the concepts inherent to the relationship between life and death were transmitted to the individual by the group through rites of passage. The elimination of all this has also removed the task of taking responsibility for educating individuals about the concepts of death and dying. Nowadays, retirement homes are not only places of healing—they have begun to have the secondary function of receiving the dying as places where death has lost much of its ritual and ceremony. They are often places where older people die, and, because of the cultural denial of death, they are rarely prepared to equip them with appropriate tools.

Indeed, what TMT studies further highlight is that although such removal dynamics allow people to live more peacefully and be more productive, since death is inevitable, the systematic exclusion of reflection on finitude produces unconscious outcomes that are not always adaptive. Among these is the social inability to give meaning to the last phase of life. The key concept that Western people have lost is inherent to the last developmental task, which it is necessary to restore.

24.3 The Last Developmental Task and Suicide Among the Elder People

Psychology adopts an ontogenetic perspective, according to which individuals change incessantly until their deaths, respecting phases influenced both by interaction with the environment and by individual genetic and psychosomatic components. Each stage keeps track of the previous ones, so that the transformations of childhood precede those of adolescence and old age retains in itself the traces of the child, the adolescent and the adult as a background. According to Erik Erikson's bio-psychosocial perspective, each step is an opportunity for growth, made possible by the resolution of crises that from time to time arise from the loss of certainties. Maturity is guaranteed by the ability to face new challenges [8] (Box 24.2).

Box 24.2 Developmental Tasks

Erikson explains this idea by taking up the concept of the 'developmental task'. Proposed for the first time by Robert J. Havighurst [9], the developmental task posits that in certain periods of growth, there are specific trials, the overcoming of which allows individuals to reach a higher stage of maturation. Havighurst's research developed a highly influential theory of human education, and the crown jewel of his research was his taxonomic model, which defines the stages of maturation throughout the cycle of individual life. Erikson further states that, preceded by seven phases that allow achieving the ability to trust, to hope, to want, to set goals, to learn, to build identity and to love, the final goal of old age is to complete the narrative plot of one's personal history. Indeed, the last stage depends on the previous one, the adult age, characterised by 'generativity', the ability to overcome selfishness and harmonise the needs of personal well-being with those of others. This is the longest phase in which intimate relationships, work and social network continually impose new duties and responsibilities. But at the turn of one's sixties, at the peak of personal realisation, the last stage begins, marked by the inevitable decline. Many previously unresolved issues may reoccur, jeopardising the success of the most difficult and important evolutionary task, which, according to Erikson, consists of knowing how to maintain one's own identity and resolve moments of despair to arrive at the most significant port of self-transcendence: wisdom.

Society is unable to manage the issues inherent both to the last developmental task and to death because healthcare professionals worry about provoking negative thoughts in people, especially in the elder people. On the contrary, in this age group, the search for the meaning of existential issues involving death is very heated, and the inhibition that is the consequence of the social inability to consider such issues does not help them [10]. The lack of a participatory language that can prepare artefacts suitable for supporting those who are heading towards retirement from the world takes away from them the symbolic tools necessary to reach the last goal of their biography with a full sense of self-realisation and completeness. In the presence of the impossibility of communicating with others about significant issues of life, the objectives of the last evolutionary task can be difficult to pursue. In this scenario, life may therefore appear to be meaningless, and suicide may suddenly acquire a salient value.

Furthermore, because of their evocation of mortality, elder persons are often alone, and among the factors that inspire the desire to die are loneliness, a sense of abandonment, existential fatigue and loss of dignity [11]. The risk of suicide in this group of people is widely described in the literature [12]. Recent studies have shown that there is a strong correlation between isolation, loneliness and mortality. It has also been shown that those who are isolated feel lonely, but those who perceive loneliness isolate themselves, and those who are and feel lonely die first or prefer to die more than those who have a network of significant relationships [13]. Another risk factor for suicide is the result of isolation and poor communication with others that causes depression, which is linked to disorders with various effects: reactive anxiety caused by awareness of being on the way to the sunset or as a result of fatigue caused by active therapies accumulated over time or in progress, metabolic disorders, physiological deficiencies and so on.

For older people, all this is experienced in conjunction with the perception of loss of dignity, resulting from the lack of autonomy and identity crisis. A fundamental objective of psychosocial intervention is therefore above all preventing such a level of discouragement, allowing the maintenance of a possibility of dialogue with others that guarantees the elder persons the recognition of their own identity and of belonging to a significant network of relationships. It is therefore important to know that to promote an authentic prevention of the suicidal desire of the aged people, it is necessary to work specifically on this psychosocial dimension, which is characterised by an intrinsic complexity that should not be underestimated.

To the extent that it is important to keep the older people from falling into depression, it is necessary to promote their agency through the valorisation of their identity and biography. The model of patient engagement may help in this regard.

24.4 The Relational Dimensions of Dignity

At the end of life, people want to die instead of prolonging their lives because living is unbearable. In the area of oncology, Harvey Max Chochinov wanted to investigate the phenomenon of euthanasia requests in relation to depression, the consequences of somatic transformations, pain and lack of social and family support. His studies have demonstrated the significance of these elements in the perception of loss of dignity and the desire for death [14]. The essential aspect for the protection of dignity and positive self-representation of oneself is the protection of personal identity. To the extent that it is maintained, it makes possible the final attainment of wisdom, that is, of the capacity generated by the relationship between what has been learned in the experiences already lived and the meaning of suffering, without this affecting the sapiential heritage previously conquered.

It is therefore necessary to know how to recognise the factors that put the identity of the sick in crisis to intervene with appropriate psychological support. Broadly speaking, three styles characterise the perception of dignity: the dynamic equilibrium, after an initial decline in the sense of dignity due to decay caused by illness or age, is followed by a process of adaptation to the situation through the redefinition of objectives and the enhancement of aspects of daily life that can still be managed; the downward trend is instead characterised by the inability to restore a satisfactory level of dignity, a strong regret for lost abilities and the desire to accelerate death; and stability is achieved when the sense of dignity remains intact because personal identity is anchored to values not necessarily linked to performance or physical characteristics. These paths therefore highlight how much the concepts of identity and self-esteem play a central role in the advancement of the evolutionary tasks that lead to the last stage of self-transcendence. Chochinov et al. [14] have focused precisely on the causes that in these three trajectories lead the sick to choose death instead of life. By conducting qualitative studies with patients with advanced cancers, the Canadian psychiatrist investigated the factors that threaten their sense of identity and personal dignity. Dignity-conserving care, i.e. the model of the dignity of the terminally ill, is composed of three themes: illness-related concerns; dignity-conserving repertoire (catalogue of dignity conservation); and social dignity inventory (inventory of social dignity) [14] (Box 24.3).

Box 24.3 Chochinov's Model

Chochinov's model can be very useful for the general practitioner. In fact, Chochinov highlights the relationships between causes related to the condition of the patient and those related to intimate and social relationships, showing how suicidal ideation develops in those who perceive themselves as hopeless, do not accept physical change and feel that they are a burden to others and depend by them and that they are treated without respect [14]. The importance of Chochinov's contribution is related to the valorisation of the biographical narratives. Indeed, sick persons often do not accept their loss of power over themselves and their own world [15], especially when they have developed a sense of intrinsic dignity based on abilities, self-esteem and autonomy [16]. The loss of certain constituent traits of the self is in fact interpreted as a disintegrative loss of individual identity. The theory of self-discrepancy [17] shows how the contrast between the real self and the ideal self (what people would like to be) and the normative self (what they perceive themselves as 'having to be') inevitably causes negative effects on psychological well-being. The difference between the three dimensions is a source of anxiety (discrepancy between the real and normative selves) or sadness and depression (discrepancy between the real and ideal selves). When ill persons no longer recognise themselves because they no longer feel valued by others, they feel mortified because of the loss of continuity with their own biography. Then, the role of social support and confirmation in preventing this outcome is very important. In fact, society can support or make possible the construction and maintenance of a positive identity even in the most severe conditions of illness. The community can intervene especially when the sense of dignity is jeopardised by the identity crisis caused, on the one hand, by dying or elder persons' loss of functionality and control over their own bodies and therefore over the common actions of daily life and, on the other hand, by the fact that all this is also perceived by others, who can treat them as if they are children. All this is inevitably humiliating.

Chochinov coined an effective acronym to orient the components of health-care professionals towards the patient: the abecedary/ABCD. 'A' stands for the appropriate attitude, not influenced by prejudices, opinions or subjective deductions. 'B' stands for the good behaviour that transmits attention, respect, kindness and humanity. 'C' stands for compassion, understood as a deep awareness of the suffering of the other. Finally, 'D' stands for the dialogue that must be characterised by authenticity. The ability to communicate is therefore always the basis of a supportive care relationship with respect to the experience of loss of the older persons, and for the relationship not to be mortifying, people must know how to enter into its existential context by recognising the biographical depth [14]. Chochinov borrowed from Erickson the concept of constructing identity, understanding it as a process that continues throughout life through the consciousness of being oneself and the perception that others also recognise it. The maintenance of individual identity is essentially acquired through two types of recognition: primary social (determined by intimate emotional, family and friendly relationships on which personal and social trust depend) and secondary social (determined by social relationships based on roles, rights and duties) that is linked to the ability to cooperate and develop relationships of trust [18]. If, on the one hand, the construction of identity is a process that continues through various phases of life and does not concern a set of traits or characteristics permanently belonging to the person but rather a flexible organisation within which the self develops through crises and resolutions that occur in more or less relevant domains of life never definitively concluded, on the other hand, the ability to give meaning (meaning-making), especially in the face of negative experience, plays a crucial role. Jerome Bruner [19] shares this idea that identity is always a narrative process that unfolds within autobiographical reflection through a tale about the self that integrates the changes that have taken place over time and brings them back to a congruent logic.

The general practitioner should recognise moments of rupture and turning points of their patients, helping them face the transition between continuity and existential discontinuity, to perform the task of recomposing and redefining their current identity. In particular, this kind of relationship can help develop an authentic dialogue with the elder persons to permit them to reconstruct the line of all their life in the past and to open the trajectory of spirituality, through which it is possible to think about the future in another dimension.

24.5 Narratives of the Past for the Future to Improve the Last Developmental Task

Chochinov's model could help general practitioners reduce psychosocial-existential suffering, reactivating agency and the sense of dignity of their dying and elder patients. In particular his contribution may be very useful to support people who have to face death by redefining the essential features of their biographies. It is an approach that has taken its cue from different orientations, in particular from the psychology of life stories, with the aim of reviewing past experiences and successes to give meaning and purpose to the current condition, pivoting on the strong point of the narrative to strengthen self-esteem and start in the direction of the last step. Chochinov has named this intervention 'dignity therapy' (DT), which is a dialogue based on Carl Rogers' patient-centred approach [20] that specifically emphasises the therapists' ability to show themselves as authentic and real persons, able to reflect (mirroring) to the patients a complete image beyond their current condition of suffering. It is structured on 11 answers, and all the sessions—which run between 30 and 60 min—are transcribed and edited by the therapist together with the patient/elder person. The fully transcribed text must be read and modified according to the will of the sick person whenever necessary until its final edition. After this process, the 'generativity document' is returned to the patient/elder person to bequeath to a friend or family member. This procedure is particularly relevant because it activates the 'generativity/leaving' factor because the conversation is recorded and its contents are transcribed to create a final document that must be handed over to someone as a moral legacy. A very delicate moment of the therapy is when the text is delivered to the designated persons. If the therapist has been able to enter into the life of the elder people, orienting them to resolve their suspensions at least with their closest people, the generative document can finally be a valid tool for the further elaboration of the grief of the family members after the exitus [14].

Taking up the psychological contribution of Erikson and Bruner, other authors developed the idea that the elements that make up the identity of the self harmonise with each other, assuming the structure of the myth that the person recognises as his or her own and thanks to which he or she can feel unique [21]. The psychology of life stories helps us understand these narrative structures and listen to them without taking for granted anything of their semantic significance because they permit reflection on the personal history and past experiences in relationship to the present and the future. The geropsychologist is able to recognise different narrative styles to follow in a coherent way the narration by older people, who could use an informative style, typical of those who still try to reflect on themselves in the surrounding world; a normative style, assumed by those who strictly orient the meaning of life on the basis of certain values; or a widespread or avoiding style, typical of those who do not want to deal directly with problems and who make clear decisions [22] (Box 24.4).

Box 24.4 Hero's Journey

A good strategy that can help the narrators reconstruct their own identity at a time of crisis can be that of the 'hero's journey', which is widely used in creative writing. This narrative structure represents the symbolic path of the self to achieve self-realisation. The term was introduced by scriptwriter Christopher Vogler [23], who is searching for the success story for the construction of his own film plots. He came across Joseph Campbell's book [24] *The Hero with a Thousand Faces*, the result of research into fairy tales and legends. Vogler assumed such a structure, the archetypal one that allows outlining a 'monomite', i.e. a way in which, starting from an ordinary situation, a character recognises a call to change or is forced to abandon normality, falling into a situation of crisis in which he or she suffers pain and despair (*catabasis*) and then finds the way to liberation through various tests that, once overcome, allow him or her to begin the ascent (*anabasis*) until he or she reaches the true identity. In this narrative scenario, it is possible for the elder person to recover the deepest roots through which humanity has represented dying, within which they can recognise themselves and undertake the path of ascent.

24.6 Conclusions

Dignity therapy and the methodologies of narrative psychology may be useful to help general practitioners talk to their patients about the past as a function of the future even when they are facing death. Being able to talk about trials that have been overcome in the past and remembering how difficulties that have been overcome have had a future helps us think beyond death. In particular, dignity therapy has proven effective with cancer patients, but this model is increasingly used in other fields. In fact, some studies confirm that the narrative methods and in particular Chochinov's dignity model have the potential to improve well-being in older people in care homes, although this context is very different compared to the one in which dignity therapy was developed [25]. The few studies that have used DT in these contexts have demonstrated its feasibility, adequacy and acceptability for the elder person, caregivers and nurses [26] and its effectiveness in reducing the stress related to the loss of dignity and depressive symptoms, thereby improving the quality of life. DT helps elder patients regain the meaning and purpose of their lives and is a useful tool for their families [26]. Offering the opportunity to focus on the most significant episodes of their lives and emotionally charged events, DT contributes to rediscovering the meaning of existence, helping participants describe their perception of dignity. However, despite DT having such positive effects, one important issue should be considered with respect to this population of patients. In fact, the high prevalence of cognitive problems and the different timing of deterioration and disease trajectory may interfere with the elaboration of memories. Of course, it is important to consider this limitation in the elaboration of the generative document.

At the same time, it is necessary to evaluate accurately the applicability of the method to certain patients.

Furthermore, particular attention should be paid to the kind of biographies emerging from the generative document. In fact, when cognitive problems emerge, it is important to help elder persons transform their biographies into an evocation of a fully lived life, therefore rendering them capable of transmitting gratitude, good wishes and hopes to those who will receive the text. In fact, sad and painful narratives, which bring into play regrets and disappointments, could be linked to false memories and perhaps to recent and generalised negative experiences. In these cases, the role of the psychotherapist is to help the elder people understand what are really the last words he or she wants to leave in memory of him- or herself to those who will come after.

References

1. Testoni I, Lazzarotto Simioni J, Di Lucia Sposito D. Representation of death and social management of the limit of life: between resilience and irrationalism. Nutr Therapy Metab. 2013;31(4):192–8.
2. Solomon S, Testoni I, Bianco S. Clash of civilizations? Terror management theory and the role of the ontological representations of death in contemporary global crisis. Testing Psychom Methodol Appl Psychol. 2017;24(3):I379–98.
3. Testoni I, Di Lucia Sposito D, De Cataldo L, Ronconi L. Life at all costs? Italian social representations of end-of-life decisions after President Napolitano's speech—margin notes on withdrawing artificial nutrition and hydration. Nutr Therapy Metab. 2015;32(3):121–35.
4. Elias N. The loneliness of the dying. Oxford: Blackwell; 1982.
5. Testoni I, Parise G, Visintin EP, Zamperini A, Ronconi L. Literary plastination: from body's objectification to the ontological representation of death, differences between sick-literature and tales by amateur writers. Testing Psychom Methodol Appl Psychol. 2016;23(2):247–63.
6. Testoni I. Psicologia del lutto e del morire: dal lavoro clinico alla death education [The psychology of death and mourning: from clinical work to death education]. Psicoterapia e Scienze Umane. 2016;50(2):229–52.
7. Galantin LP, Natati L, Testoni I. Phenomenology of agony: a qualitative study about the experience of agony phenomenon in relatives of dying patients. Ann Palliat Med. 2019;8(5):542–50.
8. Erikson EH, Erikson JM. The life cycle completed. Extended version. New York: W. W. Norton & Company; 1998.
9. Havighurst RJ. Developmental tasks and education. Chicago: University of Chicago Press; 1948.
10. Testoni I, Iasella A, Ronconi L. Rappresentazione della morte e attitudine al suicidio nell'anziano. Considerazioni sulla prevenzione [Representation of death and attitude to suicide in the elderly. Considerations on prevention]. Psicologia Della Salute. 2002;2:103–19.
11. Lerner BH. Euthanasia in Belgium and the Netherlands: on a slippery slope? JAMA Intern Med. 2015;175(10):1640–1.
12. Oyama H, Koida J, Sakashita T, Kudo K. Community-based prevention for suicide in elderly by depression screening and follow-up. Community Ment Health J. 2004;40(3):249–63.
13. Beller J, Wagner A. Loneliness, social isolation, their synergistic interaction, and mortality. Health Psychol. 2018;37(9):808–13.
14. Chochinov HM. Dignity therapy. Final words for final days. New York: Oxford University Press; 2012.

15. Rodriguez-Prat A, Monforte-Royo C, Porta-Sales J, Escribano X, Balaguer A. Patient perspectives of dignity, autonomy and control at the end of life: systematic review and meta-ethnography. PLoS One. 2016;11(3):1–18.

16. van Gennip IE, Pasman HRW, Oosterveld-Vlug MG, Willems DL, Onwuteaka-Philipsen BD. Dynamics in the sense of dignity over the course of illness: a longitudinal study into the perspectives of seriously ill patients. Int J Nurs Stud. 2015;52(11):1694–704.

17. Higgins ET. Self-discrepancy theory: what patterns of self-beliefs cause people to suffer? In: Berkowitz L, editor. Advances in experimental social psychology, vol. 22. San Diego, CA: Academic; 2018. p. 93–136.

18. Honneth A. Recognition or redistribution? Changing perspectives on the moral order of society. Theory Cult Soc. 2001;8:2–3, 43–55.

19. Bruner J. The remembered self. In: Ulric Neisser E, Fivush R, editors. The remembering self: construction and accuracy in the self-narrative. Cambridge: Cambridge University Press; 1994.

20. Rogers CR. The basic conditions of the facilitative therapeutic relationship. In: Cooper M, O'Hara M, Schmid PF, Bohart AC, editors. The handbook of person-centred psychotherapy and counselling. 2nd ed. New York: Palgrave Macmillan; 2013.

21. McAdams DP. The stories we live by: personal myths and the making of the self. New York: William Morrow & Co.; 1993.

22. Berzonsky MD. Individual differences in self-construction: the role of constructivist epistemological assumptions. J Constr Psychol. 1994;7(4):263–81.

23. Vogler C. The writer's journey: mythic structure for writers. San Francisco: Michael Wiese Productions; 1992.

24. Campbell J. The hero with a thousand faces. Princeton University Press: Princeton, NJ; 1973.

25. Hall S, Goddard C, Opio D, Speck P, Higginson IJ. Feasibility, acceptability and potential effectiveness of dignity therapy for older people in care homes: a phase II randomized controlled trial of a brief palliative care psychotherapy. Palliat Med. 2012;26(5):703–12.

26. Hall S, Goddard C, Speck P, Higginson IJ. It makes me feel that I'm still relevant: a qualitative study of the views of nursing home residents on dignity therapy and taking part in a phase II randomised controlled trial of a palliative care psychotherapy. Palliat Med. 2013;27(4):358–66.

Family Physicians' Relationship with Older Patients Between Palliative Care and Advance Care Planning Management

25

Ines Testoni, Simone Cernesi, Federica Davolio, Marta Perin, Mariagiovanna Amoroso, Chiara Villani, and Jacopo Demurtas

Abstract

The general practitioner is increasingly called upon to deal with complex bio-ethical issues arising from chronic life-limiting illnesses or the chronicization of once rapidly lethal diseases. Among these, oncological, neurodegenerative, and cardiovascular diseases emerge for importance, but those linked to infections with a long terminal period, such as AIDS, cannot be underestimated. The end-of-life conditions of older people or of patients with sicknesses that have become

I. Testoni (✉)
FISPPA Department, University of Padova, Padova, Italy

Emili Sagol Creative Arts Therapies Research Center, University of Haifa, Haifa, Israel
e-mail: ines.testoni@unipd.it

S. Cernesi
Modena, Italy

F. Davolio
Infermiere Cooperativa Sociale Domus Assistenza, Modena, Italy

M. Perin
Clinical and Experimental Medicine PhD Program, University of Modena and Reggio Emilia, Modena, Italy

Bioethics Unit, Azienda USL-IRCCS di Reggio Emilia, Reggio Emilia, Italy

M. Amoroso · C. Villani
Società Italiana di Medicina Generale (SIMG) and Movimento Giotto, Firenze, Italy

J. Demurtas
Primary Care Department, USL Toscana Sud Est, Grosseto, Italy

© Springer Nature Switzerland AG 2022
J. Demurtas, N. Veronese (eds.), *The Role of Family Physicians in Older People Care*, Practical Issues in Geriatrics, https://doi.org/10.1007/978-3-030-78923-7_25

advanced, progressive, and/or incurable require a range of decisions that general practitioners should be able to manage.

The chapter considers the role of the family doctor in relation to the self-determination of the elderly and palliative care, also taking into account the role of the nurse. Particular attention is given to the international norms that place this field of care within the space of inalienable human rights, while the bioethical dimension is taken into account in relation to the legislative one, taking Italian legislation as an exemplary case.

Keywords

General practitioner · Family doctor · Nurse · Palliative care · Self-determination
End of life

25.1 Introduction

The end-of-life is a condition of great suffering for the patients and presents an important complexity for the general practitioner to manage. In fact, it imposes to the physician to face the decision-making process, the transfer of the patient to the palliative care system, the recognition, and the respect of the patients' right to self-determination [1, 2]. Often the challenge for the physicians consists especially in the management of ethics problems related to extraordinary or hazardous interventions [3]. This complex of issues is often linked to chronic or lethal diseases that therapies have chronicized, such as cancer, heart disease, AIDS, and neurodegenerative diseases, but it also involves the elder persons [4, 5]. Furthermore, in these situations, it may happen that the general practitioner has, on the one hand, to face dysfunctional or fragmented families unable to make decisions that respect the patient's wishes and values. Furthermore, today, there are not popular traditions that help people to manage the end of life, and then family members are uncertain what they can do when a beloved person is dying. On the other hand, one of the greatest difficulties is to understand whether, for example, patients with a serious neurodegenerative disease suffer and whether or not want to continue to be treated [6]. The resolution of these difficulties requires a careful management of the long therapeutic path from the very first steps of the treatment after the inauspicious diagnosis or during the same assessment of the aging decline [5].

To better manage all these kinds of problems, recently, in Western countries the enhancement of individual autonomy in medical decision-making at the end of life is widely growing. In fact, advance care planning (ACP), also named living wills, that are designed to document patients' preferences in case of the loss of their decision-making capacity, are legally admitted in the most civilized countries. The legal devices adopted for their promotion have been advocated as a means to enhance patient autonomy. This perspective was born as a need in the most technologically advanced countries, where the boundary between life and death is no longer natural and increasingly assigned to medical technologies. In Europe the cultural choice to defer decisions to the patient the willingness to undergo any medical treatment has been enshrined by the so-called Oviedo Convention, that is, the "Convention for the Protection of Human Rights and Dignity of the Human Being with regard to the Application of Biology and Medicine: Convention on Human Rights and Biomedicine" (ETS No 164), opened for signature on 4 April 1997 in Oviedo (Spain). This convention is particularly important because it is still the only international legally binding instrument for the protection of human rights in the biomedical field, and its focus is on fundamental and inalienable respect of individual dignity. The first aim is the protection of the dignity and the identity of all people, guaranteeing them respect for their integrity and freedoms with regard to the medical interventions. The countries which recognize this document officially declare that a patient's advanced request for a death with dignity should be respected and that persons forgoing and terminating life support are immune from legal liability [7].

The discussion on the rights of people at their end of life runs in parallel with the worldwide development of palliative care (PC), which interests not only patients with terminal severe illnesses but also older people.

The World Health Organization (WHO) definition of PC affirms that it is an approach that improves the quality of life of patients and their families facing the problem associated with end of life [8]. It is important to underline that PC provides liberation from pain and other distressing symptoms, considering death and dying as a normal process, neither hastening nor postponing its advent. A particular attention is paid to the dignity of patients or older people, and the intervention is especially focused on psychological and spiritual aspects, offering a parallel support system to help patients live as actively as possible until death. Furthermore, a specific support should be offered to help the family cope during the patients end of life and in their own bereavement [9].

Despite in the last decades PC is widely considered as a human rights issue that should be available for anyone suffering from moderate or severe pain or at the end of life, unfortunately many PC programs are either unavailable or inaccessible for some categories of patients. In particular, the United Nations Committee on Economic, Social, and Cultural Rights states a special attention should be paid for older people in parallel with chronically and terminally ill persons enabling them to die with dignity [10]. As this population grows incessantly in size, PC programs and ACP management will have to be developed to address their specific needs. Despite its importance, this kind of intervention is still guaranteed only to a limited number of sick persons, because of some cultural barriers, among which the ignorance of how they work, how they are arranged in health services, and how to access them. Among those who still benefit less from this service are the older and among the healthcare professions that more properly can remove this limit are family doctors.

25.2 The Family Physician's Role in the Management of Palliative Care and Advance Care Planning with Older People

The older persons and children, as well as other groups of people defined as vulnerable (prisoners, people with psychiatric problems, people living in economic poverty, LGBT people, etc.) have little access to PC. This difficulty depends on sociocultural issues, systemic difficulties, and partly organizational models. In Europe, still uneven training in PC often remains worker-dependent even in the countries of the Global North, with modern legislation. Rooted in the belief that this form of treatment is a perfect synonym for end-of-life care, this often implies late care that does not involve multidimensional interventions as well as insufficient symptom control. Indeed, the provision of PC in older non-oncological patients living with dementia and/or advanced renal failure and/or advanced heart failure is still largely deficient, because of the lack of well-defined prognostic criteria and studies specifically oriented in this direction.

The Special Rapporteur on the Right to Health of the UN Human Rights Council [11] highlights the necessity to overcome the inequity caused by the fact that older persons are less likely to receive palliative care. Despite literature on death education [12–20] and on the general public's growing interest in death and dying [21, 22] showing the growing interest in discussing the end-of-life issues, health systems of many countries are not yet able to guarantee an appropriate competence to physicians and nurses in this field in order to remove the obstacles that impede the provision of and access to palliative care to all those facing the end of life. Recently, scholars highlighted the central role of topics regarding death and dying, not only from a technical and operational point of view [23] but also from a first-person elaboration of stressful experiences for both physicians and nurses [24]. Indeed, the study of Noguera et al. [25], which considered PC courses in European Universities, showed how the situation is quite variegated and irregular. Some problems arise from this uncertainty, because it can negatively affect the professional coping skills [26]. Specifically, in the field of end of life and ACP, it is important that the ground competencies offer some elements pertaining to the psychological field. Among them, as indicated by the European Association for Palliative Care recommendations [27], issues concerning existential distress and suffering, psychosocial needs, religious beliefs, communication, teamwork, and self-reflection ability emerged [28].

Running in parallel with PC, the ACP is composed, on the one hand, by a document that provides instructions for the medical caregivers as to medical care desired by people incapable of advising the doctor due to lack of consciousness or other reasons, and, on the other hand, by the path of elaboration that produces this document, possibly in collaboration with the family physician. The document usually contains directions to cease providing or not provide life-sustaining medical treatment or equipment, and when the person is conscious, it does not supersede the instructions of the person. If such a document is absent, the health system is ethically and legally required to provide all means possible to keep a person alive, always respecting the principles of proportionality, fairness, and not malice. But often people don't want to deal with it when they ignore the prospect of death, because they consider it remote. Especially with older people, it is important to remove this obstacle and start planning with them in advance the possibility of managing the end-of-life contingencies.

The importance of the psychological preparation of physicians and nurses to manage end of life and ACP has been underlined by many authors, among whom Masuda et al. [29], who surveyed concerns about ACP from the physicians' point of view and who mentioned both positive and negative effects of the reflection on living wills. The most common concern that they described was inherent to the physicians' feelings that they needed to take into account. In particular they felt not completely able to recognize the patient's state of mind at the end of life, pointing out that patients might change their mind in the face of impending death and raised concerns about the stability of such advance decisions [29]. From their point of view, it was first of all necessary to ensure an excellent information with family members in order to set up a genuine positive relationship in the management of their loved one's end of life, and this was not always easy. Unfortunately, it has been widely pointed out that doctors elude the arguments that deal with death and that they are in great difficulty when they have to manage the breaking bad news [30, 31]. The ability to manage shared care planning such as the ACP implies first and foremost the ability of the doctor to communicate both diagnosis and prognosis in a correct and comprehensible way. The relationship with the older requires the same skill and the ability to prepare the older for the loss of function that will progressively lead to death [32]. In fact, the document expressing willingness to manage care at the end of life is not the sole objective of the ACP. Indeed, the planning of care may respect the patient engagement model, promoted by WHO [33] and replacing the outdated compliance model. The PEM is based on the active involvement of patients in their care process. It provides for the active involvement and empowerment of patients or the older as well as their family members, who must be made aware of every step in the care process and also manage their choices. The ability to accompany and guide patients, older, and family members in this negotiation process requires great attention and empathic sensitivity, as well as preparation with respect to the management of the therapeutic path.

Masuda et al. [29] evidenced as further significant concern the one related to the insufficient communication of the patient's preference to limit end-of-life care to the family and the family's subsequent insistence on care incompatible with the patient's directive. From this lack of authenticity, some confusion may derive, as happened in some cases when family members requested treatments such as cardiopulmonary resuscitation even though the patient had requested a natural death. Actually, the family doctor is the one who enters people's homes and is the one who can realize the real difficulties in which families can find themselves. This implies a particular sensitivity to the problems that both patients and family members may encounter in managing the decline of the older and their end of life.

Although people want to die at home, in fact in many cases, the older are at risk of being simply abandoned or ignored in relation to their needs. The family doctor is precisely the one who can plan the best accompanying pathway with family members, who can also provide for hospitalization in a nursing home, where a sector dedicated to palliative care has been set up. All this requires a great deal with communicative skills. Despite many psychological instruments useful to manage the prediction of the decline leading to death, such as the "surprise question" [34], and how to prepare the patient and the older to face this path serenely [35], at the moment in many countries, it is still very rare for family doctors to take on the task of accompanying their patients along this path.

25.3 General Practitioner Between Palliative Care and Anticipated Care Planning with Terminal III Patients

Palliative care improve the quality of life for terminal patients or with chronic life-limiting illnesses, and older persons, who need multiple more or less specialist interventions. Since they are often the first point of call for this kind of patients, GPs play a key role in providing palliative care and support in the end of life. Indeed, they are the closest to family life, since they have built up a significant relationship with them for years. Such a form of relationship permits to family physicians to provide maximum support and care, in every kind of pathologies and settings. In fact, they can constantly follow-up their patients until the end of life, assuming the role of bridge in the different places of care, from home to hospital, hospice, and nursing home [36, 37], whereas ineffective communication may result in a bad pain and symptom management, in increased psychological distress, and insufficient knowledge concerning patients' preferences; on the contrary, good end-of-life communication permits patients understanding of their condition and treatment options, facilitating informed participation in decision-making, and involving the family members [38]. Furthermore, this capability is particularly significant because general practitioners can communicate and coordinate with other medical specialists, who are able to develop a time-limited relationship with the patients. Often, this time limit adversely affects the relationship and the psychological dimension of the patient, so the family doctor's mediation can be extremely valuable to optimize the specialistic treatments and the palliative care. In this perspective, they can provide extended care through the coordination of other resources between the different hospital wards, the hospice, and home, involving nurses, physiotherapists, psychologists, and social workers [39].

However, patients with chronic life-limiting illnesses experience complex symptoms and care needs.

The end-of-life decision-making process requires that psychological distress, which is common among people needing palliative care, is correctly managed by someone who has earned the trust of the dying patient and his family. The various trajectories of physical decline are very difficult to plan for in advance because of its unpredictability. However, patients want to discuss these issues with their healthcare professionals and often find the reluctance of doctors who dislike to raise the issue of planning for death because of fear of destroying hope. The relational history set up with the family allows general practitioners to know both the patients' personality and the way they view death, tailoring on their psychological instances the discussion on the treatments.

If all this characterizes especially the oncological pathologies, the situation in neurology diseases is really more complicated. Certainly, end-of-life decision-making in the context of advanced neurology disease is a complex challenge for patients and health professionals [40–42]. In such situations, advance care planning should be encouraged through the discussion with patients on their preferences in some form of an advance directive as soon as the diagnosis is communicated, that is before their physical and cognitive decline. Since not all countries have legislation allowing life-sustaining treatments such as nutritional support or noninvasive ventilation to be suspended, even when patients so wishes, it would be better that this operation occurred prior to starting them. Also in these situations, the issues should be primarily discussed with the general practitioners, since they know in the best way their patients. The ACP discussions may facilitate the offer information reflecting the evolving course of the neurology disease and permit patients to become aware of the more desirable solutions [43, 44]. The situation is more difficult in the case of dementia. The typical evolution of patients suffering from dementia follows a period of progressive decline in functional and mental capacity before death. However, the long-term relationship between general practitioners and their patients is the ideal context for introducing the subject and starting the decision-making process before the patient loses the self-awareness, that is, before time-critical situations occur [45].

25.4 Nurses' Collaboration with the Family Doctor for the Patient Engagement

Some well-established models for the functioning of the care provided by the family doctor require him/her to be supported by one or more nurses, who are able to provide care to patients according to his/her indications. The importance of this figure is essential, as the assistance and the care work in the home are particularly valuable, especially with the older and the chronically ill approaching the end of life. In fact, palliative care networks guarantee a specific home intervention, but given the current lack of functioning in this area, at the moment it is still and mainly the family doctor and his nurse who can make up for basic palliative interventions. Being also the family doctor who knows the medical history of his patients is also the one who can act as a link between specialist services for active care and the second-level palliative care team. This requires that the work of family doctors and nurses who work with them be set up as part of a network of interventions able to offer home care to the older, the chronically ill, and the dying. In fact, the specialistic PC team may find in this basic nucleus the fundamental ground of knowledge to approach the sick person and his family. Patient engagement is already considered as a fundamental part of healthcare and a critical component of safe people-centered services. Engaged patients are better able to make informed decisions about their care options

[33]. In most Western countries, primary care is often the first point of contact of patients with the healthcare system. This means that the family doctor offers are the starting point for any possible engaging patients throughout their further contact with the health system. Since patients have well-being as a primary aim considering this as a priority in the healthcare they receive, a good process of engagement may promote mutual accountability and understanding between them and the physicians' work. In this process, the work of nurses who collaborate with family physicians may be a valid resource that can facilitate the management of responsiveness and transparency in the ACP process. They can engage older and terminally ill patients in the decision-making process, paying attention to the possible substantial variations in preferences for such involvement. Indeed, following the contact of family doctors, nurses can be ideally placed to engage patients in a dialogue about their health conditions, needs, and personal values and preferences. Whether the previous communication with the physician was clear, and reliable, older persons as patients are more likely to feel confident to report both positive and negative experiences and have increased concordance with mutually agreed care management plans [33].

As indicated by literature [46], the work nurses with family doctors for the promotion of the patient and family engagement not only improves health outcomes but also advances learning and improvement, while reducing adverse events and the following critical incidents.

25.5 A Bioethical Note

A final reflection must be made with respect to the bioethical discussion on this topic, understood as an ethical reflection that aims to promote the humanization of the health field by placing the person, his values, and the choices that derive from them at the center [47, 48]. In this context, bioethics focuses on the centrality of the person and the meaning of the choices related to the individualized care path, making as an integral part of the clinical judgment the ability to make a choice and to justify it from a moral point of view. Specifically, Italian legislation is very attentive to this aspect, and law 219/2017 (art. 1) states that "the relationship of care and trust between patient and doctor (…) in which the patient's decision-making autonomy and the competence, professional autonomy and responsibility of the doctor are met" [49]. Therefore, the care relationship does not presuppose a simple meeting of two "absolute" moral agents but a relational autonomy (where) instead of practical reason, communicative reason takes over [50]. We cite this law, because it is able to take on the most delicate and complex aspects of the healing relationship before death. Actually, it takes as its foundation the Barcelona declaration, according to which the concept of absolute autonomy does not hold up in the face of the fragility and vulnerability of existence affected by illness. Faced with illness, in fact, "autonomy cannot express the full meaning of respect for and protection of the human being. Autonomy remains merely an ideal, because of the structural limitations given to it by human finitude and dependence on biological, material and social conditions, lack of information for reasoning etc." [51]. In the clinical context, the principle of self-determination should therefore be thought of as "a capacity that requires reasoning through complex sets of circumstances to reach the most appropriate autonomous decision" [52]. In other words, it is a question of considering autonomy within a real, concrete, lived process, in which the patient is supported in revealing his own reference values and in reaching decisions capable of reflecting his own concept of quality of life. Making precisely this assumption, Italian law is based on vulnerability as "object of a moral principle requiring care for the vulnerable. The vulnerable are those whose autonomy or dignity or integrity are capable of being threatened" [51]. In clinical practice it means introducing a model of care where the people involved collaborate with each other in clarifying and co-constructing the meaning of what is happening [52].

On this basis, article 5 of L.219 [49] dedicated to the definition of advance care planning as a decisive tool to pursue the aim of taking seriously the rights of the most vulnerable people. Advance care planning is carried out "in the relationship between patient and doctor" and "with respect to the evolution of the consequences of a chronic and disabling pathology or one characterized by unstoppable evolution with an inauspicious prognosis." What is described in the ACP is binding, as "the doctor and the healthcare team are obliged to comply if the patient is unable to give consent or is incapacitated". It also presupposes that the patient (or the person indicated by him/her) receives adequate information "on the possible evolution of the pathology in progress, on what the patient can realistically expect in terms of quality of life, on the clinical possibilities of intervention and on palliative care" but different from the advance directives (AD) [53]; through the CPC the patient not only leaves his or her own consent with respect to what the doctor proposes with respect to possible treatments but also and above all "his or her own intentions for the future, including the possible indication of a trustee," where the reference to intentions means a very broad spectrum of concepts, including the concept of quality of life, autonomy, health and well-being, dignity, and so on. By focusing on the patient's meanings, the CCP serves to adapt (and orient) the course of treatment with respect to those meanings and to his needs and wishes if he is no longer able to identify them in the future due to the evolution of the disease [54]. In other words, the ACP "enables individuals who have the decisional capacity to identify their values, to reflect upon the meanings and consequences of serious illness scenarios, to define goals and preferences for future medical treatment and care, and to discuss these with family and health-care providers." ACP addresses individuals' concerns across the physical, psychological, social, and spiritual domains. It encourages individuals to identify a personal representative and to record and regularly review any preferences, so that their preferences can be taken into account should they, at some point, be unable to make their own decisions [55].

Although it is now widely adopted as a tool to enforce patients' rights in situations of future and/or possible unconsciousness and/or incompetence, gray areas remain in the use of CCP. Among these, the most significant concerns the identification of the "right moment" in which to start planning, a question closely linked to the physician's ability to involve his patient as soon as possible in the decision-making process. Early and early recognition of the pathology and a solid communication competence on the part of the professional to also manage the emotional burden connected to the diagnosis of the disease play a fundamental role at this juncture. The clear and comprehensible communication of the diagnosis becomes a fundamental and delicate moment for the physician who finds himself caught between the professional duty to inform the patient and a moral feeling that pushes him to have an eye on the often devastating effects that that communication brings with it, an approach that often leads to paternalistic attitudes [56]. On the other hand, there is also a lack of training on the part of professionals not only on the contents of a fundamental law such as L.219/17, but also on the specific methods and skills needed to build a path of this kind with their patients. Given the delicacy of the issues at stake, in fact, not only communicative skills are needed, but also other skills, cultural, spiritual, and ethical, to know how to manage the meanings at stake in the most competent way possible.

However, given the exponential increase in chronic and degenerative pathologies, the challenge of the near future is to guarantee individualized and attentive accompaniment to the personal dimension of each one, combining it with ethically and clinically correct choices, with an optimal care integration and with criteria of economic sustainability, so that "the terminal phase of life can be perceived by all as a further and last occasion of meaningful existential experience and not as a silent and distressing wait for death" [57].

The bioethical reflection on Italian legislation that we have taken as an example, since it is particularly adherent to the demands of the Oviedo Convention and the Barcelona Convention, shows how the path that integrates the principles of the palliative model with that of self-determination in respect of human rights is the basis of an essential discourse for the work of family doctors and nurses who collaborate with them.

25.6 Conclusions

The relationship between palliative care and early care plans is a constant challenge for health practitioners because the different expressions of disease and aging make it very difficult to predict the course of decline. Since death is the most terrifying thought, it is inevitable that patients will try to keep the thought of the end far away. This fear makes it very difficult to manage the decision-making process, especially after the communication of the unfortunate diagnosis or critical events that signal the inevitable terminal path. Since historically we have come to the social awareness that it is necessary for individuals to prepare themselves responsibly to manage the last tract of life, they must be given the opportunity to talk about it with professionals they trust. The general practitioner is this figure, because he/she is the one who knows the patient's history and has developed a long relationship with him.

References

1. Svenaeus F. To die well: the phenomenology of suffering and end of life ethics. Med Health Care Philos. 2019.
2. Chessa F, Moreno F. Ethical and legal considerations in end-of-life care. Prim Care. 2019;46(3):387–98.
3. Price DM, Strodtman LK, Montagnini M, Smith HM, Ghosh B. Health professionals perceived concerns and challenges in providing palliative and end-of-life care: a qualitative analysis. Am J Hosp Palliat Care. 2019;36(4):308–15.
4. Lim RB. End-of-life care in patients with advanced lung cancer. Ther Adv Respir Dis. 2016;10(5):455–67.
5. Le Calvé S, Somme D, Prud'homm J, Corvol A. Blood transfusion in elderly patients with chronic anemia: a qualitative analysis of the general practitioners' attitudes. BMC Fam Pract. 2017;18(1):76.
6. Laryionava K, Pfeil TA, Dietrich M, Reiter-Theil S, Hiddemann W, Winkler EC. The second patient? Family members of cancer patients and their role in end-of-life decision making. BMC Palliat Care. 2018;17(1):29.
7. Council of Europe. Oviedo convention and its protocols. 1997.
8. World Health Organization. National cancer control programmes: policies and managerial guidelines. 2002.
9. World Health Organization. Cancer control knowledge into action: who guide for effective programs. 2007.
10. Office of the High Commissioner for Human Rights. CESCR general comment no. 14: The right to the highest attainable standard of health (Art. 12). 2000.
11. United Nations General Assembly. Thematic study on the realization of the right to health of older persons by the Special Rapporteur on the right of everyone to the enjoyment of the highest attainable standard of physical and mental health. Anand Grover. 2011.
12. Fonseca LM, Testoni I. The emergence of thanatology and current practice in death education. OMEGA. 2011;64(2):157–69.
13. Testoni I. Psicologia del lutto e del morire: Dal lavoro clinico alla death education. Psicoterapia e Scienze Umane. 2016;50(2):229–52.
14. Testoni I, Cordioli C, Nodari E, et al. Language re-discovered: a death education intervention in the net between kindergarten, family and territory. Italian J Sociol Educ. 2019;11(1):331–46.
15. Testoni I, Biancalani G, Ronconi L, Varani S. Let's start with the end: Bibliodrama in an Italian death education course on managing fear of death, fantasy-proneness, and alexithymia with a mixed-method analysis. OMEGA. 2019:1–31.
16. Testoni I, Piscitello M, Ronconi L, Zsák É, Iacona E, Zamperini A. Death education and the management of fear of death via photo-voice: an experience among undergraduate students. J Loss Trauma. 2019;24(5–6):387–99.
17. Testoni I, Iacona E, Fusina S, et al. "Before I die I want to …": an experience of death education among university students of social service and psychology. Health Psychol Open. 2018;5(2):1–9.
18. Testoni I, Ronconi L, Palazzo L, Galgani M, Stizzi A, Kirk K. Psychodrama and moviemaking in a death education course to work through a case of suicide among high school students in Italy. Front Psychol. 2018;9:1–9.
19. Testoni I, Parise G, Zamperini A, et al. The "sick-lit" question and the death education answer. Papageno versus werther effects in adolescent suicide prevention. Human Affairs. 2016;26(2):153–66.
20. Testoni I, Ancona D, Ronconi L. The ontological representation of death: a scale to measure the idea of annihilation versus passage. OMEGA. 2015;71(1):60–81.

21. Testoni I, Di Lucia Sposito D, De Cataldo L, Ronconi L. Life at all costs? Italian social representations of end-of-life decisions after president Napolitano's speech - margin notes on withdrawing artificial nutrition and hydration. Nutr Therapy Metab. 2015;32(3):121–35.

22. Testoni I, Lazzarotto Simioni J, Di Lucia Sposito D. Representation of death and social management of the limit of life: between resilience and irrationalism. Nutr Therapy Metab. 2013;31(4):192–8.

23. Rodenbach RA, Rodenbach KE, Tejani MA, Epstein RM. Relationships between personal attitudes about death and communication with terminally ill patients: how oncology clinicians grapple with mortality. Patient Educ Counsel. 2016;99(3):356–63.

24. Cripe LD, Hedrick DG, Rand KL, et al. Medical students' professionalism narratives reveal that experiences with death, dying, or palliative care are more positive than other experiences during their internal medicine clerkship. Am J Hospice Palliat Med. 2017;34(1):79–84.

25. Noguera A, Bolognesi D, Garralda E. How do experienced professors teach palliative medicine in European universities? A cross-case analysis of eight undergraduate educational programs. J Palliat Med. 2018;21(11):1621–6.

26. Cevik B, Kav S. Attitudes and experiences of nurses toward death and caring for dying patients in Turkey. Cancer Nurs. 2013;36(6):58–65.

27. European Association for Palliative Care (EAPC). Curriculum in palliative care for undergraduate medical education. Milan, Italy: EAPC; 2007.

28. Centeno C, Sitte T, De Lima L, et al. White paper for global palliative care advocacy: recommendations from a PAL-LIFE expert advisory group of the pontifical academy for life, Vatican City. J Palliat Med. 2018;21(10):1389–97.

29. Masuda Y, Fetters MD, Hattori A, et al. Physicians's reports on the impact of living wills at the end of life in Japan. J Med Ethics. 2003;29:248–52.

30. Testoni I, Bottacin M, Fortuna BC, Zamperini A, Marinoni GL, Biasco G. Palliative care and psychology education needs in nursing courses: a focus group study among Italian undergraduates. Psicologia della Salute. 2019;2:80–99.

31. Testoni I, Carafa ML, Bottacin M, Zamperini A, Galgani M. The nursing hospice care: Critical incidents in managing the relationship with patients and their families. Professioni infermieristiche. 2018;71(3):151–9.

32. Rietjens JA, Sudore RL, Connolly M, et al. Definition and recommendations for advance care planning: an international consensus supported by the European Association for Palliative Care. Lancet Oncol. 2017;18(9):e543–51.

33. World Health Organization. Patient engagement: technical series on safer primary care. 2016.

34. Elliott M, Nicholson C. A qualitative study exploring use of the surprise question in the care of older people: perceptions of general practitioners and challenges for practice. BMJ Support Palliat Care. 2017;7(1):32–8.

35. Baile WF, Buckman R, Lenzi R, Glober G, Beale EA, Kudelka AP. SPIKES—a six-step protocol for delivering bad news: application to the patient with cancer. Oncologist. 2000;5(4):302–11.

36. Borasio GD. Entscheidungen am Lebensende. Der Hausarzt spielt eine zentrale Rolle [End-of-life decisions: the general practitioner plays a decisive role]. MMW Fortschr Med. 2011;153(37):28.

37. Rhee JJ, Teo PCK, Mitchell GK, Senior HE, Tan AJH, Clayton JM. General practitioners (GPs) and end-of-life care: a qualitative study of Australian GPs and specialist palliative care clinicians. BMJ Support Palliat Care. 2018.

38. Brighton LJ, Bristowe K. Communication in palliative care: talking about the end of life, before the end of life. Postgrad Med J. 2016;92(1090):466–70.

39. Tran M, Grant M, Clayton J, Rhee J. Advance care decision making and planning. Aust J Gen Pract. 2018;47(11):753–7.

40. Thurn T, Borasio GD, Chiò A, et al. Physicians' attitudes toward end-of-life decisions in amyotrophic lateral sclerosis. Amyotroph Lateral Scler Frontotemporal Degener. 2019;20(1–2):74–81.

41. Danel-Brunaud V, Touzet L, Chevalier L, et al. Ethical considerations and palliative care in patients with amyotrophic lateral sclerosis: a review. Rev Neurol (Paris). 2017;173(5):300–7.

42. Slachevsky Ch A, Abusleme LMT, Arenas Massa Á. Cuidados paliativos en personas con demencia severa: reflexiones y desafíos [Palliative care of patients with severe dementia]. Rev Med Chil. 2016;144(1):94–101.
43. Lennard C. Best interest versus advance decisions to refuse treatment in advance care planning for neurodegenerative illness. Br J Nurs. 2018;27(21):1261–7.
44. Kent A. Advance care planning in progressive neurological conditions. Nurs Stand. 2015;29(21):51–9.
45. Bosisio F, Jox RJ, Jones L, Rubli Truchard E. Planning ahead with dementia: what role can advance care planning play? A review on opportunities and challenges. Swiss Med Wkly. 2018;148:w14706.
46. Beernaert K, Deliens L, De Vleminck A, et al. Early identification of palliative care needs by family physicians: a qualitative study of barriers and facilitators from the perspective of family physicians, community nurses, and patients. Palliat Med. 2014;28(6):480–90.
47. Malherbe JF. Elementi per un'etica clinica. Condizioni dell'alleanza terapeutica. Trento: FBK Press; 2014.
48. Reich WT. Encyclopedia of bioethics, vol. 1. New York: The Free Press; 1978.
49. Gazzetta Ufficiale della Repubblica Italiana. Legge 22 dicembre 2017, n. 219: Norme in mate-ria di consenso informato e di disposizioni anticipate di trattamento. In: Gazzetta Ufficiale della Repubblica Italiana. 2018.
50. Lalatta Costerbosa M. Una bioetica degli argomenti. Torino: Giappichelli; 2012.
51. Partners in the BIOMED-II Project. The Barcelona declaration on policy proposals to the European Commission basic ethical principles in bioethics and biolaw. In: Istituto Italiano di Bioetica. 1998.
52. De Panfilis L, Di Leo S, Peruselli C, Ghirotto L, Tanzi S. "I go into crisis when …": ethics of care and moral dilemmas in palliative care. BMC Palliat Care. 2019;18(1):70.
53. Jaworska A. Respecting the margins of agency: Alzheimer's patients and the capacity to value. Philos Public Affairs. 1999;28(2):105–38.
54. Jordens C, Little M, Kerridge I, McPhee J. From advance directives to advance care planning: current legal status, ethical rationales and a new research agenda. Intern Med J. 2005;35:563–6.
55. Alzheimer Europe. 2015: Ethical dilemmas faced by health and social care professionals pro-viding dementia care in care homes and hospital settings: a guide for use in the context of ongoing professional care training. 2015.
56. Sampson EL, Burns A. Planning a personalised future with dementia: 'the misleading simplic-ity of advance directives'. Palliat Med. 2013;27(5):387–8.
57. Zaninetta G. Muoio, quindi sono. In: L'esperienza del futuro. Janus. 2009; 33.

Educating Physicians for the Aging World: A Humanistic Approach in Doctoring

Pablo González Blasco, Graziela Moreto, and Maria Auxiliadora C. De Benedetto

Abstract

Outcomes, guidelines, and clinical trials are at the forefront of the current medical training. However, we observe well-trained technological physicians with a reduced humanistic perspective which leads to attitudes that lack ethics and professionalism. There is a growing concern about the human dimension of the future physician and how it can be taught or reinforced in the educational environment allowing to integrate technical science with the humanism that medical practice requires.

Although human suffering and death are a constant presence in medical practice, it is quite common to observe healthcare professionals having difficulties to deal with this subject. A training that goes beyond technique is needed, on know how to face death professionally. It takes attitudes, values, how to deal with the meaning of life, understanding the vital moment, as well as modern techniques, procedures, and resources for the proper performance of this function. Palliative medicine is the modern approach to managing human finitude, and it should be incorporated into medical education. Family doctors, as specialists in people, have deserved participation in palliative training, because of their focus on continuity of care, prevention, and family study. Narratives in the suffering context led trainees to recognize how doctors can create and make the entire difference, and they learn that there is always something to do.

Empathy has a broad and varied spectrum and has two main attributes: emotional and cognitive. A prerequisite for developing both affective and cognitive empathy is that an individual should not be overly preoccupied with himself and his own concerns, because the willingness to help the other person decreases.

P. G. Blasco (✉) · G. Moreto · M. A. C. De Benedetto
SOBRAMFA—Medical Education and Humanism, São Paulo, Brazil
e-mail: pablogb@sobramfa.com.br; http://www.sobramfa.com.br

© Springer Nature Switzerland AG 2022
J. Demurtas, N. Veronese (eds.), *The Role of Family Physicians in Older People Care*, Practical Issues in Geriatrics, https://doi.org/10.1007/978-3-030-78923-7_26

Empathy could bridge the gap between patient-centered medicine and evidence-based medicine. Role modeling and caring carefully for the emotional dimension of medical students are possible resources for preventing the erosion of empathy.

Humanities and arts help in building a humanistic perspective of doctoring because they enable doctors to understand patients in their whole context. The inclusion of humanities in the curriculum occasions deep rethinking of what it means to be sick and what it means to take care of the sick. They also portray a tremendous spectrum of attitudes required for building ethics and professionalism, and they illustrate complex moral choices and stimulate comments and reflection.

Because usually feelings arise before concepts in the learners, the affective path is a critical way to the rational process of learning. Medical educators need to recognize that learners are immersed in a popular culture largely framed through emotions and images. Life stories and narratives enhance emotions and therefore lay the foundation for conveying concepts. Cinema is useful in teaching the human dimension of medicine. Movies provide a quick and direct teaching scenario in which specific scenes point out important issues, emotions are presented in accessible ways where they are easy to identify, and students are able to understand and recognize them immediately. The purpose of the film methodology is not only to evoke emotions but to help the audience reflect on these emotions and figure out how to translate what they learn into attitudes and actions. Reflection is the necessary bridge to move from emotions to behavior. Our experience affirms the effectiveness of using the movie clip methodology because of their brevity, rapidity, and emotional intensity. Bringing clips from different movies, to illustrate or intensify a particular point, fits well with this modern living state. By allowing reflections on emotions, participants in these sessions can learn to develop their reflective abilities and attitudes. These skills and attitudes, in turn, can help create more humanistic, and presumably more ethical, physicians.

Keywords

Medical humanism · Empathy · Palliative care · Narrative medicine · Cinema education · Humanities

26.1 Technology and Humanism: Finding a New Balance

We live in an era where outcomes, guidelines, and clinical trials are at the forefront of medical training. We observe well-trained technological physicians with a reduced humanistic perspective which leads to attitudes that lack ethics and professionalism. Maybe this is because objective knowledge is considered scientific and valuable, whereas subjective information is thought to be "soft" and second-rate. For the relief of suffering, that conflict is not only false but an impediment [1].

Doctors exist to care for patients. Nevertheless, the frequent dissatisfaction of patients points more to the human deficiencies of medical professionals than to their technical shortcomings. Complexity comes mostly from patients, not from diseases. While technical knowledge helps in solving disease-based problems, the patient affected by these diseases remains a real challenge for the practicing doctor.

There is a growing concern about the human dimension of the future physician and how it can be taught or reinforced in the educational environment [2]. Emerging technology tends to monopolize students' attention and learning efforts, often at the expense of other important aspects of medicine. In addition, medical students are, in general, young people who are learning to be physicians at the same time as they are developing their adult personas. Medical educators must recognize this and provide ways for students to reflect on general subjects related to culture and the humanities from the medical perspective. Although technical knowledge and skills can be acquired through training with a little reflective process, it is impossible to refine attitudes, acquire virtues, and incorporate values without reflection.

Researchers on this subject [3] comment on the balance that always existed in medicine, between the two inseparable facets that compose it: medicine as science and medicine as an art. The vertiginous scientific advances would require, to maintain that balance, an extension of the scope of humanism, that is, a humanism at the height of scientific progress. And it would be this expansion of humanism, adapted to the current days, in a modern version.

When this humanist update is missing, it falls into a disproportion that is reflected in technically trained professions but with serious human deficiencies. Deformed professionals, with hypertrophy, without balance, who naturally do not conquer the confidence of the patient who expects a balanced doctor. It would be, therefore, a function of the university and the academic institutions, to expand the humanist concept in modern molds, without the aroma of mothballs, knowing how to open horizons and new perspectives. For achieving this goal, methodology, systematics, and relearning to do things are required; specially when these things are too many, wrapped in high technology, and commanded by the scientific progress that advances for seconds [4].

The French thinker Gustave Thibon [5] brings together in a volume a set of essays, to which he gives the title "Balance and Harmony." The balance is the composition of opposing forces, compromise solution, resulting from vectors that cancel each other out. Harmony is the perfect fit of the parts into a whole, so that they collaborate for the same purpose. And, quoting Victor Hugo, he comments: "Above balance is harmony, above the balance is the harp."

When we look at the actions that seek to humanization—without achieving it— we realize that the mistake is, perhaps, in seeking balance and not harmony. The balance assumes that the forces are antagonistic and that modern science supported by evidence has to be seasoned with humanitarian attitudes, for example, hearing the patient's history with love and feeling compassion. We recognize that this is already an enormous progress and an advance on what, unfortunately, we contemplate daily, where the patient is a mere adjuvant that often disturbs the doctor's practicing. But that balance is insufficient; it lacks consistency. They are still two attitudes that do not mix, like water and oil: the clear water of the evidence, and the comforting oil. But each of them with its own density and applied each to its time and in its moment. This "medical performance schizophrenia" is unsustainable in itself, it lasts for a short time, and when the doctor gets tired, he will pay attention to one to the detriment of the other.

Medical science, cutting edge medicine, demands a new humanism [6]. A position that knows how to place liver function and neurological sequelae in the same reasoning, with the meaning of life, transaminases and albumin combined with humiliation, suffering, and loss. A science that is art and therefore manages to place in the same equation dimensions so different that apparently do not mix. In truth, they are completely mixed in life: prothrombin and discouragement, neurotransmitters and tiredness of living, and hepatocytes and indignation.

This seems to be the time to invoke the construction of harmony, and know how to play, with different strings to get the perfect chord. Balance is to assume a monotonic composition, science, art, a bit of albumin, and measured doses of affection. Harmony is to put each competence in its place and have the soul of an artist to know how to play in the harp of life—of that person who is unique—the strings of different shades. These are the chords that allow the doctor to travel the path between the sick person and the meaning that the disease has for the patient, which is way of being in life. A way of life that has its own language and must find, in the sensitive physician, the receiver necessary to properly decode the meanings. This implies for the doctor to have an attitude of active anthropology: humanism and anthropology are possibilities of his self-demand, challenges to his rational thought, levels of knowledge in style, and ascending aspiration of non-conformity [7].

Humanism is thus a source of knowledge that the doctor uses for his profession [8]. Knowledge as important as those acquired by other paths that help you in the desire to take care of the human being who is sick. Humanism in medicine is not a temperamental question, an individual taste, not even an interesting complement. All that would lead to place "humanist attitudes" on the scale, to compensate for the excesses of science. Humanism as harmony, as musical virtuosity, is, for the doctor, a true work tool, not a cultural appendix. It is a scientific attitude, weighing the result of a conscious effort of learning and methodology [9, 10].

The doctor's inspiration will often come from the cord of compassion that vibrates easily in a heart willing to help. That will be the note that will give the tonality for the further development of its performance, for the harmonic chords of clinical reasoning. Gregorio Marañón, a humanist doctor and a profound connoisseur of this harmonic symbiosis, warns: "The doctor, whose humanity must always be alert within the scientific spirit, must first count on individual pain; and although he is full of enthusiasm for science, he must be willing to adopt the paradoxical position of defending the individual, whose health is entrusted to him, against his own scientific progress" [11].

In this context, the narratives and life stories, now complete and harmonious—transaminases and distresses, albumin, and heartbreak—have their true space and function: to approach the human being who suffers and awaits our care. Once more

Marañón gives us a reflection in perfect chord: "On several occasions I noted to those who work by my side, that a pure diagnostic system, deduced exclusively from analytical data, dehumanized, independent of the direct and endearing observation of the patient, it implies the fundamental error of forgetting the personality, which is so important in the etiologies and to stipulate the prognosis of the patient and teach us doctors what we can do to alleviate their sufferings" [11]. We know well from our own experience how difficult this harmony of action is: how to govern technique and humanism with expertise so we can offer a true symphony of health care [6].

The first step that the doctor must take if he wants to humanize medicine is admitting that he must humanize himself first. And for this, he cannot give up his efforts to reflect, to look for solutions, and to find resources that allow him to integrate technical science—which grows every second—with the humanism that medical practice requires [12].

Hans Jonas, with his ethics of responsibility [13], points out that what distinguishes human beings from animals is a tripod constituted by the tool, the image, and the tumulus. The tool is the technique, and in this there is no doubt that we distinguish ourselves from animals, because when we are born, we quickly incorporate all the techniques accumulated in the history that precedes us. Animals lack a scientific heritage, and each one has to be built from scratch, without taking advantage of the experiences of the ancestors of their species. We can evoke Ortega [14] when he says that the current tiger is the same tiger of thousands of years ago and that only the human being is born on a history that precedes him, a history that sets together the technique and the corresponding progress.

The second element that distinguishes us from animals is the image, which includes the ability that mankind has to represent reality through art. Art and humanities are ways to better know the reality in which the human being is immersed and to know himself, in his bodily and spiritual dimension. Finally, the third leg of the tripod is represented by the tumulus. Only the human being has an awareness of transcendence, and the representation of death is what puts him in contact with a dimension that extends beyond his own being.

It is not difficult to conclude that if, as far as technique and progress are concerned, being noticeable the distance between mankind and animals, the other two elements of the tripod have been atrophied; and if not for that reason we necessarily become animalized; there is no doubt that the human equilibrium presents itself with dangerous instability. The man—the doctor, in the case at hand—stops frequenting the arts and humanities and deprives himself of ways of knowing the world and loses the ability to admire and feel that most of the phenomena that surround him are independent of him. And, not least, he loses the sense of transcendence, the spiritual dimension, the sense of eternity, and the duration of time around him and his own. The consequences are alarming, because of not frequenting "the tumulus, door of transcendence," it becomes difficult to maintain the sense of mission, and the need to feel useful in this world, as part of the happiness we pursue. This reflection opens the way to the next point: the necessary contingency of the human being, surrounded by suffering and death.

26.2 Regarding Suffering and Death: Are We Educating Doctors for Immortal Patients?

Human suffering and death are a constant presence in medical practice. However, it is quite common to observe healthcare professionals having difficulties to deal with this subject. Death is a phenomenon that disrupts medical practice. However, it can't be seen just as an unhappy event that keeps doctors from having a good performance [15]. Doctors commonly forget that death is a real possibility and usually consider it a failure. We can observe physicians that, although able to use high-level technology, do not feel comfortable in dealing with incurable patients, in which the scientific knowledge does not work and their technical skills are not enough. As a result of our predominant model of teaching and practice of medicine, the idea that there is nothing to do for terminal patients can be deeply rooted in some medical students and doctors. Nevertheless, clinical experience with such patients is essential in medical education because doctors will commonly face this situation in their activities [16].

While we ask ourselves why this happens in medical education, the reflection raises a paradoxical theme: will we be training future doctors to take care of immortal patients, in which the possibility of suffering and death are contradictions that are not considered?

This paradox leads us to the classical aphorism that represents the doctor's mission. "Heal a few times, relieve often, always comfort," a famous statement, repeated countless times and credited to professors, leading exponents of medicine, and even Hippocrates himself. However, it is reasonable to think that the father of medicine would not have simplified the function of the physician, much less spelled out the known postulate in that order. In ancient Greece there was little that could be healed and much that could be relieved with comfort. I like to imagine that Hippocrates would have formulated the aphorism in reverse order: always comforting, relieving when it is possible, and sometimes—very few—provide the cure, a more Copernican than Hippocratic turn that sheds light on these considerations.

Of course, people keep dying. This is the destiny of the human being. However, technical progress inevitably makes us think that we have gained ground in the fight against death. In fact, it is true. We won more battles, we postponed the invasion, but in the end, we will always lose the war. It's a matter of time. After all, who is the doctor to whom patients do not die? Death is the only certain thing about human happening, and the doctor is in the way of this obligatory exit. All his skill will be in knowing how to "dilute his technique" in a humanitarian vehicle so that everyone—patient, family, and himself—can digest, with meaning and transcendence, the natural contingency of life, for which the more accurate science will always be insufficient [15].

Let's return to our aphorism. What can one expect when the doctor's recommended order is to heal, relieve, and ultimately comfort? It is logical to think that I am moving from the most important to the least, to the detail. When I can't heal, I must relieve. And when I can't even relieve, I have just to provide comfort.

Proceeding in this sequence inevitably presents relief and comfort as a consolation prize (to the doctor) that has come across an incurable, painful, terminal illness.

The basic mistake is not to contemplate the epidemiology (incidence, prevalence) of these terms. While comfort is something that should always be done, due to the very high prevalence, healing has a much lower prevalence. It would be logical then that the process of medical practice contemplates this proportion to produce better doctors. Doctors who always know how to comfort—because they have learned that this comes first—and depending on the case and the illnesses they face, also know how to cure when it is possible. That is to say, since healing is not so frequent and life is inexorably moving to its end, it would be necessary to demand from the doctor the other skills, which are much more frequently used. A doctor who does not know how to comfort or relieve cannot be credited as such, should not have a medical degree, or cannot be able to act professionally. In short, the order in which the factors are taught does alter the final product [17].

A recent work [18] explains these shortcomings in the education of medical students and, consequently, of the doctors who enter the labor market. The author, a renowned surgeon, talks about the misunderstanding of the medical student who joins college wanting to take care and over time forgets the patients because he is too busy with medicine. Gawande explains the reasons for the distraction: "What concerned us was knowledge. Although we knew how to show compassion, we could not be sure that we would be able to properly diagnose and treat our future patients. We paid college tuition to learn about the body's internal processes, the complex mechanisms of its pathologies, and the wide range of discoveries and technologies accumulated throughout history to prevent them. We had no idea we needed to think more than that. (…). Be helpful to others, but also technically competent and able to solve intricate problems. Competence brings us security, a sense of identity. I dedicate myself to a profession whose success is based on its ability to fix. If your problem can be fixed, we know exactly what to do. But what if you can't? The fact that we do not have adequate answers to this question is disturbing and causes insensitivity, inhumanity and great suffering."

Medicine is not an exact science and necessarily has flaws that can only be repaired with love and dedication. When this is not understood, when a doctor presents medicine in its technological fantasy as an exact science, it must also pay the consequences of failure. In the case of an engineer, a bridge he builds will not fall (unless earthquakes or unforeseen occur) if his calculations are accurate, and such accuracy is not difficult to achieve. If the doctor wants to present himself as a technician, such as a people mechanic, he must accept the punishment if he does not make the right calculations to "fix the damage."

Medical error is above all a shortcoming in the humanistic field. What protects the doctor is the patient's confidence; but the patient loses it when the professional appears as a brilliant technician but unable to approach the patient and tune with his affection. When the patient notices that the doctor lacks the human dimension and presents himself as an expert concerned solely with repairing the malfunctions, he will ask for satisfaction and demand compensation if the practitioner cannot keep his promises. When we explore the patient's complaints about the doctor's attention, we always find insufficiency in the affective ground. We then found that all that "medical error" started because "the doctor didn't even examine me" or "the doctor didn't explain anything about what could happen" and "didn't pay attention to what I was talking about." The blow that is accused is always in the soul, not the technical deficiency: this comes later, to embody the process. It is worth recalling an example cited by Mendel in his classic book, *Proper Doctoring*: "The patient may stop taking a medication because he realizes that it is bad for him. We must take into account these intuitions of the sick. The doctor who is not humble and does not pay attention to patients is the best candidate for a lawsuit." [19]

In a correct synthesis, Marañón [20] clarifies the theme further: "The sin of doctors in recent years has been to abdicate all that our mission had of fullness, generosity, and priesthood—to use a commonplace—and try to convert it in a scientific profession, that is, as exact as that of the engineer or the architect. [...]. In the end, everything will turn against the doctor himself, because, even if he wants to, his science will be embryonic, full of gaps and inaccurate aspects. These flaws can only be filled by love. Its exclusively scientific prestige will inevitably be subject to serious and continuous breakdowns. And that is why the doctor will be deprived of the cordial respect of his patients and of society itself, who will not accept his mistake generously but will peek at his flaws, pursuing him wherever he is."

A training that goes beyond technique is needed, to know how to face death professionally. It takes attitudes, values, how to deal with the meaning of life, understanding the vital moment, as well as modern techniques, procedures, and resources for the proper performance of this function. The physician must have a "healthy nonconformity" with the technique, an attitude that pushes him to seek, in his training and professional practice, other dimensions that will be essential to face situations that are beyond technical boundaries. This is how the structure of the professional, technical, and humanist is built at the same time, capable of taking on these challenges.

Death management is a technical function of the physician to prepare for and the wrong order in which the factors of the aphorism previously mentioned are usually presented does not help. This is a peculiar technique as it should not modify the final outcome of the intervention. It does change the process of how the situation evolves. In other words: everyone will die someday; the difference is in the way they die. Then comes the technical, managerial function of the doctor [21].

Death management always means asking yourself what is best for the patient before taking "usual" measures such as unnecessary hospitalizations, ICU transfers, obstinate, and naturally ineffective therapies when the dying process occurs. Ask yourself, before taking it, what I expect from this measure, this prescription. And, in dialogue with the family, make the decision personally, without dividing responsibilities, assuming the conduct with professional character. Managing death implies the simultaneous care of the patient and the family. The family raises questions that are "of little technical character" but of vital importance. They want to know, for example, if the patient is suffering and if anything else can be done. And they always require explanations of what is happening.

The physician cannot get tired of repeating the explanations knowing that it takes time for the family to digest the situation [22]. The doctor's words are a resource that facilitates this process of adaptation, and he cannot spare them. It is not a question of explaining a pathophysiological problem but of making a vital understanding, with all the burden of normal feelings in the situation, which is happening to the dying relative. It takes time and patience. Letting the family participate in the process of dying with the patient eliminates many doubts and burdens of conscience a posteriori. When the family is participating, seeing, and touching the patient, one does not wonder after he passed away if he could have done anything more for him, as they experienced the whole evolution. Consider here a reflection on the unnecessary distance from the family in ICUs, limited visits, and all this universe that deserves a particular approach.

Patients know more than the doctor thinks they know. It is an added sense of vital realism that the condition of dying gives them. That's why you expect from the doctor realism, comfort, and professional support. Both the patient and the doctor are harmed by their attitude that they "give up" because it is a "terminal case," as well as the one who intends to deceive the patient as if nothing serious was happening. The physician requires a thoughtful, realistic attitude, imbued with the virtue of prudence in true paradoxical balancing. And, considering that, be active, participate in the process. That is why it is worth remembering the words of a humanistic doctor, an expert in ethical questions: "A truly dignified death is not only the absence of external tribulation. Dignity in the face of death is not conferred by something external but arises from the greatness of mood with which one faces this unique situation. Therefore, to die with dignity means not just being patient, but being an agent. Be active, participate in the process" [23].

It is not superfluous to warn that, curiously, those who technically try all the resources to prolong life, "even against common sense," are the first to give up the patient when he/she goes into terminal phase and "refer the case to someone else." It is increasingly rare to see "super specialists" with the dying patient when there are no more therapeutic resources to employ. This attitude can be justified by feeling a certain discomfort of "not doing anything for the patient," which is not true. In fact, with their presence the doctors are doing a lot. It turns out that simply doing something that, while not being quantifiable, seems not to be useful. This is logical, as the utility was wrongly evaluated with purely technical parameters. The fact that this attitude cannot be measured in milligrams and therapeutic doses does not speak against the importance of it. A mother's love for her sick child cannot be represented in therapeutic dosages, but its efficacy is undeniable. The doctor should be there with love, but as a doctor—not like the mother—and here is the key to his professionalism.

To perform this function professionally requires realism and competence: competence to eliminate pain, control symptoms, and offer a quality of life. These are the elements that introduce us to palliative medicine, a modern approach to managing human finitude, which presents itself as the best antidote to the easy and unethical solution of euthanasia. When a patient who suffers says, "Doctor, I don't want to live," he is basically saying, "Doctor, I don't want to live this way."

26.3 Palliative Care: A Humanistic Approach to Human Contingency

Palliative medicine is the study and management of patients with illness in which cure is no longer possible and an end point of death is expected within a finite period of time. The focus is on the control of symptoms and maximizing patient' self-defined quality of life [24, 25].

The complex goal of relief suffering can't be one-dimensional but must include the four human dimensions of human experience: physical (pain, dyspnea, cough, constipation, delirium), emotional (anxiety, depression, grief), social (financial concerns, unfinished business), and spiritual (guilt, sadness, worthlessness). To provide this complete assistance, palliative care is usually made by an interdisciplinary team [24].

According to World Health Organization, palliative care is an approach that improves the quality of life of patients and their families facing the problem associated with life-threatening illness, through the prevention and relief of suffering by means of early identification and impeccable assessment and treatment of pain and other problems, physical, psychosocial, and spiritual. Palliative care provides relief from pain and other distressing symptoms; affirms life and regards dying as a normal process; intends neither to hasten or postpone death; integrates the psychological and spiritual aspects of patient care; offers a support system to help patients live as actively as possible until death; offers a support system to help the family cope during the patient's illness and in their own bereavement; uses a team approach to address the needs of patients and their families, including bereavement counseling, if indicated; will enhance the quality of life and may also positively influence the course of illness; is applicable early in the course of illness, in conjunction with other therapies that are intended to prolong life, such as chemotherapy or radiation therapy; and includes those investigations needed to better understand and manage distressing clinical complications [26].

The evidence shows that the lack of palliative care training can be negative to doctors and patients. Medical educators agree about the need of teaching such a discipline, which has been introduced in some medical schools' curricula around the world. In the USA a survey had demonstrated that most medical schools do not provide palliative care knowledge during graduation. The researchers suggested the implementation of a palliative guideline in the medical curriculum [27]. In our country, Brazil, palliative care is an "emergent specialty," that is performed by clinicians, a few oncologists, or family doctors. We believe that, because of the inherent characteristics of family medicine, the training of residents of this specialty in palliative care is indispensable [28].

Experts agree that experientially based and developmentally appropriate ethics education is needed during medical training to prepare medical students to provide excellent end-of-life care [29].

Because many doctors did not receive any kind of formal training in communicating skills and palliative care, they are not able, for example, to give bad news properly. Medical students don't learn anything about how to deal with the feelings that emerged in such a context. On the contrary, they are told to keep distance from the patient and relatives, never touch or kiss them, not sit on their beds, and just use technical gesture [30]. Realizing that such attitude does not work, the trainees became receptive to the new approaches they were presented to and could, day by day, learn to face death, pain, and suffering as naturally as possible, as events related to human life, but without losing a respectful attitude.

The medical educators noted a necessity or the importance to teach palliative care and are trying to improve this in medical school. There are evidences showing that the lack of palliative care training can be negative to doctors and patients. For example, an ineffective doctor-patient communication can affect the patient's satisfaction [27]. The barriers for an adequate care are from three types: no specific training, personal attitudes against death, and political disinterest [31].

26.3.1 Family Doctors and Life Stories in Palliative Care: A Successful Educational Scenario

The reason to have a family doctor in a palliative care service becomes clear if we understand the principles of family medicine that is a specialty focused on the person. The field of action of family medicine is primary care, medical education, and leadership. The family doctor is a specialist in people [32]. Family medicine participation in palliative care occurs because both specialties focus on continuity of care, prevention, and family study. Family medicine's philosophy promotes doctors that have the objective to improve health and quality of life. The doctor-patient relationship doesn't end with some incurable and death disease, even with the patient's death, because the relationship with the family goes on after that [31].

Medical students and residents usually do not learn how to deal with the feelings that emerge when caring for dying patients. On the contrary, they are more likely to be told to keep a certain distance from the patient and their relatives [33]. Realizing that this kind of attitude is harmful, the trainees are usually receptive to new approaches.

A lived experience in a didactic palliative care ambulatory clinic (PCAC) addressed to medical students and residents showed us that such a clinical setting can provide a unique training apprenticeship. The teaching involved specific issues like controlling pain symptoms but went beyond to include the more subtle aspects of caring for dying patients. Residents and students could learn that family physicians need skills in palliative care since they frequently encounter dying patients. They realized that family members play an important role in a patient's end-of-life period and must also receive support. They could learn to face death, pain, and suffering as naturally as possible as events that are part of human life but without losing a respectful attitude.

The young doctors usually started the training in the PCAC in a fearful way, feeling that there was nothing to do in the situations they are about to face. Nevertheless, their evolution in such scenery was surprising. The PCAC promoted a very special apprenticeship and brought deep and wide insights for SOBRAMFA's educational projects. Such an apprenticeship could be also extended to other settings of practice and improved the student's and resident's performance in circumstances not so complex. The learning was related to technical issues like the control of symptoms but went far beyond. This included being attentive to the subtle aspects involved in patients' care. Residents learned that, concerning family doctors, to get skills related to palliative care is a very important task since they frequently must face patients in such conditions. They developed discernment for recognizing the proper moment to send terminal patients to hospital or hospice and could realize that family members play an important role in patient's end-of-life period and must receive the proper support in order to help them effectively [34].

It was evident that the outcomes outlined here, in some way, were a consequence of the application of a narrative approach at the PCAC. Beyond the technical and pharmacological support offered to patients, the application of narrative as a therapeutic and didactical tool is one of the resources explored. A text recommended for reading was considered fundamental and clarifying—"Just Listening: Narrative and Deep" Illness by Arthur Frank. In this article, the author teaches us that by listening to terminal patients with empathy and compassion, we can make them feel they are not alone, a frequent sentiment they experience, which allows them to transform their chaos stories into quest stories, in which their illness becomes a teaching condition for all involved in the situation. For him, quest stories are stories of transcendence. When terminal patients find an attentive listener and a compassionate witness, they have the opportunity to organize the chaos produced in their lives by the illness and to find a meaning that allows them to accept life unconditionally. At the first readings of the mentioned article, some of the trainees manifested an apparent doubt and thought that those conceptions could not be effective in real life. But, in the course of time, they could realize that Frank's ideas are actually applicable in palliative care. And, for them, the author became very appreciated, a model to be followed [35].

For all participants in that scenario of practice, it was difficult to deal with so many emerging chaos stories, exactly the ones that the doctors would like to ignore, because such stories make them feel a sensation of incapacity and emphasize the questions that have no answer. After such experiences, the students and doctors often need to share narratives and to tell their own stories in order to transcend chaos into quests of their own. After a discussion related to the technical aspects of consultations, the activities in the clinic were closed with an exercise of reflective writing. Such exercise was effective in promoting reflection and an excellent tool for dealing with chaos stories [36]. The reflective writing [37]—an element of narrative methodology—played a key role in promoting reflection and demonstrated to be an excellent instrument for helping trainees to deal with pain, suffering, and death.

Nowadays, more and more authors agree that the use of talking and writing in prose or poetry to express feelings that one has difficulty to deal with has a healing effect [38, 39], which is entirely consistent with our practice in palliative care clinic.

This approach has motivated the creation of many stories during the 3 years of palliative care ambulatory' activities, stories told, written and rewritten by patients, students, patients' family members, doctors, and residents. The feelings, interpretation, and points of view of each involved in a story certainly influence the way he/she will present it. The different people involved in a given story experienced it according to their own perspectives and interpretations. The same situation can acquire unexpected meanings for each one of us and usually provides unbelievable lessons of life. When health professionals listen to their patients with empathy and compassion, they participate in the creation of a new script in which one can detect elements of overcoming and transcendence demonstrating that the course of the story was changed. Even though the end of a palliative care story is immutable—the inexorable death—it can be written in diverse ways. Certainly, the drift of the changes can depend on the way the patient-doctor and family-doctor relationships are constructed. And a great apprenticeship was that when there is apparently nothing to do, one can still listen [36].

Narratives in the suffering context led trainees to recognize little facts and changes and how doctors can create and make the entire difference. And first of all, they need to learn that there is always something to do. Doctors can help their patients with their technical knowledge and experiences. But we can do more, being really present and interested in patients; use our honesty, humility, and compassion; listen with attention; and fight for our patients; they know how to utilize our help [40].

The objectives of providing skills for an initial approach to terminal patients and families, promoting reflection about difficult themes, and breaking blockages that prevent students to deal properly with terminal patients were fulfilled. Trainees could learn that when doctors act with goodwill, humility, compassion, and honesty, patients and their families always benefit. The medical educators noted the need to foster reflection among young doctors, and this could be done through narratives, especially in a palliative care setting since the lack of palliative care training can be negative to doctors and patients [41]. The technical knowledge provided in palliative care ambulatory clinic allied to the creation of an ambiance propitious to reflection made it, in an educational way, a unique setting to a continuum learning that is essential for family doctors' schooling.

The proper management of terminal outpatients in a holistic way; the abolition of the idea that palliation is not a failure of treatment and an uninteresting demand; the understanding that when prolonging life and healing patients with interventional approaches is no longer indicated and palliation is the only possible conduct, to work under such a perspective is a very significant objective; and the apprenticeship that, concerning terminal patients and their families, there is always something to do are the lessons that all participants in this didactic life experience will take to live. It is important to remember that for us, SOBRAMFA's doctors who supervised the activity, the learning was also enormous. And over the years, we could get many teachings about life, death, pain, suffering, transcendence, empathy, compassion, friendship, peace, and liberation which inspire us still today in the practice and teaching scenarios of palliative care in which we work today. And it is necessary to emphasize that, over the years, we have been able to incorporate many teachings about life, death, pain, suffering, transcendence, empathy, compassion, friendship, peace, and liberation, which still inspire us today in the scenarios of palliative care practice and teaching in which we act today.

26.4 Meeting Patients' Needs Through Empathy: An Educational Challenge

Empathy, from the Greek *empatheia*, means understanding someone else's feelings. In the English vocabulary, empathy was used initially to describe the observers' feeling when interfacing with artistic expression. Afterwards, the term was related to understanding people, and in 1918, Southard incorporates the word empathy into the doctor-patient relationship, as a resource for facilitating diagnosis and therapeutics [42]. Empathy has to do with deeply understanding the other and is a path to bridge scientific knowledge with compassion for better caring.

Empathy, one of the most studied humanistic attitudes today, is the cornerstone of ethical and humanized behavior and medical professionalism. Empathy has also been considered an essential element in any humanization strategy [43]. It is a personal quality necessary for understanding the inner experiences and feelings of patients. It represents the essence of the doctor-patient relationship. Developing meaningful interpersonal relationships between patients and physicians is important even for improving clinical outcomes [44].

Before entering into the concept of empathy in the context of the patient-physician relationship, it is worth pausing to understand the term from a philosophical point of view. In this field, we cannot fail to cite the work developed by Edith Stein (1891–1942), a philosopher who developed his doctoral thesis on empathy. Macintyre [45] in his book on the philosophical action of Edith Stein comments that an essential feature of empathic awareness is the awareness of the feelings of others. The relationship we have with the feelings of others is analogous to the relationship we have with our own past feelings. We may notice what the other is feeling, but we don't have to feel the same as him/her. The same is true; when we remember our own feelings—even clearly—it does not mean that we will feel the same way we have in the past. A deep understanding, real understanding, no need to incorporate it. We can fully understand what we feel on one occasion, but we do not have to feel it equally at this time.

It takes caution to state that "I am putting myself in another's shoes." Yes, it is possible to do so but with our own patterns (our feelings, our reactivity, our understanding of vital reality, our own biographical history) and not his own, so that I cannot truly understand. It is not enough to put ourselves hypothetically in the other's place and continue to be ourselves experiencing this place in which I place myself. One must also be detached from one's own standards to arrive at empathic knowledge. Regarding this perspective Stein reminds us that empathy is not simply intuition, but an attitude that requires reflection, to turn back and again on ourselves and others, a course that enriches one's own and others' knowledge. It is not a spasm of knowledge but something worked.

In the context of medical education, the concept of empathy has a broad and varied spectrum. Some authors consider empathy to be a predominantly cognitive quality: it would encompass the understanding of the patient's experiences and concerns combined with communication skills [46]. Irving and Dickson [47] define it as an attitude that contemplates behavioral ability along with the cognitive and affective dimension.

Most authors place empathy on the affective dimension, giving it the ability to experience the other person's experiences and feelings. In this case it can be deduced that the ability to be empathic implies a spontaneous feeling of identification with the suffering person, a process in which emotion is involved.

The majority of the authors with an affective-oriented approach presuppose that, during the empathic event, there is something that can be characterized as a partial identification of the observer with the observed. This aspect also becomes clear especially in Carl Rogers' definition, which describes empathy as being the ability "to sense the client's private world as if it were your own, but without losing the 'as if' quality." According to this definition, the differentiation between one's own experience and the experience of another is the decisive criterion for defining effective empathy [48].

Other authors [49] stress the importance of making a distinction between sympathy and empathy; in particular, arguing that such a distinction has significant implications for the relationship between patients and clinicians because joining with the patient's emotions can impede clinical outcomes. Moreover, a clinician who is merely sympathetic in the clinical encounter can interfere with clinical objectivity and professional effectiveness. The sympathetic doctor cares about the quantity and intensity of the patient's suffering, while the empathetic doctor cares about understanding the quality of the patient's experience [46]. These authors' general conclusion is, therefore, that sympathy must be restrained in clinical situations, whereas empathy does not require a restrictive boundary [50].

In practice, separating emotional from cognitive attributes is very difficult. However, two conclusions might be drawn from our discussion of definitions and our questions regarding the right location (affective, cognitive, or both) in which empathy occurs.

First is that a prerequisite for both affective and cognitive empathy is that an individual should not be overly preoccupied with himself and his own concerns, because, if the experience is to a greater extent focused on the individual himself, then the willingness to help the other person decreases [51]. Only through self-awareness is it possible to see the behavior of the observed person as an expression of his emotional state and to make a mental distinction between oneself and the "other self." The second conclusion is that empathy could bridge the provide gap between patient-centered medicine and evidence-based medicine, therefore representing a profound therapeutic potential.

And here we come to the educational issue. Can empathy be taught? Is it possible to establish a learning process for empathy? The constant question is always if empathy can be taught [52, 53].

26.4.1 Teaching the Non-teachable Issues

A classic study published years ago comes to mind [54]. This study was mainly designed to help medical school admission committees to better select college students for medical school. The authors of the study emphasized that it is probably more important to select college students who will be superior physicians than to select those who will be excellent medical students. Based on a previous publication, subjects were asked to rank order list of 87 characteristics of a superior physician considering the importance of each characteristic and how easily it could be taught. Those ratings were validated by high correlations across several subgroups. The importance and the teachability ratings were combined into a non-teachable important index (NTII) that provides a rank order of traits that are important but cannot be taught easily.

This study aimed to determinate the important qualities of a superior physician that cannot easily be taught in medical school or later training. The authors proposed to select college students for medical school not only on the basis of academic achievements, but also on the basis of characteristics identifiable in the college student that predict excellence in the physician who many years later will emerge from our educational system.

The NTII generated by this study gives equal weight to the importance and to non-teachability. The top of the list comprises qualities closely related to empathy: understanding people, sustaining genuine concern for patients, motivated primarily by idealism, compassion, and service; oriented more toward helping people than making income; enthusiasm for medicine and dedication to his work; and ability to get the heart of a problem and to separate important points from details and adaptability. All those qualities score high in the NTTI index, which means very important and difficult to teach. This is the real challenge for teaching empathy.

Some neurophysiological studies bring certain clues [55, 56] to solve the dilemma of how to teach something that is difficult to teach. Even though empathy is a nontraditional teaching content, it might be promoted through examples and role-taking through which the neurophysiological indicators of empathy could be activated. There are some neurons in the brain which can control certain actions (e.g., behavior or emotion) in the body and can even be activated if the same action is observed in another person. Known as mirror neurons, these nerve cells respond spontaneously, involuntarily, and even without thinking [57]. Mirror neurons use the neurobiological inventory of the observer in order to make him feel what is taking place in the person that he/she is observing by way of inner simulation. Various experiments conducted by the so-called "social neurosciences" document the functioning of the mirror neurons with regard to the empathic perception of the other person [58, 59]. The functioning of mirror neurons is, therefore, an essential prerequisite for empathy [60].

Nevertheless, another question rises up in this mirroring role model theory: is a subsequently learned empathic ability authentic, or does it give a patient the impression that it is an artificial and superficial behavior (i.e., a routine checklist of empathic actions that a clinician is simply required to go through)? Do clinicians need to have previous experience being patients themselves or to witness their family/friends being patients in order to be more empathic? These questions can have great implications for medical education and medical care considering that empathy seems to be a determinant of quality in medical care because it enables the clinician to fulfill key medical tasks more accurately, thereby leading to enhanced health outcomes.

Those who are involved in medical education know that a broad range of biographical experiences and situational factors influence the development and promotion of empathy. Part of these experiences could be the role model teaching scenario, in which students and young doctors are inspired by the teacher's attitudes in dealing with patients. The tag-along model allows medical students to incorporate attitudes, behaviors, and approaches to real patients and identify emerging issues useful for their professional future [61].

Beside tag-alongs, some authors emphasize the importance of art, literature, cinema, and reflecting over one's own life in developing empathy [62]. Literature has plenty of examples and choosing appropriately is always a dilemma. In *A Fortunate Man* [63], a classic book about the story of a country doctor, there is a broad description of empathy, here called recognition. "The task of the doctor is to recognize the man. (…) I am fully aware that I am here using the word *recognition* to cover whole complicated techniques of psychotherapy, but essentially these techniques are precisely means for furthering the process of recognition. (…) In order to treat the illness fully, the doctor must first recognize the patient as a person. Good general diagnosticians are rare, not because most doctors lack medical knowledge, but because most are incapable of taking in all the possible relevant facts—emotional, historical, environmental as well as physical. They are searching for specific conditions instead of the truth about a patient which may then suggest various conditions. (…) A good doctor is acknowledged because he meets the deep but unformulated expectation of the sick for a sense of fraternity. He recognizes them. Sometimes he fails, but there is about him the constant will of a man trying to recognize."

Role modeling, giving the right example to follow, caring carefully for the emotional dimension of medical students, and for that using arts and humanities are possible resources for preventing the erosion of empathy. Because, at the end, it is not just about teaching how to be empathetic—people that enter a medical school already have quite a degree of empathy—but, mainly, to prevent of losing empathy through the so-called educational process that in many cases lacks this perspective [64, 65].

On the other hand, to teach ethics implies setting rules, guidelines, and rational decision-making. But it also requires creativity and acknowledgment of the affective aspects of our decision-making processes. We need, as teachers, to go beyond instructions and perform a caring model pursuing excellence. Is it possible to get together prudence, wisdom, and creativity for a new ethics teaching model? [66]. Usually, ethical inquires come involved in emotions, and those emotions cannot be ignored. Actually, they should be included in the learning process as an essential tool. To share emotions, in an open discussion surrounded by a friendly learning scenario, creates the path for affective education and fosters empathy that empowers patient care [67].

Teaching reflection is a goal for educators who want to move beyond transmitting subject matter content. These teachers believe that they will better understand their students and the nature and processes of learning if they can create more supportive learning environments. Effective teaching is often both an intellectual creation and a performing art [68]. Excellence in teaching requires innovation and risk-taking in dealing with sometimes unanticipated learner response. This is at the core of education and where the humanities and the arts have a place in responding to the challenge of teaching.

26.5 Why We Need Humanities for Educating Patient-Centered Doctors?

26.5.1 Humanities in Medical Education: From Emotions to Ethical Attitudes

To care implies comprehending the human being and the human condition, and for this endeavor, humanities and arts help in building a humanistic perspective of doctoring. They provide a source of insight and understanding and enable doctors to understand patients in their whole context. For this reason, arts and humanities are not just appendages of the medical knowledge but necessary tools and sources of information for proper doctoring. They should be as much a part of medical education as training in differential diagnosis or medical decision-making [69].

Without humanism doctors would not be physicians but simply mechanics [15] (technicians who try to fix the immediate presenting problem, and nothing else). Teaching how to effectively take care of people requires creating methods that address the human aspects of medicine [70]. Humanities also offers a counterpart to the necessary reductions of the natural sciences. The unit of medicine is the particular patient, always irreducible. We know that medicine runs into trouble when individual persons are examined only with instruments that reduce specific meanings to simplistic data [71]. A new balance is needed to incorporate a modern perspective in medical humanism.

Arts and humanities, because they enhance an understanding of human emotions, are useful resources when incorporated into medical education. The students' emotions easily emerge through arts like movies, music, poetry; and teachers can impact student learning by broadening their perspectives of student development. In life, the most important attitudes, values, and actions are taught through role modeling and example, a process that acts directly on the learner's emotions. Because people's emotions play a specific role in learning attitudes and behavior, educators cannot afford to ignore students' affective domain. Certain types of learning have more to do with the affection and love teachers invest in educating people than with theoretical reasoning [72]. Usually feelings arise before concepts in the learners. Understanding emotionally through intuition comes in advance. First, the heart becomes involved, and then a rational process clarifies the learning issue. Thus, the affective path is a critical way to the rational process of learning.

To educate through emotions doesn't mean that learning is limited to values and attitudes exclusively in the affective domain. Rather, it comes from the position that emotions usually come before rational thinking, especially in young students immersed in a culture where feelings and visual impact prevail. Thus, medical educators need to recognize that learners are immersed in a popular culture largely framed through emotions and images [73]. Since emotions and images are privileged in popular culture, they should be the front door for learners' educational processes. Emotions are a kind of bypath to better reach the learners, a type of track for taking off and moving more deeply afterwards, which requires fostering reflection on the learners. The point is to provoke students to reflect on those values and attitudes [74], with the challenge here to understand how to effectively provoke students' reflective processes.

Life stories and narratives enhance emotions and therefore lay the foundation for conveying concepts. When strategically incorporated into the educational process and allowed to flow easily into the learning context, emotions facilitate a constructive approach to understanding that uses the learners' own empathetic language. Furthermore, in dealing with the students' affective domain, the struggle in learning comes close to the pleasure felt, and it is possible to take advantage of emotions to point out attitudes and foster reflection over them.

The instructor's role consists not just in pouring out emotions but in catalyzing the process by which the audience moves from the emotions to immerse themselves in personal reflection and begin to generate concrete ideas for how, in specific and concrete ways, they can incorporate the lessons they've learned from the emotional experience into their daily lives. These experiences are real educational footprints and become open doors for generating attitudes that modulate behavior [75]. The first step in humanizing medical education is to keep in mind that all humans, including medical students, are reflective beings. They need an environment that supports and encourages this activity to refine attitudes, construct identities, develop well-rounded qualities, and enrich themselves as human beings.

Likewise, faculty members use their own emotions in teaching, so learning proper methods to address their affective side is a complementary way to improve their communication with students. Therefore, excellent teachers develop their teaching skills through constant self-evaluation, reflection, the willingness to change, and the drive to learn something themselves [76]. Faculty face challenges when they teach and have few opportunities to share them and reflect with their peers. Usually when teachers discuss educational issues with their colleagues, they often spend most of the time talking about problems instead of nurturing themselves. As teachers, we need to state new paradigms in education, learn how to share our weaknesses and frustrations, and find resources to keep up the flame and energy for a better teaching performance. Humanities could be incorporated in faculty development strategies because they provide a useful peer reflective scenario [77].

26.5.2 Narrative Medicine: Reloading a Millenary Resource for Caring

A predominantly biomedical focus attributed to teaching and practice in health sciences contributes to a dehumanization process. Any strategy that intends to address the issue depends on the presence of well-educated health professionals from both the technical and humanistic point of view. The greatest deficits concern humanistic education. Research about the effectiveness of using narratives as a didactic resource in humanistic education point out issues related to the concealed curriculum and the importance of medical students' exposure to a patient-centered teaching model that gives priority to ethical reflections [78].

It is true that narratives are an important educational topic in the context of family medicine. Narrations, life stories, which allow us to contemplate the patient's world, meet him as a person, so that we can take care of him in a competent manner. There is also a tendency to think that the narrations are just a complement to positive science, which is not possible to measure with laboratory results. Thus, it would be just a methodology that broadens a way of aiming to reach out to the person and focus on her care, without deterring the illness that affects her. That perspective takes the risk of being "complementary," that is, the soft edge of what really matters. The dissociation between science and art remains, as two forces that act synergistically, but in parallel, and therefore never found themselves. The medical action that would fall would be condemned to these complementary positions, in which competency and compassion never meet.

Medicine as art recognizes that each patient is unique. Not only from the perspective of the disease that attacks him/her, but in the way that pathology "becomes incarnate and concretized": this is an illness, being sick [79]. The disease is always personalized, installed in someone who will become sick "in their own way," according to their personal being. A bifocal perspective is necessary, which manages to unite in artistic symbiosis the attention to the disease—with all the technical evolution—and to the patient who feels sick, with the vital understanding that entails. This is a person-centered medical performance, simultaneous exercise of science and art [9].

To listen carefully is a skill that the doctor needs to heal [80]. This requires the rescue of the ancient resources of medical art [81]. Patients show subtle clues about their experience with the condition, but doctors often ignore them because we hear only "the voice of medicine" and have trained us to ignore the emotional side, that is, the "voice of the patient's life" [82].

Already in the middle of the twentieth century, Gregorio Marañón [11]—paradigm of art and science—warned off the danger of using purely technical tools without knowing the patient, without listening carefully, without really caring about him: "It must be admitted that ordinary medicine is usually reduced, or to problems that are easy to solve, or completely insoluble for the most gifted man of wisdom. The fundamental thing in any case is that the doctor be with his five senses in what he is, and not thinking about other things." When the doctor sits and listens to the patient, he is communicating a humanistic attitude par excellence. Today we have sophisticated technology—important—but we are losing the pleasure of sitting down and hearing narratives of life. We lack chairs or, perhaps, patience to sit and listen.

The inclusion of humanities in the curriculum occasions deep rethinking of what it means to be sick and what it means to take care of the sick. They also portray a tremendous spectrum of attitudes required for building ethics and professionalism. We need to be creative in using arts and humanities to effectively reach our students. This is why brief readings, pieces of art, music, and movie clips have a proper place in medical educating. They illustrate complex moral choices and stimulate comments and reflection. A well-known researcher in medical humanities quotes: "we are midwifing a medicine that makes contact with the mysteries of human experience along with its certainties—a medicine that appreciates the deep beauty of health, the silence of health, the wisdom of the body, and the grace of its genius. It is an arch to far times and places, a site for all the living and the dying that go on; it is a link to what it means to be human" [83].

Teaching through humanities includes several modalities in which art is involved [84]. Literature and theater [85], poetry [86], and opera [87] are all useful tools when the goal is to promote learner reflection and construct what has been called the professional philosophic exercis [88]. Teaching with movies is also an innovative method for promoting the sort of engaged learning that education requires today [89, 90]. For dealing with emotions and attitudes, while promoting reflection, life stories derived from movies fit well with the learners' context and expectations. Teaching with films engages the emotions and could serve as a great launching point for discussions of both the emotions and ethical scenarios [91–93]. The crucial role of teaching is to help frame these discussions in such a way as to foster reflective practice among clinicians and clinicians in training.

26.6 Teaching with Movies to Foster Reflective Practice

As film is the favored medium in our current culture, teaching with cinema is particularly well-suited to the learning environment of medical education. Cinema is the audiovisual version of storytelling. Movies provide a narrative model framed in emotions and images that is also grounded in the student's familiar, everyday universe and stimulates a reflective attitude in the learner. We know that in the clinical setting, the life histories of patients are a powerful resource in teaching. Similarly, when the goal is promoting reflection that includes both cognitive and emotional components, life histories derived from the movies are well-matched with the students' desires and expectations.

Life stories are a powerful resource in teaching. In ancient cultures, such as classical Greece, the art of storytelling was often used to teach ethics and human values [94]. Stories are one reasonable solution to the problem that most people, especially young people, can only be exposed to with a limited range of life experiences. Storytelling, theater, literature, opera, and movies all have the capacity to supplement learners' understanding of the broad universe of human experience. Exposure to life experience—either one lived or one lived through story—provides what Aristotle called catharsis. Catharsis has a double meaning, each of which deals with human emotion. Catharsis literally means to "wash out" the feelings retained in the soul. It also implies an organizing process in which the person sorts through orders and makes sense of emotions. In short, in the normal course of events, people keep their feelings inside, storing them in an untidy fashion, but don't think about them. Catharsis helps empty one's emotional drawers and reorganizes them in ways that provide a pleasant sense of order and relief.

Cinema is useful in teaching the human dimension of medicine [95] because it is familiar, evocative, and nonthreatening for students. Movies provide a quick and direct teaching scenario in which specific scenes point out important issues, emotions are presented in accessible ways where they are easy to identify, and students are able to understand and recognize them immediately.

In addition, students have the opportunity to "translate" movie life histories into their own lives, and into a medical context, even when the movie addresses a non-medical subject. Movie experiences act like emotional memories for students' developing attitudes and remain with them as reflective reference points while proceeding through their daily activities, including those related to their role as future doctors. Students identify easily with film characters and movie "realities" and through a reflective attitude gain new insights into many important aspects of life and human relationships. The educational benefit also is expanded by the phenomenon of students' "carrying forward" into their daily lives the insights and emotions initially generated in response to cinema experience. In other words, the movie teaching scenario acts like "an alarm" to make learners more aware when similar issues and situations occur in their daily lives.

For teaching ethics and the human matters of doctoring, which implies refining attitudes, acquiring virtues, and incorporating values, one can employ the purely rational method favored by ethics lectures and deontology courses. But movies offer another path: exposing learners to particular examples with strong emotional consequences to either follow or reject. The movie scenes lead the learners to reflect on where their own attitudes and responses will lead, not only intellectually but emotionally, both for themselves and others. In this way, bringing examination of emotional responses and their consequences into the discussion serves as an effective shortcut that helps reconnect learners with their original idealistic aspirations and motivations as physicians.

This learning scenario stimulates learner reflection. In life, important attitudes, values, and actions are taught using role modeling, a process that impacts the learner's emotions. Since feelings exist before concepts, the affective path is a critical shortcut to the rational process of learning. While technical knowledge and skills can be acquired through training with little reflection, reflection is required to refine attitudes and incorporate values. The purpose of the film methodology is not only to evoke emotions but to help the audience reflect on these emotions and figure out how to translate what they learn into attitudes and actions. Reflection is the necessary bridge to move from emotions to behavior. The goal is to move beyond a specific medical solution to reach a human attitude in life that requires integrity and wholeness [96]. To foster reflection is the main goal in this cinematic teaching set. The purpose is not to show the audience how to incorporate a particular attitude, but rather to promote their reflection and to provide a forum for discussion. And this works for any kind of audience, despite cultural background or language [97].

Fostering reflection stimulates discussion about the interaction of health with the breadth of human experience, and this discussion often elicits profound conflicts and concerns about their future professional roles and as human beings. A new learning process is created, and through it the students are involved in an ongoing process of learning spread into their daily life. The movie teaching methodology stimulates their reflection and, through accessing learners' emotions, offers new paths to the rational process of learning. This is how we can foster reflective practice for the future doctors. A process that is at the core of ethical decisions: never giving up with reflection and never giving in with mediocrity, which in Hannah Arendt's words leads to the banality of evil [98].

Dealing with cinema education is also useful to lead clinicians and students in getting familiar with their own emotional responses, an issue often neglected in medical education. Little effort is exerted to develop emotional honesty in medical students or residents, either in terms of their own affective responses or in terms of their awareness of others' emotions. When students experience negative emotions and nothing is done to construct a real affective education, learners sometimes decide to adopt a position of emotional detachment and distance, and this comes to attitudes lacking professionalism [99]. Narrative films can provide valuable access to viewers' affective lives by "lighting up" disruptive or disturbing parts of the self that might otherwise be ignored or neglected. Because the characters portrayed in movies are "not real," learners can be more honest about their reactions than if they were discussing actual patients. This emotional honesty becomes a starting point for exploring emotional responses.

Movies allow us to go beyond the illustrations of theories and principles, so that we might develop not only a range of rational and analytic skills but also a range of emotional and interpretative ones, including those habits of the heart. The standard models of ethical decision-making so commonly taught in medical school classrooms, the step-by-step approach seeking for an answer, maybe one answer to a particular dilemma are someway disrupted by the films, opening doors to multiple questions and may never fully resolve an issue [100]. Discussions among and with students and colleagues, independent of their level of knowledge and experience, are thought-provoking and can be intensely personal, transforming ethics education into a pendulous experience that oscillates from scientific debate to an exciting and often uneasy voyage of moral inquiry. This educational scenario forces us to reflect on who we are, who we have become, and who we long to be. Before doctors we are human beings, and this is what lies at the bottom of any ethical decision.

In this sense, film, as art, can affect the root of our being. Using film clips in a structured way allows for new opportunities in ethics education. Here comes the specific methodology using movie clips.

26.6.1 The Movie Clip Methodology: Using Wisely Short Time Teaching

Which movies are useful for teaching this or that point? This is a common question people ask. The answer could be something like this: "What you get out of a film often depends upon what you bring to it." Useful movies for teaching whatever you want are those that are valuable to you and those that touched you and lead you to reflect. I can share what movies touched me and why, but I am not able to say what will impress you and be part of your life. When a movie seems remarkable for the educator, we always find the way to incorporate our teaching set. So you need to build your own experience before sharing it with your audience. Keep in mind what you want to teach, the specific ethical dilemma.

Using medical movies is similar to presenting a specific case—like problem-based learning—and discussing it. This is valuable, but not what we are trying to achieve. In our method [101], what matters is not the case or the situation that demands a particular answer. Our goal is to move beyond a specific medical solution to reach a human attitude in life that requires integrity and wholeness. We move from technical responses to deep reflection on how to call forth the best learners have inside themselves. The specific translational process is intentionally left up to learners as they encounter their own lives as doctors and as people.

Do you use a whole movie or just some scenes? Here comes another usual question. The answer depends on what you want to point out, the time you have at your disposal, and the outcomes you expect. Our experience affirms the effectiveness of using the movie clip methodology in which multiple movie clips are shown in rapid sequence, along with facilitator comments while the clips were going on [102]. Teaching with clips in which several, rapid scenes, taken from different movies are all put together, works better than viewing the whole movie. Nowadays, we live in a dynamic and fast-paced environment of rapid information acquisition and high emotional impact. In this context it makes sense to use movie clips because of their brevity, rapidity, and emotional intensity. Bringing clips from different movies, to illustrate or intensify a particular point, fits well with this modern living state.

The value of instructor commentary during the viewing of clips is a conclusion based on our own experience. Although the sudden changing of scenes in the clips effectively evoke participants' individual concerns and fosters reflection in them, making comments while the clip is playing acts as a valuable amplifier to the whole process. Because learners are involved in their personal reflective process, they may at times disagree with the facilitator's comments and form their own conclusions. But this doesn't matter and may even be desirable. In fact, participants note that divergent comments are particularly useful to facilitate the reflecting process. The effect is a rich generation of perspectives and points of view, which in turn trigger multiple, often, contradictory emotions and thoughts in the viewers. In this context, learners' have an intensely felt need for reflection about what they have just seen.

A model involving film clips might foster a more holistic approach to ethics education. Using films, specifically short clips of films, to prompt and frame discussions would be of value for medical ethics education. By allowing reflections on emotions, participants in these sessions can learn to develop their reflective abilities and attitudes. These skills and attitudes, in turn, can help create more humanistic, and presumably more ethical, physicians. There is a selection of movies, time counting scenes, and comments in the appendix from some of these publications.

The academic community requests proof of the effectiveness of a new technique before advocating or even supporting its widespread application. Educators have long ago learned that the measurement of success in teaching remains an elusive, controversial, and at the least quite an ambiguous goal. We should not confuse quality teaching with successful teaching, one that produces learning as is understood exclusively in its achievement sense. At this point, we can envision why those "intangibles" topics, difficult to teach and to assess, in which ethics, empathy, compassion, and commitment are included, could be endorsed through the cinema education methodology. What we can say is that acquiring a taste for the aesthetic provides an additional dimension to medical learning and that even when morality is at issue, a reason is an ideal tool for understanding. Maybe, in Pascal's words, this has something to do with those "reasons from the heart, those reasons that our mind is not able to understand."

In cinema education the educational outcomes don't materialize simply from watching movies. People attend cinema all the time, and see the same scenes, and while they might have similar emotions, the reflective process is lacking. This is where the competence and the teaching skills of the facilitator come into play, that is, by putting all the scenes together and fostering reflection through comments and personal thoughts, even as unanswered open questions are introduced. That is the teacher's role.

There is still a remaining question. Does this movie teaching methodology depend on the charisma of the presenter, or can it be well developed by anyone? There is no definitive answer. All we can say is, if you love movies and if you like to teach deep from your heart, you deserve to try this. Try it and wait for the surprises!

References

1. Cassell EJ. Diagnosing suffering: a perspective. AnnIntern Med. 1999;131:531–4.
2. Moyer C, Arnold L, Quaintance J, Braddock C, Spickard A, Wilson D, et al. What factors create a humanistic doctor? A nationwide survey of fourth-year medical students. Acad Med. 2010;85:1800–7.
3. Robb D. Ciência, Humanismo e Medicina. Rasegna. 1985;3:21–32.

4. Blasco PG, Benedetto MAC, Reginato V. Humanismo em Medicina, vol. 100. São Paulo: SOBRAMFA-Educação Médica e Humanismo; 2015. p. 437.
5. Thibon G. El equilibrio y la armonía. Barcelona: Belacqua; 2005.
6. Blasco PG, Janaudis MA, Levites MR. Un nuevo humanismo médico: la armonía de los cuidados. Aten Primaria. 2006;38(4):225–9.
7. Monasterio F. Planteamiento del Humanismo Médico. Humanismo y Medicina. Murcia: II Encuentro Cultural de la Sociedad Española de Médicos Escritores; 1982.
8. Correa FJL, Blasco PG. (organz).La Humanización de la Salud y el Humanismo Médico en Latinoamérica, vol. 1. Santiago de Chile: FELAIBE, SOBRAMFA y Facultad de Ciencias de la Salud de la Universidad Central de Chile; 2018. p. 253.
9. Roncoletta AFT, Moreto G, Levites MR, Janaudis MA, Blasco PG, Leoto RF. Princípios da Medicina de Família. São Paulo: Sobramfa; 2003.
10. Blasco PG. De los principios científicos para la acción: el idealismo práctico de la Medicina de Família. Aten Primaria. 2004;34(6):313–7.
11. Marañón G. La medicina y nuestro tiempo. Madrid: Espasa; 1954.
12. Levites MR, Blasco PG. Competencia y Humanismo: La Medicina Familiar en Busca de la Excelencia. Archivos de Medicina Familiar y General. 2009;6:2–9.
13. Jonas H. El Principio de Responsabilidad: ensayo de una ética para la civilización tecnológica. Barcelona: Herder; 1995.
14. Ortega y Gasset J. La rebelión de las masas. Madrid: Revista de Occidente; 1930. p. 38–9.
15. Blasco PG. O médico de família hoje. São Paulo: SOBRAMFA; 1997.
16. Jubelier SJ, Welch C, Babar Z. Competences and concerns in end of life care for medical students and residents. W V Med J. 2001;97:118–21.
17. Blasco PG. A ordem dos fatores altera o produto. Reflexões sobre educação médica e cuidados paliativos. Educación Médica. 2018;19:104–14.
18. Gawande A. Being mortal. Illness, medicine and what matters in the end. New York: Holt & Company; 2014.
19. Mendel D. Proper doctoring. Berlin: Springer; 1984.
20. Marañón G. Vocación y ética. Buenos Aires: Espasa-Calpe; 1946.
21. Blasco PG. O Médico Perante a Morte. RevBrasCuidados Paliativos. 2009;2(4):7–12.
22. Blasco PG. O Paciente e a Famillia perante a morte: o papel do médico de familia. Revista Meaning. 2009;2:12–5.
23. Kass LR. Human life review, vol. XVI. New York: The Human Life Foundation, Inc.; 1990.
24. Melvin AT. The primary care physician and palliative care. Palliat Care. 2001;28(2):239–45.
25. Mahoney MC, Yates JW. Oncology. In: Rakel RE, editor. Textbook of family medicine. 6th ed. Philadelphia: Saunders; 2002. p. 1193–4.
26. World Health Organization. WHO definition of palliative care. Cancer.
27. Van Aalst-Cohen ES, Riggs R, Byock IR. Palliative care in medical school curricula: a survey of United States medical schools. J Palliat Med. 2008;11(9):1200–2.
28. Pinheiro TRP, De Benedetto MAC, Levites MR, Del Giglio A, Blasco PG. Teaching palliative care to residents and medical students. Fam Med. 2010;42(8):580–2.
29. Lloyd-Williams M, Macleod RDM. A systematic review of teaching and learning in palliative care within the medical undergraduate curriculum. Med Teach. 2004;26(8):683–90.
30. Torke AM, Quest TM, Branch WT. A workshop to teach medical students communication skills and clinical knowledge about end-of-life care. J Gen Intern Med. 2004;19:540–4.
31. Irigoyen M. El paciente terminal: Manejo del Dolor y Cuidados Paliativos em Medicina Familiar. Medicina Familiar Mexicana: México DF; 2002.
32. Moreto G. Cuidando do Paciente. In: Blasco PB, Janaudis MA, Leoto RF, Roncoletta AF, Levites MR, editors. Princípios de Medicina de Família. São Paulo: SOBRAMFA; 2003. p. 121–36.
33. Hennezel M, Leloup JY. A Arte de Morrer. Petrópolis: Editora Vozes; 2005.
34. Pinheiro TR, Blasco PG, De Benedetto MAC, Levites M, Del Giglio A, Monaco C. Teaching palliative care in a free clinic: a Brazilian experience. In: Chang E, Johnson A, editors.

Contemporary and innovative practice in palliative care. 1st ed. Rijeka: InTech—Open Access Company; 2012. p. 19–28.

35. Frank A. Just listening narrative and deep illness. Fam Syst Health. 1998;16:197–212.
36. De Benedetto MAC, Castro AG, Carvalho E, Sanogo R, Blasco PG. From suffering to transcendence: narratives in palliative care. Can Fam Physician. 2007;53:1277–9.
37. Wald HS, Reis SP. Beyond the margins: reflective writing and development of reflective capacity in medical education. J Gen Intern Med. 2010;25(7):746–9.
38. Carroll R. Finding the words to say it: the healing power of poetry. Evid Based Complement Alternat Med. 2005;2(2):161–72.
39. Smyth JM, Stone AA, Hurewitz A, Kaell A. Effects of writing about stressful experiences on symptom reduction in patients with asthma or rheumatoid arththritis. JAMA. 1999;281(14):1304–9.
40. Coulombe L. Talking with patients: it is different when they are dying? Can Fam Physician. 1995;41:423–37.
41. Taylor L, Hammond J, Carlos R. A student initiated elective on end of life care: a unique perspective. J Palliat Med. 2003;1:86–9.
42. Hojat M. Empathy in patient care. Antecedents, development, measurement, and outcomes. New York: Springer; 2007.
43. Costa SC, Figueiredo MRB, Schaurich D. Humanization within adult intensive care units (ICUs): comprehension among the nursing team. Interface (Botucatu). 2009;13(1):571–80.
44. Hojat M, Gonnella JS, Mangione S, Nasca TJ, Veloski JJ, Erdmann JB, et al. Empathy in medical students as related to academic performance, clinical competence and gender. Med Educ. 2002;36:522–7.
45. MacIntyre A. Edith Stein. Un prólogo filosófico. Granada: Ed Nuevo Inicio; 2008.
46. Hojat M, Vergare MJ, Maxwell K, Brainard G, Herrine SK, Isenberg GA, et al. The devil is in the third year: a longitudinal study of erosion of empathy in medical school. Acad Med. 2009;84:1182–91.
47. Irving P, Dickson D. Empathy: towards a conceptual framework for health professionals. Int J Health Care Qual Assur Inc Leadersh Health Serv. 2004;17:212–20.
48. Neumann M, Bensing J, Mercer J, Ernstmann N, Ommen O, Pfaff H. Analyzing the "nature" and "specific effectiveness" of clinical empathy: a theoretical overview and contribution towards a theory-based research agenda. Patient Educ Couns. 2009;74:339–46.
49. Stephan WG, Finlay KA. The role of empathy in improving inter-group relations. J Soc Issues. 1999;55:729–43.
50. Hojat M, Gonnella JS, Nasca TJ, Mangione S, Vergare M, Magee M. Physician empathy: definition, components, measurement, and relationship to gender and specialty. Am J Psychiatry. 2002;159:1563–9.
51. Aderman D, Berkowitz L. Self-concern and the unwillingness to be helpful. Soc Psychol Q. 1983;46:293–301.
52. Bayne HB. Training medical students in empathic communication. J Spec Group Work. 2011;36:316–29.
53. Moreto G, González-Blasco P, De Benedetto MAC. Reflexiones sobre la enseñanza de la empatía y la educación médica. Aten Fam. 2014;21(3):94–7.
54. Sade R, Stroud M, Levine J, Fleming G. Criteria for selection of future physicians. Ann Surg. 1985;201:225–30.
55. Decety J, Jackson P. A social-neurosience perspective on empathy. Curr Dir Psychol Sci. 2006;15:54–8.
56. Gallese V. The roots of empathy: the shared manifold hypothesis and the neural basis of intersubjectivity. Psychopathology. 2003;36:17180.
57. Rizzolatti G, Sinigaglia C. So quell che fai: il cervello che agisce e I neuroni specchio. Milano: R Cortina Ed.; 2006.
58. Decety J, Jackson P. The functional architecture of human empathy. Behav Cogn Neurosci Rev. 2004;3:71–100.

59. Wicker B, Keysers C, Plailly J, Royet JP, Gallese V, Rizzolatti G. Both of us are disgusted in my insula: the common neural basis of seeing and seeking disgust. Neuron. 2003;40:644–55.
60. Bauer J. Warum ich fühle, was Du fühlst. Intuitive Kommunikation und dasGeheimnis der Spiegelneurone (Why I feel what you feel. Intuitive communication and the mystery of the mirror neurons). Hamburg: Hoffmann und Campe; 2005.
61. Blasco PG, Roncoletta AFT, Moreto G, Levites MR, Janaudis MA. Accompanying physicians in their family practice: a primary care model for medical students' learning in Brazil. Fam Med. 2006;38(9):619–21.
62. Larson EB, Yao X. Clinical empathy as emotional labor in patient-physician relationship. JAMA. 2005;293(9):1100–6.
63. Berger J, Mohr J. A fortunate man. The story of a country doctor. New York: Vintage; 1997.
64. Moreto G, Santos I, Blasco PG, Pessini L, Lotufo PA. Assessing empathy among medical students: a comparative analysis using two different scales in a Brazilian medical school, vol. 19. Spain: Educación Médica (Ed. impresa); 2018. p. 162–70.
65. Moreto G. Avaliação da empatia de estudantes de medicina em uma universidade na cidade de São Paulo utilizando dois instrumentos. Tese Doutoral em Medicina (Ciências Médicas) Universidade de São Paulo, USP, Brasil. Disponível em. 2015.
66. Christianson CE, McBride RB, Vari RC, Olson L, Wilson HD. From traditional to patient-centered learning: curriculum change as an intervention for changing institutional culture and promoting professionalism in undergraduate medical education. Acad Med. 2007;82:1079–88.
67. Marcus ER. Empathy, humanism, and the professionalism of medical education. Acad Med. 1999;74:1211–5.
68. Bain K. What the best college teachers do. Cambridge, MA: Harvard University Press; 2004.
69. Mullangi S. The synergy of medicine and art in the curriculum. Acad Med. 2013;88:921–3.
70. Blay Pueyo C. Como evaluar el desarrollo profesional continúo. Evaluación de la competencia: métodos y reflexiones. Jano Extra; 2006. pp 36–42.
71. Belling C. Sharper instruments: on defending the humanities in undergraduate medical education. Acad Med. 2010;85:938–40.
72. Ruiz-Retegui A. Pulchrum – Reflexiones Sobre La Belleza. Madrid: Rialp; 1999.
73. Ferres J. Educar en una cultura del espectáculo. Barcelona: Paidós; 2000.
74. Blasco PG, Alexander M. Ethics and human values. In: Alexander M, Lenahan P, Pavlov A, editors. Cinemeducation: a comprehensive guide to using film in medical education, vol. 2005. Oxford, UK: Radcliffe Publishing; 2005. p. 141–5.
75. Blasco PG, Moreto G, Janaudis MA, Benedetto MAC, Altisent R, Delgado-Marroquin MT. Educar las emociones para promover la formación ética. Persona y Bioética. 2013;17:28–48.
76. Palmer PJ. The courage to teach. San Francisco: Jossey-Bass; 1998.
77. Blasco PG, Moreto G, González-Blasco M, Levites MR, Janaudis MA. Education through movies: improving teaching skills and fostering reflection among students and teachers. Creative Educ. 2015;11:145–60.
78. De Benedetto MAC. O Papel das Narrativas como Recurso Didático na Formação Humanística dos Estudantes de Medicina e Enfermagem. Tese (PhD). São Paulo: Universidade Federal de São Paulo (UNIFESP). 2017.
79. Kleinman A, Eisenberg L, Good B. Culture, illness, and care. Clínical lessons from anthropologic and cross-cultural research. Ann Intern Med. 1978;88:251–8.
80. Greenhalgh T. Narrative based medicine: why study narrative? BMJ. 1999;318:48–50.
81. Greenhalgh T. Narrative based medicine in a evidence based world. BMJ. 1999;318:323–5.
82. Brown JB, et al. The first component: exploring both the disease and the illness experience. In: Stewart M, Brown JB, Weston WW, McWninney R, McWilliam CL, Freeman TR, editors. Patient-centered medicine. Transforming the clinical method. 2nd ed. Abingdon, UK: Radcliffe Med Press; 2003. p. 3–52.
83. Charon R. Calculating the contributions of humanities to medical practice – motives, methods, and metrics. Acad Med. 2010;85:935–7.

84. Ousager J, Johannessen H. Humanities in undergraduate medical education: a literature review. Acad Med. 2010;85:988–98.
85. Shapiro J. Literature and the arts in medical education. Fam Med. 2000;32(3):157–8.
86. Whitman N. A poet confronts his own mortality: what a poet can teach medical students and teachers. Fam Med. 2000;32(10):673–4.
87. Blasco PG, Moreto G, Levites MR. Teaching humanities through opera: leading medical students to reflective attitudes. Fam Med. 2005;37(1):18–20.
88. Decourt LV. William Osler na Intimidade de Seu Pensamento. Revista do Incor. 2000.
89. Baños JE, Bosch F. Using feature films as a teaching tool in medical schools El empleo de películas comerciales en las facultades de medicina. Educación Médica. 2015;16(4):206–11.
90. Self DJ, Baldwin DC. Teaching medical humanities through film discussions. J Med Humanit. 1990;11(1):23–9.
91. Colt H, Quadrelli S, Friedman L. The picture of health: medical ethics and the movies. New York: Oxford University Press; 2011.
92. Self DJ, Baldwin DC, Olivarez M. Teaching medical ethics to first-year students by using film discussion to develop their moral reasoning. Acad Med. 1993;68(5):383–5.
93. Searight HR, Allmayer S. The use of feature film to teach medical ethics: overview and assessment. Int J Modern Educ Forum. 2014;3(1):1–6.
94. McIntyre AC. After virtue. A study in moral theory. Notre Dame: Notre Dame Press; 1984.
95. Blasco PG. Humanizando a Medicina: Uma Metodologia com o Cinema. São Paulo: Centro Universitário São Camilo; 2011.
96. Blasco PG, Benedetto MAC, Garcia DSO, Moreto G, Roncoletta AFT, Troll T. Cinema for educating global doctors: from emotions to reflection, approaching the complexity of the human being. Prim Care. 2010;10:45–7.
97. Blasco PG, Mônaco CF, Benedetto MAC, Moreto G, Levites MR. Teaching through movies in a multicultural scenario: overcoming cultural barriers through emotions and reflection. Fam Med. 2010;42(1):22–4.
98. Blasco PG. Commentary on Hannah Arendt. Acad Med. 2016;91:675.
99. Shapiro J. Does medical education promote professional alexithymia? A call for attending to the emotions of patients and self in medical training. Acad Med. 2011;86:326–32.
100. Blasco PG. Review of Henri Colt, Silvia Quadrelli, and Lester Friedman (eds), the picture of health: medical ethics and the movies: getting familiar with the cinema education methodology. Am J Bioethics. 2011;11:9–41.
101. Blasco PG. Medical Education, Family Medicine and Humanism: Medical students' expectations, dilemmas and motivations analyzed through discussion of movies. PhD diss. São Paulo: University of São Paulo Medical School. 2002.
102. Blasco PG, Moreto G, Roncoletta AFT, Levites MR, Janaudis MA. Using movie clips to foster learners' reflection: improving education in the affective domain. Fam Med. 2006;38(2):94–6.

Part VIII

Appendix

Hints for Meta-research on Ageing for Family Doctors

Nicola Veronese and Jacopo Demurtas

Abstract

The need for major information in meta-research (i.e. the part of medicine interested in systematic reviews [SRs] and meta-analyses [MAs]) is increasing. In the last years, we are observing an exponential rate of publications as SRs/MAs in geriatric medicine, but the role of family doctors in this kind of research is poorly explored. We believe that primary care research, applied to ageing problems, is of great importance, also when talking about meta-research for several reasons such as an optimal use of primary care resources or since family doctors can underline problems not traditionally covered by geriatric medicine. Given this background, in this chapter we will briefly discuss the importance of meta-research of ageing for family doctors.

Keywords

Meta-research · Meta-analysis · Systematic review · Primary care

N. Veronese (✉)
Department of Internal Medicine and Geriatrics, University of Palermo, Palermo, Italy
e-mail: ilmannato@gmail.com

J. Demurtas
Primary Care Department, USL Toscana Sud Est, Grosseto, Italy

© Springer Nature Switzerland AG 2022
J. Demurtas, N. Veronese (eds.), *The Role of Family Physicians in Older People Care*, Practical Issues in Geriatrics, https://doi.org/10.1007/978-3-030-78923-7_27

27.1 Introduction

Systematic reviews and meta-analyses (SRs and MAs), the process of synthesizing previously published research evidence proposed for answering specific questions in clinical practice, are commonly considered as the highest evidence in the scientific pyramid [1]. It is widely known that SRs and MAs can significantly contribute to clinical practice, since they can increase knowledge and identify fields, where current evidence is still lacking. Unfortunately, many SRs and MAs have been considered redundant, misleading, serving conflicting interests or of low quality. These shortcomings, instead of improving actual evidence, multiply the limitations of primary studies, rather than objectively and critically presenting them [2, 3].

These issues are widely applicable to geriatric medicine [4] and to primary care research [5].

In this chapter we will briefly discuss the importance of meta-research of ageing for family doctors.

27.2 What Is Meta-research?

In a seminal paper, John Ioannidis defined meta-research as "the study of research itself" [6]. Science is the key driver of human progress since it improves the efficiency of scientific investigation leading to more credible and more useful research findings that can translate to major benefits for human beings [6]. Meta-research tries to use an interdisciplinary approach to study, promote, and defend robust science, without any possible bias [7].

27.3 Meta-research in Geriatric Medicine: Specific Issues

Geriatric medicine has some specific points that an investigator should consider when approaching a SR and/or MA [4]. The accurate identification/inclusion of specific groups (such as older persons pertinent to daily practice) is crucial as well as the high drop-out rate of older people observed in several randomized controlled trials (RCTs). In addition, the low reporting of older people in RCTs is another important shortcoming [4, 8, 9]. Finally, to the best of our knowledge, little is known about the interest and competence of physicians interested in older people care regarding SRs and MAs, even if the interest in meta-research is great, also among physicians interested in geriatric medicine research [10].

27.4 The Importance of Family Doctors in Meta-research Regarding Ageing

Clinically speaking, family doctors, as gatekeepers and first-line professionals, are among the first to touch and deal with the problems of older patients. Therefore, they have a great importance in geriatric medicine that, however, is so far poorly covered in research. We believe that primary care research, applied to ageing problems, is of great importance, also when talking about meta-research for several reasons. For example, primary care resources are extremely important for some problems traditionally related to geriatrics, such as frailty, indicating newer kinds of possible intervention for this condition [11]. In the same way, family physician may highlight excess of medicalization and provide useful directives for quaternary prevention. Given this background we can purpose some hints for (young) family doctors, potentially interested in geriatric medicine and (or) meta-research.

27.5 Hints for Meta-research on Ageing for Family Doctors

In a nice and topical review, Shenkin et al. reported some basilar concepts for doing SR/MA in geriatric medicine that we believe it is correct to briefly summarize for family doctors [4].

First, when approaching this argument, the importance of age should be underlined. In particular, we believe that in works treating geriatric conditions a formal cut-off for defining older age should be decided and, if possible, to use age as potential moderator of heterogenous data. Second, in older populations, medical conditions can have atypical presentations and not validated diagnoses/definitions. It is the typical case of some common conditions, for example, dementia, that can be defined as self-reported, through neuropsychological tests, medical records, or validated interviews. As expected, the choice to include all the definitions of a single medical condition can create heterogeneity and, at the same time, to exclude some participants for the definition of a condition. Another big problem encountered in meta-research on ageing regard the inclusion/exclusion criteria used in the original studies. These choices, unfortunately, lead to a significant difference between the patients included in the RCTs (and therefore in SRs/MAs) and those that we have in our daily clinical practice. Konrat et al. reported that older patients are poorly represented in RCTs of drugs they are likely to receive, making the prevision of benefits and side effects very difficult and consequently far from evidence based medicine [12].

27.6   Conclusions

In this chapter, we have briefly discussed the importance of meta-research (see also Box 27.1 for further indications) in geriatric medicine introducing the role of family doctors in this research. We believe that, as in other topics typical of geriatric medicine, the cross-talking between family doctors and geriatricians is only at the beginning, and we hope that our chapter can encourage further steps in this direction.

Box 27.1 Hints for Meta-research for Family Doctors Interested in Geriatric Medicine

Meta-research is investigation and can be seen like a sort of treasure hunt, aiming to obtain robust evidence or valuable confirmation with specific methodology and rules.

The first thing to do is to find a map, make, provide, or stick to a protocol, stating at least which population we are going to investigate, which intervention, which comparison if any, and what is the outcome/s we are looking for.

With our map, the protocol, which is better to register on one of the specific databases, we can start our quest to evidence.

In the first phase, we will need to find the documents that can help us find our treasure. Usually it is worth asking a librarian or somebody expert in searching scientific literature to launch a search on different databases (i.e. Medline/PubMed, Epistemonikos, Cinhal) to gather documents.

Many documents will be found, but are they of any use for your quest? This depends on your eligibility criteria!

1. Our suggestion is to, as well, established an explained in papers like the one on PRISMA checklist[1], to work at least in pairs, doublechecking every document you were able to find, first looking at title and abstracts, and then checking thoroughly the full paper and supplementary materials.

After this phase you will be able to find the literature you need, you have found your treasure!

Now, the hardest part, is all worthy? Does it make any sense to unearth all the treasure?

No, so you will have to dig and search just those things you were looking for and register them.

After this you will convert your treasure to current currency, and to do this you will need the help of a statistician and specific programs.

When all will be set and you have had what you were searching, you could also publish your data and tell the world about your quest!

---

[1]Liberati A, Altman DG, Tetzlaff J, Mulrow C, Gøtzsche PC, Ioannidis JPA, Clarke M, Devereaux PJ, Kleijnen J, Moher D (2009) The PRISMA statement for reporting systematic reviews and meta-analyses of studies that evaluate health care interventions: explanation and elaboration. PLoS medicine 6:e1000100–e1000100.

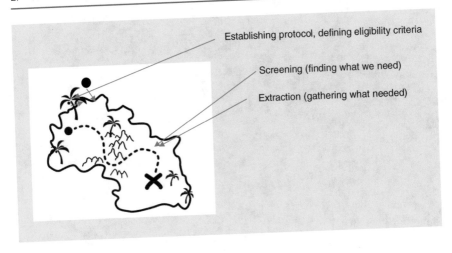

Establishing protocol, defining eligibility criteria

Screening (finding what we need)

Extraction (gathering what needed)

References

1. Stevens KR. Systematic reviews: the heart of evidence-based practice. AACN Adv Crit Care. 2001;12(4):529–38.
2. Møller MH, Ioannidis JP, Darmon M. Are systematic reviews and meta-analyses still useful research? We are not sure. New York: Springer; 2018.
3. Ioannidis JP, Lau J. Pooling research results: benefits and limitations of meta-analysis. Jt Comm J Qual Improv. 1999;25(9):462–9.
4. Shenkin SD, Harrison JK, Wilkinson T, Dodds RM, Ioannidis JP. Systematic reviews: guidance relevant for studies of older people. Age Ageing. 2017;46(5):722–8.
5. Tatsioni A, Ioannidis J. Meta-research: bird's eye views of primary care research. Fam Pract. 2020;37(3):287–9.
6. Ioannidis JP. Meta-research: why research on research matters. PLoS Biol. 2018;16(3):e2005468.
7. Ioannidis JP, Fanelli D, Dunne DD, Goodman SN. Meta-research: evaluation and improvement of research methods and practices. PLoS Biol. 2015;13(10):e1002264.
8. Cherubini A, Signore SD, Ouslander J, Semla T, Michel JP. Fighting against age discrimination in clinical trials. J Am Geriatr Soc. 2010;58(9):1791–6.
9. Crome P, Cherubini A, Oristrell J. The PREDICT (increasing the participation of the elderly in clinical trials) study: the charter and beyond. Expert Rev Clin Pharmacol. 2014;7(4):457–68.
10. Veronese N, Torbahn G, Demurtas J, Beaudart C, Soysal P, Marengoni A, et al. Interest in meta-research in geriatric medicine: a survey of members of the European Geriatric Medicine Society. Eur Geriatr Med. 2020;1(6):1079–83.
11. Macdonald SH-F, Travers J, Shé ÉN, Bailey J, Romero-Ortuno R, Keyes M, et al. Primary care interventions to address physical frailty among community-dwelling adults aged 60 years or older: a meta-analysis. PLoS One. 2020;15(2):e0228821.
12. Konrat C, Boutron I, Trinquart L, Auleley G-R, Ricordeau P, Ravaud P. Underrepresentation of elderly people in randomised controlled trials. The example of trials of 4 widely prescribed drugs. PLoS One. 2012;7(3):e33559.

Beyond Quantitative Research: How Qualitative Research Could Affect Our Understanding of Older People Needs

28

Luca Ghirotto, Mariagiovanna Amoroso, Maria Milano, and Lorenza Garrino

Abstract

Qualitative research represents a humanistic imperative in professional practice. Qualitative evidence improves care processes and takes into account the complexity of human experience. In this chapter, we highlight the importance of conducting qualitative studies in primary and older people care, clarifying the theoretical underpinnings of qualitative methodologies. Phenomena qualitative research may deepen include personal experiences and perceptions, behaviours within a specific context, and psychosocial processes. We summarize the relevant qualitative research involving older assisted persons and family physicians: available qualitative evidence informs clinical practice by identifying needs older people are not aware of or repress, understanding the complex treatment paths from the patients and physicians' perspectives and outlining decision-making processes dynamics. Finally, we stress listening and participation as pivotal features of conducting qualitative research. From the qualitative research lesson, family physicians may learn how to listen to the assisted persons and maximise patients and caregivers' participation in treatments.

L. Ghirotto (✉)
Qualitative Research Unit, Azienda USL—IRCCS di Reggio Emilia, Reggio Emilia, Italy
e-mail: luca.ghirotto@ausl.re.it

M. Amoroso
Società Italiana di Medicina Generale (SIMG) and Movimento Giotto (Italy), Firenze, Italy

M. Milano
Medical School of Turin, Torino, Italy

Società Italiana di Medicina Generale (SIMG) and WONCA, Firenze, Italy

L. Garrino
Department of Public Health and Paediatric Sciences, University of Turin, Torino, Italy

© Springer Nature Switzerland AG 2022
J. Demurtas, N. Veronese (eds.), *The Role of Family Physicians in Older People Care*, Practical Issues in Geriatrics, https://doi.org/10.1007/978-3-030-78923-7_28

Keywords

Qualitative research · Qualitative methods · Family physicians · Older people care · Primary care · Older people · Phenomenology · Ethnography Grounded theory

28.1 What Is Qualitative Research, and Why Is It Important?

Guidelines in older people care are based on unexceptionable trials and generalizable evidence. Nevertheless, every family physician knows that they are hugely valid on selected populations: mainly men, never in old age and often with a single pathology.

Diversity is what primary care deals with: the population of patients varies by gender, age, ethnicity, and pathologies. Family physicians, therefore, work attempting to apply guidelines, trying to give them an applicable meaning and balancing evidence and uncertainty within their clinical practice. Besides, a "Silver Tsunami" is transforming primary care into a territorial geriatrics, especially for those countries where the older people population is prevalent. In Italy, for example, 8% of the inhabitants are over 85 years old and about one in four more than 65 years old [1]. Old age implies chronicity, multi-pathologies, multi-morbidity and clinical frailty, concurrently emerging and rarely tested together. Finally, the low birth rate is resulting in a shortage of young family caregivers which may help older assisted persons, leaving space for equally older people's caregivers, more often spouses or partners.

In this context, how to apply the guidelines in a population where they have not been tested? How does chronicity-related polytherapy reconcile with prescriptive appropriateness, therapeutic adherence and cognitive decline of the patient? What are the care needs of the caregivers of a chronic older patient? What if the decline involves the caregiver?

In these contexts, no trial can answer those complex questions which are pivotal for family physicians. Caring for an older adult entails numerous factors which, to be understood, require not only deepening clinical skills but also a holistic assessment. Human variability, values, culture, health-related behaviours and relationships could not be adequately described using quantitative methods. Here, the importance of relying on qualitative research evidence emerges to the fullest. The quickest way to answer the question "what is qualitative research?" would be highlighting the line that separates qualitative from quantitative research. The answer appears to be self-evident: quantitative researchers and clinical trialists use numbers, the data matrix, statistics and qualitative researchers do not. However, this is unsatisfactory and does not justify the relevance and significance of qualitative research, in particular for health professionals and, explicitly, for family physicians [2]. The main difference between the quantitative and qualitative relies on the research question and the way researchers deal with the research setting [3].

The research question circumscribes what researchers are looking for. If the research question is "what are specific behavioural indications for preventing the spread of infection?", it is necessary to conduct quantitative studies to inform international guidelines. In quantitative methodologies, researchers condition the study context to adapt it to the method and for hypothesis testing purposes. During this process, therefore, researchers manipulate reality so that it is controllable and, therefore, can be studied through a clear and shared research method. Quantitative research tries to develop generalisations that can be applied to a range of contexts.

Conversely, qualitative research focuses on the context of a phenomenon. If researchers want to understand the experiences of people affected by the disease or the emotions related to the fear of contagion in a given context, it is necessary to investigate and explore these phenomena through a qualitative approach, which assumes the participants' perspective and can address the complexity and singularity of human experiences. Phenomena refractory to quantitative methods are individual meanings, psychological and social processes, emotions, beliefs and behaviour patterns within life contexts. These cannot be gagged within a rigid hypothetical-deductive method of investigation [4]—qualitative research results in the comprehension of meanings and experiences representing the prerequisite for shared or shareable solutions. On the one hand, therapeutic adherence and chronic diseases management regard the meanings patients attribute to what they live and value.

On the other hand, the exploration of the meanings that the physicians attribute to patients and caregivers' behaviours allows investigating how diagnostic and therapeutic choices are shaped by the physicians. In other words, qualitative research entails reflection on one's perspective about the world she/he lives in and trains both the participants and researchers' reflexivity towards themselves and the care actions to take [5]. In this regard, the qualitative approach represents a real humanistic imperative in a professional practice of family physicians, and the production of qualitative evidence to improve the care processes may shed light on the existence of the person, in his/her irreducible complexity [6].

28.2 The Underpinnings of Qualitative Research

The initial phase of a qualitative research process is the compelling need to understand a phenomenon from the participants who experience a phenomenon. A growing methodological literature has therefore been produced, from manuals on participant observation, discourse and conversation analysis to handbooks for textual analysis of documents or focus groups conduction. All these strategies are a means to grasp the "voice" of participants concerning what they live and experience. In this approach, human beings are seen holistically within their social context [7]. It is becoming increasingly clear that qualitative research "is a theory-driven enterprise" [8] with specific philosophical assumptions underlying each research method. The overall logic of qualitative research includes epistemological paradigms. The paradigms' ultimate goal is the description and comprehension of phenomena rather than their explanation (as it may be noted below regarding phenomenological approach, ethnographic method, grounded theory and the consistent data collection strategies like interviews, observations, fieldwork, field observations, etc.). Patients, family members, friends and professionals' perceptions, meanings and emotions, the reasons for the decisions taken or to be taken, require respectful methods of investigation, capable of not distorting the real occurring dynamics. The researchers cannot, moreover, manipulate these phenomena but should assume them in their appearance and study them according to adequate methodologies that do not falsify or alter them. In other words, it is necessary to use strategies to understand rather than to verify hypothesis: in qualitative research, the scientific focus shifts from explanation to understanding, from a deductive reasoning (useful for hypothesis testing and verification) to an inductive approach (concerned with the generation of new theory and knowledge emerging from the data) [9]. Besides, the logic of qualitative inquiry involves also the paradigm of critical inquiry, whose intent is investigating how to change settings (action research, feminist research, discourse analysis methodologies and the consistent data collection strategies like participative group work, reflective journals, focus groups, policies' analysis, etc.) [10]. The transformative logic implicitly connotates the family physicians' care process since it requires managing changes both in health conditions and personal situations, by means of relationship and proximity with the assisted persons. Evidence from the real problems that "affect" patient care daily [11] helps family physicians to achieve the transformative goal of care practice by making qualitative-informed decisions.

28.3 Qualitative Approaches and Methods

Qualitative research seeks to study complexity [12] using strategies sufficiently descriptive not to lose the richness of the phenomena and still rigorous enough to allow intersubjective control of the data collected and their interpretation [13]. There are various approaches and methods in qualitative inquiry, ranging from historical, ethnographic to phenomenological methods. "Qualitative" phenomena mainly include personal experiences and perceptions, behaviours within a specific context and psychosocial processes. Researchers may choose many qualitative methods, consistent with the research question and phenomenon. Mainly, but not exclusively, qualitative research is used to answer questions about beliefs (but also habits and behaviours) of a given social group, personal experiences and psychosocial processes. Researchers should not follow qualitative methods to answer questions about causes or to verify hypotheses or theories. Below, we explore the main qualitative methods that respond to the phenomena listed above: ethnography, phenomenology and Grounded Theory (GT) [11].

Ethnography is a useful research approach to study a group of people, their habits, beliefs and behaviours, with their context of life. Ethnography analyses languages, symbolic codes, practices, repertoires and in situ interactions, used to describe the behaviours of a given social group as systematically as possible, starting from data collected through fieldwork, the main feature of the ethnographic method [14]. The fieldwork includes the observation, participant or nonparticipant, of a social group by a researcher, who can be an insider or outsider, resulting in a thick description. A thick description contains all the evidence observed concerning facts, comments and any interpretations of those facts by members of the social group. Geertz [15] thus lists the characteristics of an excellent ethnographic description:

- It takes into consideration not only observational data but also the study of the meaning-giving processes of individuals and the group.
- It is informative as regards the interpretations of social events.
- It uses the expressions and words of the group studied.
- It describes the behaviours that take place in a micro context.

Ethnographers study people in their life contexts by collecting those data that allow them to understand the idioms, the dictionaries in use, the behaviours and the actions of the members of a group. These emerge mainly thanks to observation, one of the main ethnography data collection techniques. The ethnographers spend a long time in the field (the research setting) to experience the group "culture". Therefore, the ethnographers not only observe what is happening but "feel" what it means to be part of that particular group. A further tool of this research method is the field notes that are the collection of details and descriptions but also comments and analytical reflections by the ethnographers. Field notes are a prelude to the thick description. When the researchers take the field notes, they do not synthesise, generalise or hypothesise. The notes capture and describe the events that, in a second moment, will allow inferring the cultural meanings of the circumstances and the behaviours of the participants.

When researchers aim at understanding intimate aspects of living specific experiences (the so-called lived experiences), they may conduct a phenomenological study. Before being a research method, phenomenology is a philosophical movement dealing with the study of phenomena (and not of objective facts). A phenomenon is what the individual (or collective) consciousness signifies. In philosophical terms, signifying is possible because of intentionality: the process through which the consciousness gives meaning to things. Consequently, phenomenology is the method that most coherently answers research questions about experiences as the persons perceive and live them [16]. Phenomenology aims to grab the "essence" or "structure" of the lived experiences, its fundamental meaning: it is the essence that makes the experience what it is, rather than the sum of its variations in everyone's life [17]. The phenomenologists try to reach the most profound comprehension possible by collecting data, preferentially, through open, semi-structured or in-depth, interviews. The sample of a phenomenological study is usually small and very homogeneous, to allow the analysis of the essences or invariants in each of the interviews collected, valid to describe the experience of that group of participants. Defining the results includes the following steps:

- The phenomenologists read the interviews' transcripts to retain the underlying sense of what the participants experienced.
- By a non-judgemental attitude (*epochè*), analysts fracture the transcripts into meaning units.
- The researchers "translate" the meaning units to make implicit and undeclared meanings explicit.
- Finally, based on the transformed units, the structure or essence of the overall experience is described [18].

Finally, if researchers need to answer research questions aiming at an explanation of what is going on within a particular setting, GT is a suitable method [19]. Conducting a GT allows researchers to construct a theoretical explanation of a process whose meanings informants negotiate. In this sense, GT is particularly useful for studying care considered a process shaped by the interplay of patients, caregivers, and professionals. This method was initially conceived by Glaser and Strauss [20], systematised in the volume *The Discovery of Grounded Theory*. The great novelty of the method lies in the possibility of operating conceptualisations and theoretical models starting from data. Essential characteristics of GT are:

- The immersion of the researchers in the research setting.
- An in-depth analysis, which implements induction, as a qualitative form of reasoning.
- The tension to understand the context, through the constant comparison of cases.
- The simultaneous collection and analysis of data.
- Theoretical sampling.

The researchers who want to use GT as a method to answer their research question must, first of all, immerse themselves in the research context and be part of those relationships that shape the processes under investigation. From the "natural" contexts, the researchers collect data, isolate the cases of analysis and define their salient features [21]. Coding is the GT data analysis strategy for reaching the general levels of theory. Coding includes three stages: open, focused and theoretical coding. During open coding, researchers index the interviews' transcripts using "codes" or labels. Then, to perform focused coding, they group the codes into conceptual categories, identifying overarching concepts at a higher level of abstraction. Lastly, through theoretical coding, researchers define the explanatory theoretical model, highlighting the relationships between the conceptual categories. The collection and analysis of data are simultaneous activities in GT: precisely based on the characteristics of the cases and the first conceptual explanations emerging from the open and focused coding, the researchers keep selecting the participants by varying the characteristics of the sample. This strategy is called theoretical sampling, a strategy for choosing the participants not according to statistical representativeness criteria but to collect data from contrary cases, to confirm or disconfirm the first explanatory hypotheses. In doing so, researchers may achieve the saturation of the conceptual categories. The collection and analysis of data are, therefore, at the service of theory construction for explaining the process under investigation [19, 21].

28.4 Examples of Qualitative Studies in the Area of Chronicity and Primary Care

What is current qualitative research involving older assisted persons and family physicians about? Qualitative research investigated the world of older patients, revealing itself as an effective means for identifying needs older persons are not aware of or repress. Studies concerning depression [22] (e.g. there are still many obstacles to the recognition of depression as a disease), sexual functioning (family physicians tend not to initiate discourse with older patients on sexuality but rather discuss sexuality mostly in conjunction with other medical conditions) [23], alcoholism [24] and ability to drive [25] are present in the literature. Qualitative strategies of research may help to understand the complex treatment paths, for example, of those suffering from rare disease [26]. They may also provide the family physicians with evidence about older patients' perceptions, experiences and social implications as in the case of a qualitative study on living with an implanted defibrillator [27]. Contextually, qualitative research addressed how diseases differ among men and women in terms of prevention, clinical signs, therapeutic approach, prognosis and psychological and social impact [28]. Marginalisation resulting from ageing with a disability and living in a foreign country or in a rural area is another qualitatively discussed topic [29–31].

Moreover, qualitative studies considered access to treatment and care [32, 33], as well as reported about the perspective on the acceptability of screening and health literacy campaigns. Stakeholders' participation in the research was essential for comprehending how to improve the level of assistance [34, 35]. In this context, qualitative research may answer questions about how to support the whole family, particularly family caregivers, especially when the assisted persons live with Alzheimer [36] or the loved ones recently acquired spinal cord injury [37].

Qualitative research concerning family physicians caring for older assisted individuals debated the decision-making processes and emotions [38], motivations [31] or prejudices [28] involved in it. The use of qualitative research has undoubtedly contributed to understanding how professionalism is interpreted [39] and put into practice. For example, Kristensen and colleagues [40] investigated patients' experiences of disease and self-care as well as perceptions of the general practitioner's role in supporting patients with impaired self-care ability and showed that patient experiences of self-care could collide with what general practitioners find appropriate in a medical regimen [40]. Therapeutic alliance [41] is another subtopic qualitatively investigated as well as managing polytherapy [42, 43] and deprescription [44]. Besides, since in the western culture, a growing number of older people live at home, family physicians are supposed to play a pivotal role in the organisation of integrated care for this patient group: networking within the community, team building and team working [45] and leadership [46] were research topic addressed by qualitative approaches in the literature.

Since enhancing the decision-making ability of older people and those with cognitive impairments is an issue every family physician faces, qualitative research studies explored experiences in such a delicate area, especially when it involves the terminal stages of life [47]. Qualitative methodology was used for understanding how to overcome barriers to advance care planning with older people [48], for example, and provided an essential contribution in encouraging adaptation processes and adherence to therapies in the care pathways [49].

Finally, qualitative research seemed to be the proper methodology to target emerging family physicians' training and support needs [50].

28.5 Conclusion: Qualitative Research as Listening and Participation

As it may be noted, many phenomena which can be inquired by qualitative methodologies are of interest to the family physicians. The capabilities requested for conducting qualitative research include careful listening to biographies and narratives. Family physicians are involved in real stories for their professionalism requires it [51, 52]. They may assume a functional and directive relationship with patients along with the risk of not being respectful of the meanings of the others. Otherwise, learning from the qualitative research lesson, they may listen to the assisted persons and improve their awareness and autonomy, respecting their freedom in life choices [53]. As to qualitative methodology, researchers listen to the narratives of older people, family members and caregivers, and, by seeking the uniqueness of that evidence, they advantage professionals in defining the most effective care strategies. Family physicians experience every day the human intertwine between clinical aspects and personal and social phenomena. Making the technical knowledge practice of listening-recognition of the priority of the nonmedical components of the life of the people is one of their specific responsibility [54]. The humanising power of qualitative research impacts on the care practices of family physicians providing them with a sort of "epidemiology of memory" [54], in which the role of protagonist and generator of knowledge is given back to the assisted persons. Qualitative evidences may change intervention into accompaniment and bring physicians to acknowledging that medical competence is best expressed in a shared, nondirective dialogue among persons rather than among a doctor and his/her patients [55]. While cure is provided by effective treatments, care is given within the relationship by co-construction of meaning [56, 57]. An authentic and circular narrative communication shapes the process of conducting qualitative studies as they are respectful of the meanings and values the participants live and prioritise. Qualitative research involves researchers deepening the doctor-patient relationship and treatments' underlying processes.

Hence, qualitative research may maximise patients and caregivers' participation in treatments. Qualitative evidence informs patient engagement that it can be an innovative and viable approach to ensuring appropriate future care. Health organisations worldwide are committed to expanding patient engagement beyond a token level of involvement [58–60].

Qualitative research teaches that clinical choices are constructs negotiated by multiple actors (by family physicians, informal caregivers and patients) and that qualitative evidence may support a more family-patient centred scientific approach. Proper qualitative research in the area of older people and primary care is still scarce but more and more desirable.

References

1. Foreman KJ, Marquez N, Dolgert A, Fukutaki K, Fullman N, McGaughey M, et al. Forecasting life expectancy, years of life lost, and all-cause and cause-specific mortality for 250 causes of death: reference and alternative scenarios for 2016-40 for 195 countries and territories. Lancet. 2018;392:2052–90.
2. Cardano M. La ricerca qualitativa. Bologna: Il Mulino; 2011.
3. Mortari L, Ghirotto L. Metodi della ricerca educativa. Roma: Carocci; 2019.
4. Denzin NK, Lincoln YS. Introduction: entering the field of qualitative research. In: Denzin NK, Lincoln YS, editors. The landscape of qualitative research. Theories and issues. Thousand Oaks, CA: Sage; 1998. p. 1–34.
5. Polit DF, Beck CT. Essentials of nursing research: appraising evidence for nursing practice. 8th ed. Philadelphia: Lippincott; 2013.
6. Mortari L, Zannini L. La ricerca qualitativa in ambito sanitario. Roma: Carocci; 2017.
7. Streubert Speziale HJ, Carpenter DR. Qualitative research in nursing: advancing the humanistic imperative. Philadelphia: Lippincott Williams & Wilkins; 2005.
8. Silverman D. Doing qualitative research. A practical guide. London: Sage; 2000.
9. Marshall PL, Koenig BA. Ethnographic methods. In: Sugarman J, Sulmasy DP, editors. Methods in medical ethics. Washington, DC: Georgetown University Press; 2001. p. 169–91.
10. Morse JM. Qualitative health research: creating a new discipline. Walnut Creek, CA: Left Coast Press; 2012.
11. Sasso L, Bagnasco A, Ghirotto L. La ricerca qualitativa. Una risorsa per i professionisti della salute. Milano: Edra; 2015.
12. Denzin NK, Lincoln YS. The SAGE handbook of qualitative research. Thousand Oaks, CA: Sage; 2011.
13. Mantovani S. La ricerca sul campo in educazione. Milano: Bruno Mondadori; 1995.
14. O'Reilly K. Key concepts in ethnography. London: Sage; 2008.
15. Geertz C. The interpretation of cultures: selected essays. New York: Basic Books; 1973.
16. Giorgi A. Introduzione al metodo fenomenologico descrittivo: l'uso in campo psicologico. Encyclopaideia. 2010;XIV:23–32.
17. Giorgi A. Phenomenological and psychological research. Pittsburgh, PA: Duquesne University Press; 1985.
18. Giorgi A. The descriptive phenomenological method in psychology: a modified Husserlian approach. Pittsburgh, PA: Duquesne University Press; 2009.
19. Charmaz K. Constructing grounded theory. 2nd ed. Thousand Oaks, CA: Sage; 2014.
20. Glaser BG, Strauss AL. The discovery of grounded theory. Strategies for qualitative research. Chicago: Aldine Publishing Company; 1967.
21. Tarozzi M. What is grounded theory? Bloomsbury: Oxford, UK; 2020.
22. Stark A, Kaduszkiewicz H, Stein J, Maier W, Heser K, Weyerer S, et al. A qualitative study on older primary care patients' perspectives on depression and its treatments - potential barriers to and opportunities for managing depression. BMC Fam Pract. 2018;19:2.

23. Levkovich I, Gewirtz-Meydan A, Karkabi K, Ayalon L. Views of family physicians on hetero-sexual sexual function in older adults. BMC Fam Pract. 2018;19(1):86.

24. Haighton C, Wilson G, Ling J, McCabe K, Crosland A, Kaner E. A qualitative study of service provision for alcohol related health issues in mid to later life. PLoS One. 2016;11:e0148601.

25. Friedland J, Rudman DL, Chipman M, Steen A. Reluctant regulators: perspectives of family physicians on monitoring seniors' driving. Top Geriatr Rehabil. 2006;22:53–60.

26. Garrino L, Picco E, Finiguerra I, Rossi D, Simone P, Roccatello D. Living with and treating rare diseases: experiences of patients and professional health care providers. Qual Health Res. 2015;25:636–51.

27. Garrino L, Borraccino A, Peraudo E, Bobbio M, Dimonte V. "Hosting" an implantable cardio-verter defibrillator: a phenomenological inquiry. Res Nurs Health. 2018;41:57–68.

28. Levkovich I, Gewirtz-Meydan A, Karkabi K, Ayalon L. When sex meets age: family physi-cians' perspectives about sexual dysfunction among older men and women: a qualitative study from Israel. Eur J Gen Pract. 2019;25:85–90.

29. Wand APF, Peisah C, Draper B, Brodaty H. Understanding self-harm in older people: a sys-tematic review of qualitative studies. Aging Ment Health. 2018;22:289–98.

30. Sagbakken M, Spilker RS, Nielsen TR. Dementia and immigrant groups: a qualitative study of challenges related to identifying, assessing, and diagnosing dementia. BMC Health Serv Res. 2018;18:910.

31. Constantinescu A, Li H, Yu J, Hoggard C, Holroyd-Leduc J. Exploring rural family physi-cians' challenges in providing dementia care: a qualitative study. Can J Aging. 2018;37:390–9.

32. Igwesi-Chidobe CN, Bartlam B, Humphreys K, Hughes E, Protheroe J, Maddison J, et al. Patient direct access to musculoskeletal physiotherapy in primary care: perceptions of patients, general practitioners, physiotherapists and clinical commissioners in England. Physiotherapy. 2019;105:e31.

33. Reddy R, Welch D, Lima I, Thorne P, Nosa V. Identifying hearing care access barriers among older Pacific Island people in New Zealand: a qualitative study. BMJ Open. 2019;9:e029007.

34. Azhar N, Doss JG. Health-seeking behaviour and delayed presentation of oral cancer patients in a developing country: a qualitative study based on the self-regulatory model. Asian Pac J Cancer Prev. 2018;19:2935–41.

35. Daker-White G, Hays R, Blakeman T, Croke S, Brown B, Esmail A, Bower P. Safety work and risk management as burdens of treatment in primary care: insights from a focused ethno-graphic study of patients with multimorbidity. BMC Fam Pract. 2018;19:155.

36. Abojabel H, Werner P. Exploring family stigma among caregivers of persons with Alzheimer's disease: the experiences of Israeli-Arab caregivers. Dementia. 2019;18:391–408.

37. Conti A, Garrino L, Montanari P, Dimonte V. Informal caregivers' needs at discharge from Spinal Cord Unit: analysis of perceptions and lived experiences. Disabil Rehabil. 2016;38:159–67.

38. Michiels-Corsten M, Donner-Banzhoff N. Beyond accuracy: hidden motives in diagnostic testing. Fam Pract. 2018;35:222–7.

39. Glette MK, Kringeland T, Røise O, Wiig S. Exploring physicians' decision-making in hospital readmission processes - a comparative case study. BMC Health Serv Res. 2018;18:725.

40. Kristensen MAT, Guassora AD, Arreskov AB, Waldorff FB, Hølge-Hazelton B. 'I've put diabetes completely on the shelf till the mental stuff is in place'. How patients with doctor-assessed impaired self-care perceive disease, self-care, and support from general practitioners. A qualitative study. Scand J Prim Health Care. 2018;36:342–51.

41. van Bussel E, Reurich L, Pols J, Richard E, Moll van Charante E, Ligthart S. Hypertension management: experiences, wishes and concerns among older people-a qualitative study. BMJ Open. 2019;9:e030742.

42. Schöpf AC, von Hirschhausen M, Farin E, Maun A. Elderly patients' and GPs' perspectives of patient-GP communication concerning polypharmacy: a qualitative interview study. Prim Health Care Res Dev. 2018;19:355–64.

43. Barton E, Twining L, Walters L. Understanding the decision to commence a dose administra-tion aid. Aust Fam Physician. 2017;46:943–7.

44. AlRasheed MM, Alhawassi TM, Alanazi A, Aloudah N, Khurshid F, Alsultan M. Knowledge and willingness of physicians about deprescribing among older patients: a qualitative study. Clin Interv Aging. 2018;13:1401–8.
45. Johansen ML, Ervik B. Teamwork in primary palliative care: general practitioners' and specialised oncology nurses' complementary competencies. BMC Health Serv Res. 2018;18:159.
46. Grol SM, Molleman GRM, Kuijpers A, van der Sande R, Fransen GAJ, Assendelft WJJ, et al. The role of the general practitioner in multidisciplinary teams: a qualitative study in elderly care. BMC Fam Pract. 2018;19:40.
47. Sharp T, Malyon A, Barclay S. GPs' perceptions of advance care planning with frail and older people: a qualitative study. Br J Gen Pract. 2018;68(666):e44–53.
48. Glaudemans JJ, de Jong AE, Onwuteaka Philipsen BD, Wind J, Willems DL. How do Dutch primary care providers overcome barriers to advance care planning with older people? A qualitative study. Fam Pract. 2019;36:219–24.
49. Torresan MM, Garrino L, Borraccino A, Macchi G, De Luca A, Dimonte V. Adherence to treatment in patient with severe cancer pain: a qualitative enquiry through illness narratives. Eur J Oncol Nurs. 2015;19:397–404.
50. Jovicic A, McPherson S. To support and not to cure: general practitioner management of loneliness. Health Soc Care Community. 2020;28:376–84.
51. Bruner J. The narrative construction of reality. Crit Inq. 1991;18:1–21.
52. Launer J. Narrative-based primary care: a practical guide. Abingdon: Radcliffe Medical Press; 2002.
53. Heidegger M. Being and time. Oxford: Basil Blackwell; 1962.
54. Tognoni G. Spunti di ricerca. In: Milano M, Bondielli G, editors. Storie di cura al domicilio sul declinare della vita. Frammenti di specchio. Milano: FrancoAngeli; 2015. p. 152–5.
55. Charon R. Narrative medicine: honoring the stories of illness. Oxford: Oxford University Press; 2006.
56. Palmieri C. La cura educativa. Milano: FrancoAngeli; 2000.
57. Mortari L, Saiani L. Gestures and thoughts of caring. A theory of caring from the voices of nurses. Milano: McGraw-Hill; 2014.
58. Jouet E, Las Vergnas O, Noël-Hureaux E. Nouvelles coopérations réflexives en santé. Paris: Edition des Archives Contemporaines; 2014.
59. Karazivan P, Dumez V, Flora L, Pomey MP, Del Grande C, Ghadiri DP, et al. The patient-as-partner approach in health care: a conceptual framework for a necessary transition. Acad Med. 2015;90:437–41.
60. Pomey MP, Ghadiri DP, Karazivan P, Fernandez N, Clavel N. Patients as partners: a qualitative study of patients' engagement in their health care. PLoS One. 2015;10:e0122499.

COVID-19: Impact of Pandemic on Older People Health and Well-Being

Nicola Veronese and Jacopo Demurtas

Abstract

Since March 2020 and the declaration of pandemic, we may consider that three categories of disease are striking worldwide, COVID-19, a surge of noncommunicable diseases which due to COVID-19 are less treated and considered, and agism.

COVID-19 is known to be sever in frail older people, with poor outcomes and often our older patients are frail. Moreover, frailty and COVID-19 share a proinflammatory cytokines cascade which may lead to an increase of mortality in these patients.

COVID-19 lockdown also has led and is leading to several psychological disorders, notably in older people and older people with cognitive impairment.

Patients in rural settings, primary care, and nursing homes with frailty were severely affected with COVID-19, also in their social and familial relationship. It is a crucial task for both general practitioners and geriatricians to assess and treat their older patients even in this context, notwithstanding the obstacles and limitations, levering eventually on e-health and ICT.

N. Veronese
Department of Internal Medicine and Geriatrics, University of Palermo, Palermo, Italy

J. Demurtas (✉)
Primary Care Department, USL Toscana Sud Est, Grosseto, Italy
e-mail: jacopo.demurtas@unimore.it; eritrox7@gmail.com

© Springer Nature Switzerland AG 2022
J. Demurtas, N. Veronese (eds.), *The Role of Family Physicians in Older People Care*, Practical Issues in Geriatrics, https://doi.org/10.1007/978-3-030-78923-7_29

Keywords

COVID-19 · Frailty · Cognitive impairment · Agism · eHealth

29.1 Introduction

In March 2020, the World Health Organization declared the coronavirus disease 19 (COVID-19) outbreak as global pandemic [1]. At 23 March 2021, more than 124 million people were officially affected by COVID-19, with more than 2.7 million deaths in the world [2]. We can actually consider COVID-19 as a condition typical of older people. Epidemiological data, in fact, suggested that the mortality rates are extremely high in older persons and that the prevalence of COVID-19 is more elevated in older persons compared to the younger ones [3]. A particular interest was given to the COVID-19 outbreak in nursing homes for several reasons [4–6]. First, nursing homes commonly include people that are particularly frail (e.g., for the presence of severe dementia) or disabled. Moreover, even if less than 10% of all COVID-19 cases are observed in nursing home, nursing home and assisted living facilities residents and staff accounted for more than one third of the all deaths recorded [7, 8].

29.2 Frailty and Agism in COVID-19

COVID-19 has indicated again the importance of frailty and agism in older people. Frailty is an age-related clinical condition associated with a decline in energy, strength, and function that increases a person's vulnerability to stressor conditions resulting in an increased risk of negative outcomes such as hospitalization, falls, admission to long-term care, and mortality [9]. Older adults are characterized by heterogeneity of health and vigor. Single aspects, such as chronological age and concurrent disease, cannot truly reflect overall health status. To solve this knowledge gap, frailty syndrome has been widely introduced in recent decades. Frailty was confirmed to be a predictor of risk with worse outcomes, such as falls, mortality, and lower quality of life in different populations [10]. Several studies have presented the association between frailty and mortality in patients with COVID-19, the majority of which have shown a clear association between increasing frailty and worse outcomes [11]. Although the mechanism relating frailty and mortality has been described by previous studies, this association has not been yet fully explained. Patients with frailty suffer from various observable deficits, namely, a reduced physiologic reserve, chronic undernutrition, and cognitive impairment, that may increase the likelihood of an adverse outcome when patients are exposed to major negative stressors, such as COVID-19 or surgery operations. Second, frailty involves the process of complex chronic inflammation. Proinflammatory cytokines, such as C-reactive protein, tumor necrosis factor (TNF)-a, interleukin (IL), or interleukin-6, exacerbate the risk of mortality in COVID-19 [12]. Recently, a huge increase in proinflammatory cytokines was reported in patients with COVID-19 [13]. Proinflammatory cytokines cause an inflammatory storm in COVID-19 patients, which may lead to lung injury and notably ARDS, heightening mortality risk [13]. Third, older adults infected with SARS-CoV-2 have an increased risk of referral to ICU and intensive medical care. This may lead to invasive ventilation, more drugs, and even extracorporeal circulation support. Critically ill patients with frailty were reported to have a 1.71-fold risk of mortality [11].

Another important problem that faced during the 2020 is agism. Agism is a complex phenomenon that encompasses stereotypes, prejudice, and discrimination against older adults, old age, and aging [14]. According to World Health Organization [15], agism is the most socially normalized of all forms of discrimination and COVID-19 perpetuated and triggered several forms of public agism [16, 17]. Subjective perceived age discrimination (PAD) has been claimed to produce detrimental effects [18] with harmful consequences for physical, mental, and social health [19, 20].

Agism and frailty are conditions that share the possibility of being associated with negative outcomes for the older people; however, very few studies included frailty as a factor potentially related to agism [21, 22], and little is known of the possible relationship between these two conditions, even if in the early 2020 some works indicated that younger people should be privileged compared to older persons for some interventions such as invasive ventilation, without considering the older person in his/her complexity [23].

29.3 Cognitive and Psychological Problems in Older People During COVID-19

Confinement and isolation were proven to be highly effective for the control of infectious diseases, including COVID-19 pandemic [6]. However, previous outbreaks of SARS and MERS showed that quarantine has negative effects on mental health, with an increase in psychiatric symptoms and syndromes, notably those related to stress reactions such as anxiety, depression, and anguish [7]. Considering findings from previous outbreaks and preliminary observations during the COVID-19 pandemic, an alarm about a possible imminent "pandemic" of psychiatric disorders was launched [8–10]. Factors triggering an increase of post-pandemic psychiatric disorders may be multiples. Among those are direct effect of isolation, with restrictions on movements, impoverishment of social contacts, affective relationships, and perceived loneliness. Anxiety may arise from the rapid need to adapt to new lifestyle and changes of routines. In addition, an increased state of alert due to fear of contagion, grief, or bereavement could impair mental health [10].

These considerations apply to the general population, and very few information is available for the most vulnerable persons in society, such as older people and those affected by dementia [11, 12]. Individuals with dementia are frail, depend on caregivers for daily living activities, and need the support of a network of social and health services resources (memory clinics, Alzheimer café, diurnal centers, physiotherapy, etc.). In this scenario, extended lockdown with imposed self-isolation and change or deprivation of usual daily activities may represent a stressor event in both patients and caregivers, with high risk to induce anxiety and depression [13]. Changes in neuropsychiatric symptoms in subjects with dementia may exacerbate the psychological effects of lockdown in their caregivers, situation which may further worsen patients' behavioral symptoms, globally increasing psychiatric burden. Finally, confinement reduces access to physical exercise or even physiotherapy, and movement restriction exacerbates symptoms of dementia [13, 14]. In turn, the lack of activities and global cognitive and physical stimulation may cause delirium in individuals with dementia, contributing further to morbidity. There is also increased evidence that psychological symptoms due to stressor events can contribute to cognitive decline [15]. In one of the most important studies regarding psychological issues during 2020 in older people, it was reported that quarantine induces a rapid increase of BPSD in approximately 60% of patients and stress-related symptoms in two-thirds of caregivers. Health services need to plan a post-pandemic strategy in order to address these emerging needs [24].

29.4 The Role of Geriatrician and General Practitioner in COVID-19

The coronavirus disease 19 (COVID-19) is surging up in older people, and it affects especially frail people in primary care settings and nursing homes in which frail people, notably with cognitive impairment and behavioral problems, are usually admitted. COVID-19 is known to affect not only our older patients' clinical state but also their relationship with families and their social life, impairing globally their functioning and eventually speeding up their decline.

GPs have also experienced the challenge of caring for their older patients in rural contexts, with a need to balance chronic disease management with the risk of virus transmission, either during health care consultations or when traveling from rural to urban areas [25].

The recent e-health and communication technologies may help mitigate this conditions, i.e., GPs, geriatricians, and other healthcare professionals may use video conferencing tools [26]. Patients should be evaluated and treated also using telemedicine and including prognostic tools in daily clinical practice.

Nevertheless, digital divide is indeed an obstacle to the realization of this, and seniors that have previously been shown to have higher prevalence of chronic conditions and greater difficulties with healthcare access are also less likely to adopt use of e-health tools [27].

29.5 Conclusions

COVID-19 pandemic represents, with its millions dead worldwide, an un prece-dented tragedy.

Hopefully, due to the massive vaccination campaign effort with extraordinarily effective vaccines, COVID-19 pandemic will eventually end or at least our systems will be able to manage the pandemic or co-exist with SARS-CoV-2. Family physicians and geriatricians will participate to the post-COVID-19 healthcare, building upon the COVID-19 experience and making use of the new tools in order to provide care to frail and older patients, both in nursing homes and community dwelling.

References

1. Jebril N. World Health Organization declared a pandemic public health menace: a systematic review of the coronavirus disease 2019 "COVID-19", up to 26th March 2020. Available at SSRN 3566298. 2020.
2. World Health Organization. Coronavirus disease 2019 (COVID-19): situation report, 45. 2020.
3. Onder G, Rezza G, Brusaferro S. Case-fatality rate and characteristics of patients dying in relation to COVID-19 in Italy. JAMA. 2020;323(18):1775–6.
4. McMichael TM, Currie DW, Clark S, Pogosjans S, Kay M, Schwartz NG, et al. Epidemiology of covid-19 in a long-term care facility in King County, Washington. N Engl J Med. 2020;382(21):2005–11.
5. Burton JK, Bayne G, Evans C, Garbe F, Gorman D, Honhold N, et al. Evolution and effects of COVID-19 outbreaks in care homes: a population analysis in 189 care homes in one geographical region of the UK. Lancet Healthy Longevity. 2020;1(1):e21–31.
6. Trabucchi M, De Leo D. Nursing homes or besieged castles: COVID-19 in northern Italy. Lancet Psychiatry. 2020;7(5):387–8.
7. Weinberger DM, Chen J, Cohen T, Crawford FW, Mostashari F, Olson D, et al. Estimation of excess deaths associated with the COVID-19 pandemic in the United States, March to May 2020. JAMA Intern Med. 2020;180(10):1336–44.
8. Eurosurveillance Editorial Team. Updated rapid risk assessment from ECDC on the novel coronavirus disease 2019 (COVID-19) pandemic: increased transmission in the EU/EEA and the UK. Eurosurveillance. 2020;25(10).
9. Clegg A, Young J, Iliffe S, Rikkert MO, Rockwood K. Frailty in elderly people. Lancet. 2013;381(9868):752–62.
10. Pilotto A, Custodero C, Maggi S, Polidori MC, Veronese N, Ferrucci L. A multidimensional approach to frailty in older people. Ageing Res Rev. 2020;60:101047.
11. Zhang X-M, Jiao J, Cao J, Huo X-P, Zhu C, Wu X-J, et al. Frailty as a predictor of mortality among patients with COVID-19: a systematic review and meta-analysis. BMC Geriatr. 2021;21(1):1–11.
12. Shenoy S. Coronavirus (Covid-19) sepsis: revisiting mitochondrial dysfunction in pathogenesis, aging, inflammation, and mortality. Inflamm Res. 2020;69:1077–85.
13. Ye Q, Wang B, Mao J. The pathogenesis and treatment of the 'Cytokine Storm' in COVID-19. J Infect. 2020;80(6):607–13.
14. Voss P, Bodner E, Rothermund K. Ageism: the relationship between age stereotypes and age discrimination. Contemporary perspectives on ageism. Cham: Springer; 2018. p. 11–31.
15. World Health Organization. Developing an ethical framework for healthy ageing: report of a WHO meeting, Tübingen, Germany, 18 March 2017. Geneva: World Health Organization; 2017.
16. Fraser S, Lagacé M, Bongué B, Ndeye N, Guyot J, Bechard L, et al. Ageism and COVID-19: what does our society's response say about us? Age Ageing. 2020;49(5):692–5.
17. Bravo-Segal S, Villar F. Older people representation on the media during COVID-19 pandemic: a reinforcement of ageism? Rev Esp Geriatr Gerontol. 2020;55(5):266–71.
18. Barnes M, Gahagan B, Ward L. Re-imagining old age: wellbeing, care and participation. Wilmington: Vernon Press; 2018.

19. Pascoe EA, Smart Richman L. Perceived discrimination and health: a meta-analytic review. Psychol Bull. 2009;135(4):531.
20. Lyons A, Alba B, Heywood W, Fileborn B, Minichiello V, Barrett C, et al. Experiences of ageism and the mental health of older adults. Aging Ment Health. 2018;22(11):1456–64.
21. Salguero D, Ferri-Guerra J, Mohammed NY, Baskaran D, Aparicio-Ugarriza R, Mintzer MJ, et al. Is there an association between ageist attitudes and frailty? BMC Geriatr. 2019;19(1):1–6.
22. Ye B, Gao J, Fu H, Chen H, Dong W, Gu M. How does ageism influence frailty? A preliminary study using a structural equation model. BMC Geriatr. 2020;20(1):1–11.
23. Medford A, Trias-Llimós S. Population age structure only partially explains the large number of COVID-19 deaths at the oldest ages. Demogr Res. 2020;43:533–44.
24. Cagnin A, Di Lorenzo R, Marra C, Bonanni L, Cupidi C, Laganà V, et al. Behavioral and psychological effects of coronavirus disease-19 quarantine in patients with dementia. Front Psych. 2020;11:916.
25. Bhatia RS, Shojania KG, Levinson W. Cost of contact: redesigning healthcare in the age of COVID. BMJ Qual Saf. 2021;30(3):236–9.
26. Daly JR, Depp C, Graham SA, Jeste DV, Kim HC, Lee EE, et al. Health impacts of the stay-at-home order on community-dwelling older adults and how technologies may help: focus group study. JMIR Aging. 2021;4(1):e25779.
27. Gordon NP, Hornbrook MC. Older adults' readiness to engage with eHealth patient education and self-care resources: a cross-sectional survey. BMC Health Serv Res. 2018;18(1):220.